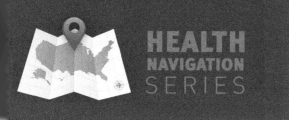

NAVIGATING HEALTH INSURANCE

Alexis Pozen, PhD

Assistant Professor, CUNY School of Public Health,
New York, New York

Jim P. Stimpson, MA, PhD

Associate Dean for Academic and Faculty Affairs, Professor,
CUNY School of Public Health, New York, New York

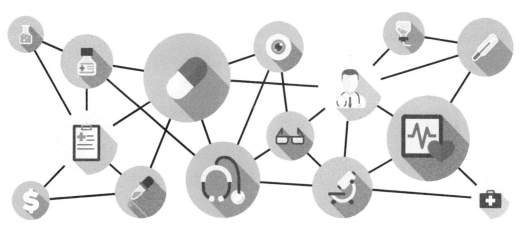

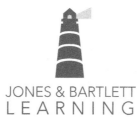

JONES & BARTLETT
LEARNING

World Headquarters
Jones & Bartlett Learning
25 Mall Road
Burlington, MA 01803
978-443-5000
info@jblearning.com
www.jblearning.com

Jones & Bartlett Learning books and products are available through most bookstores and online booksellers. To contact Jones & Bartlett Learning directly, call 800-832-0034, fax 978-443-8000, or visit our website, www.jblearning.com.

32123-4

Production Credits

VP, Executive Publisher: David D. Cella
Publisher: Michael Brown
Associate Editor: Danielle Bessette
Vendor Manager: Nora Menzi
Senior Marketing Manager: Sophie Fleck Teague
Manufacturing and Inventory Control Supervisor: Amy Bacus
Composition and Project Management: Integra Software Services Pvt. Ltd.

Cover Design: Kristin E. Parker
Director of Rights & Media: Joanna Gallant
Rights & Media Specialist: Merideth Tumasz
Media Development Editor: Shannon Sheehan
Cover Image: © Hilch/Shutterstock
Printing and Binding: LSC Communications
Cover Printing: LSC Communications

Library of Congress Cataloging-in-Publication Data
Names: Pozen, Alexis, author. | Stimpson, Jim P., author.
Title: Navigating health insurance / Alexis Pozen, Jim P. Stimpson.
Description: First edition. | Burlington, Massachusetts : Jones & Bartlett,LLC
  Learning, [2018] | Includes bibliographical references and index.
Identifiers: LCCN 2016053491 | ISBN 9781284113129 (paperback)
Subjects: | MESH: United States. Patient Protection and Affordable Care Act.
  | Insurance, Health | Health Care Reform | United States
Classification: LCC RA412.2 | NLM W 275 AA1 | DDC 368.38/200973—dc23
LC record available at https://lccn.loc.gov/2016053491&

6048

Printed in the United States of America
26 25 24 23 22   10 9 8 7 6 5 4 3 2

CONTENTS

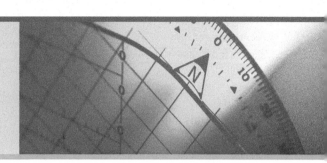

Health Navigator Applied Associate Degree and Academic Certificate Programs

"Health Navigator" is the term used by the Association of Schools and Programs of Public Health (ASPPH) and the League for Innovation in the Community College (League) for applied associate degrees and academic certificate programs that prepare students for employment in existing and emerging fields such as community health worker, patient navigator, and health insurance navigator. These programs also benefit employers and practitioners by offering opportunities for employees to obtain academic credentials that reflect the knowledge, skills, and abilities gained through job experience. As recommended by the Society for Public Health Education (SOPHE), Health Navigator programs should be designed to transfer to bachelor's Health Education degree programs should a graduate wish to do so.

The need for individuals with the skills to help patients obtain and maximally benefit from community services, clinical care, and health insurance is becoming a major issue in the increasingly complex and expensive U.S. health system. Those with Health Navigator training may assist individuals with limited health literacy as well as the elderly with accessing community services and implementing prevention. They may facilitate access to care and follow-up for sick and complicated patients with cancer, HIV, and a range of other complex and chronic health problems. In addition, Health Navigators can assist with identifying and enrolling patients in health insurance plans including those available through the Affordable Care Act exchanges, Medicaid, Medicare, as well as through community health centers.

The recommended Health Navigator applied associate degree program includes 30 semester credit hours of general education as well as 30 semester credit hours of coursework in the following areas:

- **Public Health Core:** 1) Population & Personal Health; 2) Overview of Public Health; and 3) Health Communications
- **Health Navigator Core:** 1) Prevention & Community Health; 2) Accessing and Analyzing Health Information; 3) Health care Delivery Systems; 4) Health Insurance
- Experiential learning
- Elective coursework allowing students to tailor their education to specific jobs in the field

This coursework can also form the centerpiece of academic certificate programs designed for nurses and allied health students as a complement to their clinical education. Certificate programs are well-suited for individuals with workforce experience and/or an academic degree who seek to augment their academic portfolio with a Health Navigator credential. Detailed course content outlines are available at www.league.org/ccph/ as part of the *Community Colleges and Public Health* report.

While this need has existed for a long time, until recently it has not been met through paid positions with well-defined roles. This is rapidly changing as a result of the growing commitment to develop specific Health Navigator positions and to integrate these positions into the health care and public health systems. Moreover, new funding mechanisms as part of Medicaid, Medicare's 30 day hospital readmission policy, and the Affordable Care Act have dramatically increased demand for employees with Health Navigator credentials. Salaries for Health Navigator graduates range from $30,000 to $55,000 per year. The Department of Labor estimates that by 2022 the demand for Community Health Workers—the only Health Navigator-related job classification it currently tracks—will increase by at least 25 percent.

INTRODUCING

THE HEALTH NAVIGATION SERIES

FROM JONES & BARTLETT LEARNING

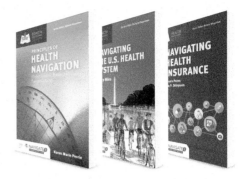

The NEW Jones & Bartlett Learning *Health Navigation* series meets the full range of Health Navigation education competencies of the League for Innovation in the Community College based on the Association of Schools and Programs of Public Health (ASPPH) Community Colleges and Public Health report.

Developed under the editorial direction of Richard K. Riegelman, MD, MPH, PhD, this series of three textbooks and accompanying digital learning materials is designed for Health Navigator associate degree and certificate programs leading to employment as community health workers, patient navigators, and/or health insurance navigators.

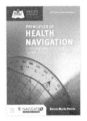

Principles of Health Navigation

by Karen Marie Perrin, PhD, MPH, CPH University of South Florida, College of Public Health

This text will provide an overview of the content and knowledge competencies expected as part of health navigation education including health services delivery and health insurance, care of the individual, and accessing and analyzing health information competencies.

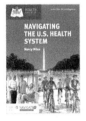

Navigating the U.S. Health System

by Nancy Niles, MPH, MS, MBA, PhD, Associate Professor, Rollins College
Available Spring 2017

This text will comprehensively cover the knowledge competency in healthcare delivery and public health expected as part of health navigation education in the United States.

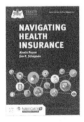

Navigating Health Insurance

by Alexis Pozen, PhD, and **Jim P. Stimpson**, PhD, MA, Both of the CUNY School of Public Health
Available Spring 2017

This text will comprehensively cover the health insurance knowledge competencies needed to understand health insurance and serve as a health insurance navigator.

Each title will serve as a free-standing text designed for a 3 semester hour course. Together the series will cover the required course work recommended for health navigation associate degree and academic certificate programs by the ASPPH Community Colleges and Public Health report.

HEALTH NAVIGATION SERIES

www.healthnavigationseries.com

PROLOGUE

Navigating Health Insurance, by Alexis Pozen and Jim P. Stimpson, is a key book in the new Jones & Bartlett Learning *Health Navigation* series. It provides a comprehensive yet engaging look at the U.S. health insurance system.

Navigating Health Insurance addresses the perspectives of the many stakeholders involved in the U.S. health care system, including providers, insurers, and the government, but focuses especially on the perspective of the consumer. By engaging readers in multiple viewpoints, the book provides future health care professionals of all types with the knowledge and tools to help consumers successfully navigate the system.

Together with *Principles of Health Navigation* by Karen Marie Perrin and *Navigating the U.S. Health Care System* by Nancy Niles, *Navigating Health Insurance* provides the core content for a health navigation certificate program or associate degree. Each book implements health navigation content recommended by the League for Innovation in the Community College and the Association of Schools and Programs of Public Health.

The authors of *Navigating Health Insurance* are exceptionally well qualified to write this textbook. Alexis Pozen, PhD, a health economist, is Assistant Professor at the CUNY School of Public Health, where she teaches health economics and quantitative methods. She has taught undergraduate- and graduate-level courses in health policy, health economics, and econometrics. Jim P. Stimpson, PhD, is Associate Dean for Academic and Faculty Affairs and Professor at the CUNY School of Public Health. He has more than 10 years of teaching and research experience focused on the social determinants of population health and inequalities as well as the role that policy plays in shaping our behavior and our health.

Navigating Health Insurance includes additional materials to help faculty engage students with the book's content. The preface carefully explains the rationale and context for the book and lays out a roadmap for the chapters that follow.

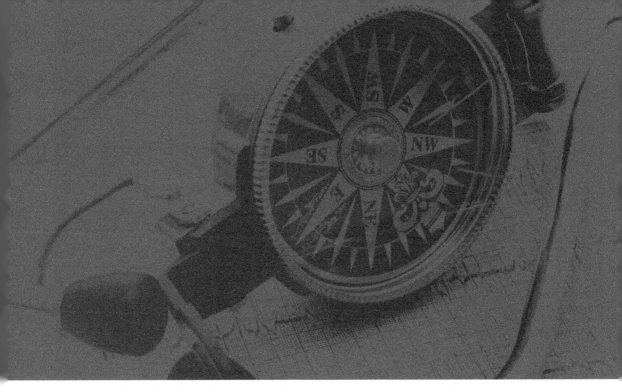

The text begins by introducing readers to the concept and history of insurance and the system of health insurance in the United States, continues by explaining basic health insurance principles and terminology, and then discusses the various systems of public and private health insurance in the United States. The text concludes with broader discussions on health insurance from the perspective of consumers and health care providers, as well as comparisons with other countries.

The text examines a full range of health insurance issues, including what health insurance covers and what it does not cover and how health insurance works for retirees, people with disabilities, and those in need of long-term care. It includes chapters on how providers make a health care claim and the rights of health care consumers. *Navigating Health Insurance* focuses on the U.S. health insurance system but also provides comparisons with health insurance systems in other countries.

The text is ideally suited to introductory health insurance courses as part of health navigation education including course work taught in nursing, social services, and a range of other disciplines in which graduates help patients navigate the U.S. health insurance system.

As editor of the Jones & Bartlett Learning *Health Navigation* series, I am delighted that *Navigating Health Insurance* is now a key component of the series.

Richard Riegelman, MD, MPH, PhD
Editor, Jones & Bartlett Learning
Health Navigation *series*

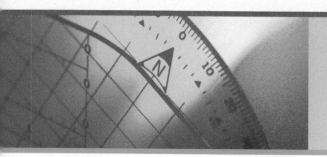

PREFACE

Originally intended to protect against large, unpredictable financial losses, health insurance in the United States has expanded over the past century to take on a more profound social role. The 2010 Patient Protection and Affordable Care Act (ACA) substantially increased the percentage of insured Americans for the first time since Medicare and Medicaid in 1965. As a result, there is an unprecedented need for public health professionals to assist their community members in navigating this new health care environment. The goal of this book is to provide a foundation for professional health insurance navigators, as well as those more generally interested in public health and health care services.

We aim to engage students in critical analysis of the U.S. health insurance system by approaching the subject from multiple perspectives, including those of the consumer, provider, insurer, and government. The text is divided into sections of related chapters. Section 1 is the Fundamentals of Health Insurance. It begins with a history of the U.S. health insurance system and the principles of health insurance (Chapter 1); options for coverage in the United States, including both private and public coverage (Chapter 2); the uninsured (Chapter 3); and the ACA (Chapter 4). Section 2 explores the perspective of consumers and includes chapters on what types of benefits are covered under different plans (Chapter 5); how much consumers are expected to pay for health insurance (Chapter 6); and consumer protections (Chapter 7). Section 3 discusses the perspective of providers and insurers, two sides of the same coin, and covers mechanisms of payment between the two parties (Chapter 8); and claims and reimbursement for providers (Chapter 9). Section 4 examines the perspectives of several different special populations, including people with disabilities (Chapter 10); those needing long-term care (Chapter 11); and retirees (Chapter 12). Finally, Section 5, Beyond the United States, compares the U.S. health insurance system to those in other high-, middle-, and low-income countries (Chapter 13).

We hope that the information and resources provided in this textbook help readers to better understand the health insurance system in the United States, and to prepare a new generation of health care professionals to navigate the health insurance system on behalf of consumers.

Alexis Pozen and Jim P. Stimpson

CONTRIBUTORS

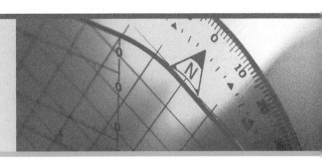

Julia K. Duch, BA
Independent Consultant
New York, NY

April Falconi, PhD, MPH, MA
Postdoctoral Research Fellow
Stanford University School of Medicine
Stanford, CA

John A. Gravina, MPH
Student, Doctor of Public Health
CUNY Graduate School of Public Health and
    Health Policy
New York, NY

Erin Hemlin, MA
National Director of Training and Consumer
    Education
Young Invincibles
Washington, DC

Sara M. Ingram, MPA
Director, Disability Affairs for Homeless Services
The Office of Client Advocacy and Access
Human Resources Administration
City of New York
New York, NY

Katie Keith, JD, MPH
Health Consultant
Keith Policy Solutions LLC
Washington, DC

Deanna Meyler, PhD
Senior Associate
Rabin Martin
New York, NY

Gordon C. Shen, PhD, SM
Assistant Professor
CUNY Graduate School of Public Health and
    Health Policy
New York, NY

Sarah Swanson, BS Ed, Certificate in Public Health
Community and Family Resource Specialist
Munroe-Meyer Institute, University of Nebraska
    Medical Center
Omaha, NE

Kate E. Trout, MPH
Research Assistant, Doctoral Candidate
Health Services Research and Administration,
    University of Nebraska Medical Center
Omaha, NE

Fernando A. Wilson, PhD
Associate Professor and Director
Center for Health Policy, University of Nebraska
    Medical Center
Omaha, NE

CHAPTER 1

Principles of Health Insurance

Alexis Pozen, PhD

LEARNING OBJECTIVES

- What is health insurance?
- How have the objectives of health insurance evolved over time in the United States?
- In what ways does the United States make health insurance a social priority?

INTRODUCTION

We call it health insurance, but it does not, in fact, insure against poor health. Insurance is a guarantee, usually a financial guarantee, against an unforeseen event. But of course, no one, much less an insurer, can guarantee against getting sick or recovering from illness. Instead, insurers write policies that provide financial protection from medical expenses. Health insurance plans pay for a portion of the bill when you are hospitalized, visit a doctor, get blood drawn, have an X-ray or MRI, or fill a prescription. You may use your health insurance even when you are not sick or injured, such as for preventive care. But health insurance is not a guarantee against bankruptcy from medical bills, nor does it compensate for pain and suffering from lost work or leisure time.

Yet even though it cannot guarantee recovery from illness or injury, health insurance serves many purposes beyond paying medical bills, and

the government has adopted policies over the years meant to increase the number of people and conditions covered. These policies' features highlight the importance of health insurance in society relative to other types of insurance, such as such as fire, automobile, and homeowners, where insurance is mainly intended to protect consumers from large financial losses.

For example, imagine that you live 20 miles from work and there is no reliable public transportation where you live. You must drive to get to work, meaning that you must be able to afford car payments, gas, maintenance, and auto insurance. If you live in New Jersey, Hawaii, or California, then you may be eligible for government-subsidized auto insurance, but in other states there is no such program. On the other hand, if you cannot afford health insurance, there are myriad programs available nationwide. Every state has a Medicaid program, and the federal Patient Protection and Affordable Care Act (PPACA)—or just the Affordable Care Act (ACA)—provides subsidies for low-income individuals and families to purchase health insurance through the state health insurance exchanges in every state.

Now suppose your sweet but stranger-shy dog, Huxley, has bitten a visitor to your home. You have just moved into an apartment and would like to purchase renter's insurance. You should not be surprised to find dog bites excluded from coverage, or coverage that includes dog bites limited up to a certain dollar amount. You should not even be surprised to find that the insurer will not write you a policy, because insurance is meant to protect you against something that might happen in the future, not something that has already happened. We will discuss this point in greater detail later. On the other hand, if you already have diabetes and you would like to purchase health insurance, then there are limitations (depending on the type of health insurance) on how long a plan may exclude diabetes from coverage, if it may even exclude this condition at all. Even if you and the insurer already know that you have diabetes when the insurer writes you a new plan, then the insurer still must cover your insulin injections, glucose meter, endocrinologist visits, and so on.

Finally, if you live near dense forests in Northern California, an area ravaged by seasonal wildfires, then you will face a much higher price for fire insurance than in other areas. Similarly, auto insurance costs more if you have been in a collision, because the auto insurer expects you to cost them more based on their experience with you. On the other hand, no matter how sick or injured you are, health insurance plans participating in state exchanges (marketplaces) may not charge you more for a plan. Prices may be adjusted for geography (to account for the higher cost of care in, say, California versus Mississippi), age (but only within limits), smoking status, and whether coverage is for an individual or for a family. Sicker individuals, however, may not be charged more for health insurance.

We prioritize health insurance in a way that we do not prioritize auto insurance, homeowners insurance, life insurance, property insurance, or long-term care insurance. Originally intended to protect consumers against large, unpredictable losses, health insurance has evolved into a system that reimburses consumers even for inexpensive, predictable medical expenses. Why do we not simply save our own money ("self-insure") to pay for physician visits, prescription

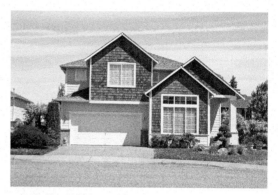

© alexmisu/Shutterstock

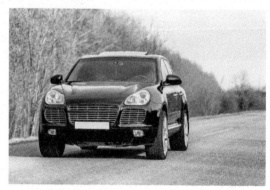

© Alexandr Shevchenko/Shutterstock

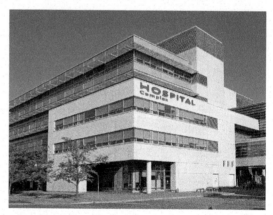

© Pete Spiro/Shutterstock

medications, and routine laboratory tests? Why instead do we pool our money and pay every month to have these services and supplies covered by insurance? This chapter will trace the history and development of health insurance in the United States that led to the system we have in its current form. It will also discuss the principles of insurance and explain why we have a system of health "insurance" that deviates significantly from the traditional definition.

DEVELOPMENT OF HEALTH INSURANCE IN THE UNITED STATES

The historical context of health insurance is critical to understanding its strong ties to employment and the private sector, and its importance in society over other types of insurance. As we know it today, health insurance is protection against costly, unpredictable medical bills; if medical care is neither costly nor unpredictable, however, then health insurance is not necessary. Indeed, in the first half of the century, when formal medical care did little to advance health and may have done substantial harm, health insurance existed primarily to replace lost income rather than to cover medical bills. The development of health insurance into its current form corresponded with the increasing complexity and expense of medical care and the advance of scientific knowledge.

The link between health insurance and employment in the United States dates to the middle of the nineteenth century, when workers in a newly industrial America began to seek safeguards from the dangers of their jobs. Although the government had sponsored health care plans as far back as 1798, these plans were limited in scope and never intended to be part of a comprehensive, nationwide state-sponsored health insurance system. Instead, employers and unions established their own health insurance plans, primarily to replace lost wages in case of illness or injury, rather than to pay for medical services (Hoffman, 2003; Starr, 1982). In particularly risky occupations, however, such as mining and railroads, employees did purchase insurance to pay for medical services. These workers became part of the first prepaid group plans, paying physicians a fixed monthly fee in exchange for services covering the entire group of employees (Scofea, 1994).

Progressive Era

The Progressive era, from about 1890 to 1920, reinforced the employment-based structure of the U.S. health insurance system (**Figure 1-1**). In 1915 the American Association for Labor Legislation (AALL) proposed a mandatory government-sponsored bill in which low-income employees and their employers would contribute to a subsidized plan to insure against medical bills and lost wages. Higher-income employees would have the option of buying into the plan as well. But this plan was unpopular with several groups. Led by Samuel Gompers, the American Federation of Labor (AFL) opposed the bill on the grounds that labor would lose leverage in negotiations with employers by ceding part of employees' compensation package to a predetermined government benefit package. Insurers opposed the bill because it included insurance against burial expenses, a profitable sector of their business. And finally, although organized medicine, the American Medical Association (AMA), at first supported the bill, they quickly changed course and came out against it, arguing that it would impede physician autonomy and the physician-patient relationship (Scofea, 1994; Starr, 1982).

Employee "sickness funds" during the Progressive era weakened the urgency for mandatory, government-sponsored insurance. Thousands of sickness funds existed, though they covered only a minority of workers. Employees would pool a small portion of their income and distribute funds in the case of illness or injury, mostly to replace lost income rather than to pay medical bills. Though not particularly generous, these funds were effective enough to diminish support for a government plan. As actuarial methods (methods to anticipate the cost of enrollees) advanced, however, insurance plans became larger and more financially stable, and thus a more attractive alternative for employees (Murray, 2007).

Great Depression

Workers and hospitals relied on each other to endure the financial devastation of the Great Depression, further entwining employment with health insurance. In the 1920s economic prosperity had increased demand for health care services, and physicians and hospitals raised fees in response. As a result, medical care occupied an increasingly higher proportion of family income, straining even the middle class (Starr, 1982). But when the stock market collapsed in 1929, workers and hospitals came to rely on each other. They formed mutually beneficial

FIGURE 1-1 Progressive Era Cartoon Endorsing Compulsory Health Insurance in New York State

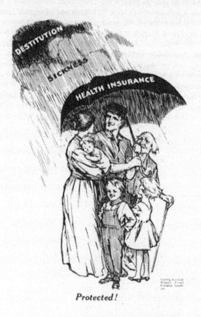

Protected!

From the *American Labor Legislation Review*, 1919, 9.

contractual arrangements in which unions prepaid for hospital services, thereby guaranteeing income to financially struggling hospitals, while insuring workers against high, unpredictable hospital costs. These contractual arrangements with hospitals were the precursors to Blue Cross plans. Toward the end of the Depression, analogous arrangements with physicians became the precursors to Blue Shield plans.

Also during the Great Depression, employees joined the first integrated prepaid group plans, which would later develop into health maintenance organizations (HMOs). Prepaid group plans differed from Blue Cross (hospital insurance) and Blue Shield (physician insurance) plans because enrollees exclusively used clinics or hospitals owned by the plan. Blue Cross did not own hospitals; rather, it contracted with area hospitals. Similarly, Blue Shield did not own medical clinics; rather, it contracted with area clinics and their physicians. Prepaid group plans, however, built their own clinics and hospitals, and only members of the plan could use these facilities; on the other hand, members could not use other area facilities. Such a plan may sound familiar to you—Kaiser Permanente (Kaiser Foundation Health Plan and Permanente Medical Group) is an example of such a plan. And in fact, Kaiser was one of the earliest integrated prepaid group plans, founded by Dr. Sidney Garber in 1933 to provide on-site care for workers building an aqueduct for shipbuilder Henry J. Kaiser.

With historic levels of unemployment, it might have seemed that the Great Depression would have severed the link between employment and health insurance, but state-sponsored insurance was not a priority for economic recovery. Emerging from the Great Depression, President Franklin Delano Roosevelt's New Deal had excluded a national health insurance option to minimize objection to other programs, especially Social Security, unemployment insurance, and welfare benefits.

World War II

Though health insurance had long been tied to employment, employers had not used it as a recruitment and retention tool until World War II, when runaway inflation, or price growth, led the War Labor Board to impose limitations on wages that employers could offer. These limitations, however, did not apply to fringe benefits, including health insurance. Consequently, while employers could not compete for the best employees by offering higher wages, they could offer more generous health insurance benefits. Under the Wagner Act of 1935, workers were guaranteed the right to collectively bargain for such benefits, and so health insurance became an integral part of employees' compensation package.

Post-War Period

After the war, national legislation further protected employee fringe benefits, strengthening the relationship between health insurance and employment. In 1954, Congress and the Internal Revenue Service (IRS) allowed employers and employees to contribute to employee insurance premiums without paying taxes on those contributions. This tax treatment remains largely in effect today, though the 2010 ACA imposed some taxes on health plans with very high premiums. Because there is such a considerable advantage to purchasing insurance through an employer versus through the individual (non-employer) market, employees may find themselves tied to a job they do not want, working when they want to retire or raise children, or purchasing a plan through their employer that is more generous than they would have purchased on the individual market without the tax advantage.

The post-war period also aligned the structures of commercial and Blue Cross plans. Previously on the fringes of the market, commercial plans began to compete more vigorously with the Blues as more unions searched for an insurance carrier, and by 1955 commercial plans covered more enrollees (**Figure 1-2**) (Conrad, 2009). While the Blues set premiums based on health care spending in the entire geographic area (community rating), commercial plans set premiums based on spending for just one group or individual (experience rating). While community rating is good for people who are sick, it is expensive for those who are healthy; experience rating, on the other hand, does not pool the healthy and the sick together as much as community rating. Experience rating allowed commercial plans to undercut prices in low-spending healthy areas,

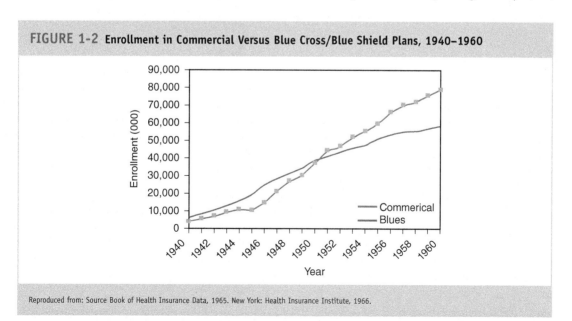

FIGURE 1-2 **Enrollment in Commercial Versus Blue Cross/Blue Shield Plans, 1940–1960**

leaving the Blues with only the highest cost (sickest) enrollees (Starr, 1982). As nonprofit organizations founded with the purpose of serving the community, the Blues were reluctant to experience rate premiums, which would have left sicker areas with higher premiums, but eventually did so to remain competitive with commercial plans.

The Blues and commercial plans began to resemble each other in how they paid providers as well. Early commercial plans provided coverage by paying indemnities—payments *to the subscriber*, usually a fixed amount per hospital day. This payment structure required workers to pay facilities directly; insurers only later reimbursed expenses. Not only were workers thus required to have sufficient cash on hand to pay for medical services but they were also left at risk for the balance of the bill if the indemnity did not cover all of the expenses. Recall that early Blue Cross plans, on the other hand, prepaid hospitals a fixed dollar amount per worker per month. Facilities were required to treat subscribers regardless of ability to pay the balance of the bill. While some Blue Cross plans also provided indemnity insurance, during the Depression the American Hospital Association encouraged all plans to move toward service benefits, paying the physicians and facilities directly for expenses after they had been incurred. The Blues were able to take on this additional risk and offer more attractive plans to subscribers because (1) as nonprofits, they did not have to pay taxes; (2) Blue plans were forbidden to compete with each other, and so local plans enjoyed geographic market exclusivity; and (3) relationships with providers were strong, and so favorable rates could be negotiated compared to commercial plans. Yet as commercial plans gained traction by experience rating premiums, the Blues could not take on as much risk and began to offer more indemnity policies (Starr, 1982). After the war, then, commercial and Blue Cross plans looked increasingly alike.

Experience rating and the growing cost of medical care in the middle of the century made health insurance for older, sicker Americans unaffordable. Mid-century was a time of rapid medical progress. Antibiotics,

discovered in 1928 and entering widespread use in the 1930s through the 1940s, protected patients against bacterial infections and thus made hospitalization much safer. Public vaccination campaigns for newly discovered vaccines reduced the spread of infectious disease. Mortality from heart attacks and strokes declined with the advent of procedures such as cardiac catheterization in 1959, and antihypertensives and cholesterol-lowering medications (Cutler, 2004). With this medical progress came a higher price tag; medical spending tripled from 1949 to 1964 (Engel, 2006).

But the disappearance of community rating meant that much of this medical progress was out of reach for the elderly and the poor. Experience rating set lower premiums for healthy, low-risk subscribers and higher premiums for sicker, high-risk subscribers. These high premiums were unaffordable for those in the highest-risk groups, and lower-income families were more likely to be uninsured (Starr, 1982).

Medicare and Medicaid

Medicare (health insurance for those 65 and older) and Medicaid (health insurance for the poor) were the public response to this lapse in the private market. President John F. Kennedy had strongly advocated for a national health insurance program for the elderly, but he did not see his legislative vision realized before he was assassinated in 1963. His successor, Lyndon B. Johnson, took up the cause, and under his presidency Congress passed Medicare and Medicaid in 1965. While insurance for the aged was the primary piece of the legislative agenda, advocates for insurance for the poor used the opportunity to pass Medicaid at the same time. But legislators designed the programs in fundamentally different ways. Medicare was an earned benefit for all Americans 65 or older who had worked. The federal government would administer the program and all enrollees would pay the same premium and receive the same benefits. In contrast, Medicaid was not a universal program; rather, only those receiving Aid to Families with Dependent Children (AFDC)—commonly known as welfare—would be eligible. Further, states and their welfare departments would be responsible for administering the program and receive federal matching funds if they met certain income threshold and benefits criteria (Engel, 2006).

These new programs contributed to substantial health care spending growth. Despite spending controls and a sluggish economy, from 1966 to 1973 health expenditures grew at an average rate of 7.2 percent per year, outpacing GDP growth by 3.2 percentage points. Medical progress, along with newly expanded insurance, contributed to this growth (Catlin & Cowan, 2015). Federal and state governments undertook many policies to rein in this spending. One of the most impactful policies during this time was the 1973 Health Maintenance Organization Act, which encouraged HMOs to enter the market by providing them with funding, overruling state laws prohibiting them, and requiring employers who offered tax-exempt health insurance to offer at least one HMO. Similar to prepaid group plans, HMOs pay a fixed fee to providers per patient per month (a capitation), thereby setting a "budget" for each enrollee. Enrollees must also consult a primary care "gatekeeper" before using specialty services. In 1970, there were fewer than two million HMO enrollees; by 1992, there were 39 million (Scofea, 1994).

Managed Care

HMOs launched the managed care era. Managed care is a set of tools used by managed care plans to reduce spending and improve the quality of health care. These tools include imposing out-of-pocket costs on enrollees, contracting with low-cost providers, and limiting coverage for some types of procedures deemed inappropriate. Throughout the 1980s and 1990s, managed care enrollment grew Figure 1-3. Traditional indemnity insurance for health care expenses now constitutes only a tiny proportion of the health insurance market. But HMOs are not the only type of managed care plan. Preferred Provider Organizations (PPO) plans, developed in the 1980s, do not prepay for services, but rather contract with "preferred" providers to pay a negotiated rate for services (a fee-for-service) after they have been provided. Any providers whose services have not been contracted are out-of-network, or "non-preferred." Point-of-service (POS) plans are somewhere in between the two—less restrictive than an HMO, but more restrictive (and thus less expensive) than a PPO.

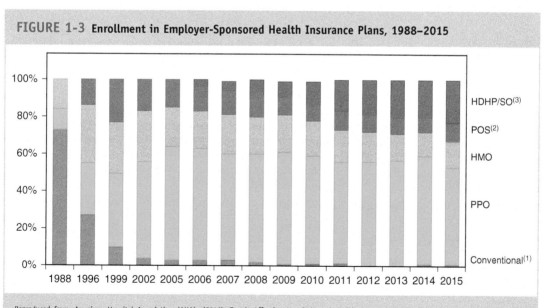

FIGURE 1-3 **Enrollment in Employer-Sponsored Health Insurance Plans, 1988–2015**

Enrollees are generally assigned a primary care gatekeeper and may use an out-of-network provider, provided they pay more out of pocket. Like HMOs, exclusive provider organizations (EPOs) have restrictive networks and limited—if any— out-of-network benefits, but unlike HMOs, they usually do not require a primary care gatekeeper. Today, plans generally have features of all three types of plans. HMOs may prepay for primary care services but not hospital services, and PPO plans may require higher out-of-pocket payments for some non-preferred providers. Table 1-1 highlights the differences among managed care plans, though it is worth repeating that the distinctions have become blurry. For example, while PPO plans pay most of their physicians' fee-for-service, some have experimented with other payment types, including capitation.

In its heyday in the late 1980s and early 1990s, managed care was successful in lowering health care spending and the price of insurance. But selective contracting of hospitals and physicians became difficult as providers responded by joining forces. From 1989 to 1996, there were 190 hospital mergers, beginning with just 6,000 hospitals, over double the number from 1983 to 1988 (Dafny, 2009). Consumers also reacted to managed care. Techniques such as primary care gatekeeping and limiting provider networks led to a managed care "backlash" by the late 1990s (Blendon et al., 1998).

Consumer-Directed Health Care

In order to attract enrollees, insurers were pushed to offer plans with larger networks and fewer restrictions on services. But with more generous plans again came higher premiums, and so another tool emerged: consumer-directed health plans (Figure 1-3). These plans are intended to limit enrollee spending by requiring large out-of-pocket payments before insurance covers expenses. The 2003 Medicare Modernization Act authorized the creation of health savings accounts (HSAs), into which an employer or employee may contribute tax-free dollars for out-of-pocket payments related to such a plan. Under the law, the employee owns the HSA and may thus take it from job to job, or in transitioning to unemployment.

The Patient Protection and Affordable Care Act

Until Congress passed the ACA in 2010, the proportion of non-elderly Americans uninsured at any given time remained steady for decades at around 15 percent. Not since the enactment of Medicare and Medicaid had the uninsurance rate declined so dramatically. The ACA was a landmark piece of legislation intended to expand coverage among non-elderly adults (elderly adults are almost universally covered by Medicare). It required individuals to purchase

TABLE 1-1 Types of Managed Care Plans

Managed Care Insurance Plans	Payment To	Physician Payment (Primary Method)	Primary Care Gatekeeper	Network Restrictiveness
Preferred Provider Organization (PPO)	Provider	Fee-for-service	No	Low
Point of Service (POS)	Provider	Fee-for-service	No	Medium
Exclusive Provider Organization (EPO)	Provider	Fee-for-service	No	High
Health Maintenance Organization (HMO)	Provider	Capitation	Yes	High
Managed Indemnity	Patient	Fee-for-service	No	Low

insurance (individual mandate), large employers to offer insurance or to pay to cover premiums for outside insurance (employer pay-or-play mandate), and gave states the option to receive federal financial assistance to expand Medicaid coverage to everyone under 138 percent of the federal poverty level (FPL), not just those receiving welfare benefits. Thirty-two states have expanded Medicaid. The law also required that each state have a virtual health insurance marketplace, called an exchange, in which people could shop for and purchase standardized plans, with subsidies for those 100–400 percent of the FPL. The federal government and states imposed regulations on health insurance plans to expand access and affordability. Key ACA provisions, including Medicaid expansions, health insurance marketplaces, and the individual mandate to purchase coverage, became effective in 2014. At the end of 2013, just before these provisions were implemented, an estimated 42.7 million people were uninsured, or approximately 15 percent of the population; by 2015, this number had dropped to 25.8 million people, or approximately 10 percent of the population (Carman, Eibner, & Paddock, 2015).

PRINCIPLES OF INSURANCE

As defined at the beginning of this chapter, insurance is a guarantee against an unforeseen event, but health insurance, of course, does not guarantee against unforeseen illness or injury, and covered medical expenses are often anticipated well in advance. In this section, we will discuss the ways in which health insurance in the United States violates many of the principles of "ideal" insurance.

Why purchase health insurance at all? Why not "self-insure"—put aside savings to cover personal, unforeseen expenses? In fact, we all self-insure for at least some events. We save money for when our car breaks down, for when our water heater must be replaced, and for when Huxley makes an unexpected trip to the veterinarian. But the more unpredictable and costly these events become, the more it makes sense to pool our savings with others to cover these expenses—in other words, to purchase insurance. Imagine if it cost

$100,000 to fix your car or $40,000 to replace your water heater, or $50,000 to pay Huxley's veterinarian. Very few people could afford these bills, even if they happened infrequently. But if we pooled our money together, then we could collectively afford them—as long as most people's cars did not break down.

Insurers rely on the fact that not all enrollees will actually use their insurance, but sometimes it is difficult—both for the insurer and the enrollee—to know how much care will be used. As the quotable baseball player Yogi Berra famously said (or is attributed to have said), "It's tough to make predictions, especially about the future." Insurers charge a premium based on two components: one component, the actuarially fair premium, is based on enrollees' predicted costs (the frequency and costliness of their medical care); the other component is the loading charge, an additional cost that the insurer charges to administer claims and make a profit.

Insurers can charge loading costs because enrollees are risk averse—they dislike unpredictability and prefer a certain outcome over an uncertain one. The more risk-averse enrollees are, the more they are willing to pay to avoid risk—in other words, the higher a premium beyond the actuarially fair premium they are willing to pay. Premiums are a small but certain financial loss that risk-averse people would prefer to pay rather than to gamble on a potentially catastrophic hospitalization. Note that there are reasons beyond a low degree of risk aversion that people are unwilling to pay for health insurance every month. People may not be able to afford premiums, or they may underestimate their expected medical costs. Insurers rely on risk aversion to charge a high enough premium to cover administrative expenses and earn a profit; there are not too many risk-loving people who prefer a gamble when it comes to their health care finances.

We expect sicker people to join plans with more generous benefits and higher premiums, and healthier people to join plans with skimpier benefits and lower premiums. This phenomenon, the sorting into plans based on health status, is called selection. Insurers attempt to price plans accurately based on enrollees' prior health costs and family histories, such that plans with sicker enrollees have higher premiums and plans with healthier enrollees have lower premiums. But two factors prevent insurers from pricing plans entirely accurately: (1) enrollees generally know more about their health than insurers; and (2) regulations and other organizational factors may prohibit insurers from charging higher premiums for sicker enrollees. Adverse selection is a type of selection in which health plan sorting is *caused* by such incomplete or asymmetrical information between insurers and enrollees. What makes this selection *adverse* is that, without enough information about enrollees' health costs, insurers cannot accurately price premiums. Costly enrollees may sign up for a plan whose premium is too low to cover the costs of the plan.

Adverse selection happened in the post–World War II era when commercial plans began to experience rate premiums, drawing off healthier enrollees to whom they could offer lower rates. The Blues, whose mission limited them to community rating, were not able to cover the costs of the remaining, sicker enrollees, and eventually had to follow suit and experience rate premiums as well. The ACA requires plans in the state exchanges to community-rate their premiums, but at the same time states may limit insurers' premium increases. As a result, adverse selection may prevent some insurers from offering health insurance under ACA regulations.

In an attempt to prevent adverse selection, many insurers previously limited coverage for pre-existing conditions—illness or injury present even before coverage begins. Limiting such coverage is consistent with the traditional definition of insurance. What if you wanted to purchase insurance for a car that had already broken down, for a water heater that needed replacement, and for a dog that had broken its leg? Would an insurer sell you coverage for these events? Not likely. Insurance is protection against events that have not yet happened.

So why do insurers offer coverage for diabetes, chronic heart disease, and lower back pain to enrollees who already have these conditions?

In fact, the ACA required that almost all plans—with the exception of older, individual (non-employment-based) plans—cover pre-existing conditions. We previously noted that health insurance has expanded beyond its original function—to protect against unpredictable financial losses—because of the importance that society places on health. The requirement that insurers community-rate premiums and cover pre-existing conditions at the risk of adverse selection is an example of this expansion.

We require people to sign insurance contracts for only one year, so if someone becomes sick or knows that they will need a medical procedure in the upcoming year, then they can sign up for a plan that covers these expenses during the next open enrollment period. A hypothetically "ideal" insurance contract would begin at birth, bind the enrollee for life, and cover every potential health condition that currently exists and that could exist in the future. In this case, there would be no "pre-existing" conditions and no selection into more generous health plans based on illness (Arrow, 1963).

Another puzzle is why health insurance covers such small claims (requests from providers for payment)—$50 for an office visit, $100 for a blood test, $80 for a 30-day supply of generic medication. Premiums include not only the cost of medical care but also the cost of administering claims, so for inexpensive services like office visits and blood tests, wouldn't it be cheaper to just self-insure? If it costs $10 to administer each claim, then administration accounts for 20 percent of an office visit claim ($10 divided by $50), 10 percent of a claim for a blood test ($10 divided by $100), and 8 percent of a claim for a 30-day supply of generic medication ($10 divided by $80). In contrast, $10 is a negligible proportion (0.03 percent) of a $30,000 knee surgery. The larger the medical bill, the smaller the proportion of that bill that is attributable to administration.

One explanation for why insurance covers small claims is that insurers negotiate prices with providers (hospitals, physicians, and pharmacies) that individuals do not have the power to negotiate themselves, so even for small claims like office visits and blood tests, consumers rely on insurance for payment. Consumer-directed health insurance is in part intended to save money on these small claims by giving enrollees the benefit of the negotiated rate but requiring large out-of-pocket payments before insurance covers expenses. The role of the health insurer as a negotiator is another example of its expansion beyond its original function of collecting premiums and paying out benefits.

Finally, precisely because insurance protects enrollees against risk, having insurance may encourage enrollees to use more care or behave more recklessly, a phenomenon called moral hazard. Health insurers thus have yet another role—to design benefits and review utilization to limit moral hazard. Many tools are available: insurers can impose copayments (a fixed cost per episode of care, such as a doctor's visit for hospitalization), coinsurance (a fixed percentage of the cost of care, such as 10 percent or 20 percent of the cost of a doctor's visit), deductibles (a fixed amount that the enrollee must pay before insurance covers expenses, commonly used in consumer-directed health plans), and annual and lifetime limits on covered expenses. Insurers can also restrict patients to a narrow network of providers that is willing to offer a lower price to the insurer. Other tools include utilization review, an evaluation of the cost and medical necessity of care. An example of utilization review is prior authorization, a requirement that enrollees seek approval from an insurer before obtaining medical services (**Table 1-2**).

Health insurance in the United States is far from the hypothetical ideal in which only large, unpredictable health conditions are covered. It has expanded beyond its original role replacing lost income, and now resembles a gym membership more than traditional insurance such as auto or homeowners, which have adhered more closely to the ideal. At a gym, dues are paid every month. In return, you can visit the gym—or not. If you would like to join a fancier gym with gleaming new equipment and nice showers, then you must pay more. Some gyms offer additional services à la

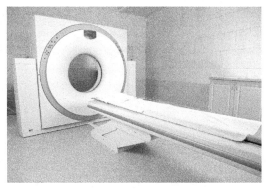

© Sergey Rusakov/Shutterstock

TABLE 1-2 Insurer Tools to Manage Two Major Market Failures

Moral Hazard	Adverse Selection
Out-of-pocket payments	Experience rating
• Deductible	Limit coverage for pre-existing conditions
• Coinsurance	Open enrollment
• Copayments	
Annual and lifetime limits	
Utilization review	
• Prior authorization	

carte—you may pay extra for yoga classes, massage, towel service, or for a smoothie at the café downstairs. Gyms curb overuse by limiting use of machines to 30 minutes and restricting attendance in classes. Analogously to a gym membership, you (or your spouse, parents, or the government) must pay a premium to join a health insurance plan. Generous plans with more in-network providers and covered services are more expensive. You may purchase additional services or supplies à la carte, such as a prescription drug that is not covered or services from an out-of-network provider. Some plans even have add-ons such as dental and vision services. The origins and development of health insurance in the United States help to clarify why it adopted such peculiar features and a pivotal place in U.S. society.

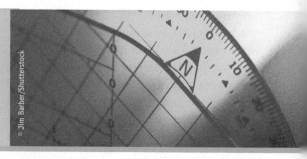

Summary

It is not feasible to offer insurance against the possibility of getting ill, or even to guarantee full recovery for someone who has become sick or injured. In many cases, such as with chronic disease and the gradual decline that comes with age, illness is not a well-defined event, and medical care is not the only factor that contributes to good health. Social, environmental, political, and genetic factors are also predictive of illness and injury, but insurance cannot guarantee a safe and healthy life. Thus health insurance is not really health insurance at all but actually *medical care* insurance—a guarantee against unpredictable, costly medical care bills. Because of the importance that society places on health, however, medical care insurance also covers predictable, not-so-costly bills as well, despite the risk of adverse selection and moral hazard.

There are tradeoffs in health insurance as with any limited resource. Premiums can be equally distributed across the population, as with community rating, or can be efficiently distributed across the population proportionate to expected cost, as with experience rating. Insurance benefits can be generous, covering a large number of people and conditions, or can be less costly. The trend in the United States has been toward emphasizing premium equality and generosity of coverage, rather than efficiency and affordability. Insurance has become the mechanism by which society transfers money from the healthy to the sick.

References

Arrow, K. J. (1963). Uncertainty and the welfare economics of medical care. *The American Economic Review, 53*(5), 941–973.

Blendon, R. J., Brodie, M., Benson, J. M., Altman, D. E., Levitt, L., Hoff, T., & Hugick, L. (1998). Understanding the managed care backlash. *Health Affairs (Project Hope), 17*(4), 80–94.

Carman, K., Eibner, C., & Paddock, S. (2015). Trends in health insurance enrollment, 2013–15. *Health Affairs, 34*(6), 1044–1048.

Catlin, A., & Cowan, C. (2015). *History of health spending in the United States, 1960–2013.* Retrieved from https://www.cms.gov/Research-Statistics-Data-and-Systems/Statistics-Trends-and-Reports/NationalHealthExpendData/Downloads/HistoricalNHEPaper.pdf

Conrad, P. (Ed.). (2009). *The sociology of health & illness: Critical perspectives* (8th ed.). New York, NY: Worth.

Cutler, D. (2004). *Your money or your life: Strong medicine for America's health care system* (1st ed.). New York, NY: Oxford University Press.

Dafny, L. (2009). Estimation and identification of merger effects: An application to hospital mergers. *Journal of Law & Economics, 52*(3), 523–550.

Engel, J. (2006). *Poor people's medicine: Medicaid and American charity care since 1965.* Durham & London, United Kingdom: Duke University Press.

Hoffman, B. (2003). Health care reform and social movements in the United States [abstract]. *The American Journal of Public Health, 93*(1), 75.

Murray, J. E. (2007). *Origins of American health insurance: A history of industrial sickness funds.* New Haven, CT: Yale University Press.

Scofea, L. A. (1994). Health care reform and social movements in the United States [abstract]. *Monthly Labor Review, 117*(3), 3–10.

Starr, P. (1982). *Social transformation of American medicine: The rise of a sovereign profession and the making of a vast industry.* New York: Basic Books.

CHAPTER **2**

Public and Private Coverage in the United States

April M. Falconi, PhD, MPH, MA

LEARNING OBJECTIVES

- What are the different types of health insurance offered in the United States?
- Who is covered by the different types of health insurance?
- What are the strengths and weaknesses of private versus public coverage?

INTRODUCTION

In the United States, health insurance coverage is offered through an array of public and private sources (Table 2-1), although more people have private health insurance than government-provided coverage. In 2014, 66 percent of the civilian, non-institutionalized population had private health insurance and 37 percent had government-sponsored insurance at some point during the year; 10 percent were uninsured for the entire year. Note that the totals do not add up to 100 percent of the population because some people have more than one type of health insurance or they are covered by public and private coverage at different points in the year (Smith & Medalia, 2015).

Private health insurance coverage is most often provided through an individual's employer, although individuals sometimes purchase their own health coverage independently. Public sources of health insurance include Medicare,

Medicaid, the Children's Health Insurance Program, TRICARE, and federal and state health plans (Claxton & Lundy, 2008).

Certain characteristics, such as age, income, and disability status, influence the type of coverage an individual is likely to have. Nearly all (99 percent) individuals aged 65 years or older, for example, reported having health insurance in 2014, because most are covered by Medicare. Children under age 19 also had relatively high rates of coverage (94 percent), because Medicaid and the Children's Health Insurance Program cover most children from low- and even moderate-income families. In contrast, only 86 percent of working-age adults aged 19 to 64 years had health insurance in 2014 (Smith & Medalia, 2015).

People in low-income households (i.e., household income less than $25,000 per year) are also more likely to have government coverage than people in higher-income households, because Medicaid covers many low-income families. Individuals in households earning less than $25,000 per year, for example, were 17 percent more likely to have government coverage than individuals in households earning between $25,000 and $49,999 (Smith & Medalia, 2015).

Lastly, adults with a disability are less likely to have private health insurance than adults without a disability, because public programs

TABLE 2-1 Distribution of Health Insurance in the United States, 2014

	% of Population
Private	
Employer/Group	55.4%
Individual/Non-Group	14.6%
Public	
Medicare	16.0%
Medicaid/SCHIP	19.5%
TRICARE	4.5%
Uninsured	10.4%

Note: Some individuals had multiple sources of insurance, so percentages add up to more than 100 percent.

Data from 2015 Current Population Survey. Available at http://www.census.gov/content/dam/Census/library/publications/2015/demo/p60-253.pdf

such as Medicare and Medicaid assist people with qualifying disabilities. Among adults age 18 to 64, 41 percent of those with a disability had private health insurance, compared to 74 percent of adults with no disability (Smith & Medalia, 2015).

This chapter will explain the different types of health insurance coverage provided in the United States, comparing sources of private insurance to public insurance, and will conclude with a discussion of the strengths and weaknesses associated with each.

PRIVATE HEALTH INSURANCE

Private health insurance is an agreement that a state-licensed health insurer or a self-funded employee health benefit plan will take on financial risk for health care costs, administer benefits, and pay claims, or contract these functions to a third party, for individuals or groups of individuals, and their families. Smaller employers and individuals generally pay state-licensed insurers not only to administer benefits but also to take on financial risk; this arrangement is called a fully insured plan. On the other hand, larger, especially cross-state, employers generally take on risk in-house by collecting premiums and paying out benefits in-house; this arrangement is called a self-funded (self-insured) plan. Self-funded employers may purchase administrative services from a third-party insurer, but that insurer will not take on any financial risk.

Outside of employment, options for coverage include public insurance (for those who qualify) or fully insured coverage either directly from a state-licensed health insurer or through a state health insurance exchange, set up by the 2010 Affordable Care Act (ACA).

The group market sells insurance to employers, and the individual market sells insurance to individual subscribers and their families. More formally, the group market is the online or brick-and mortar place where individuals, insurers, and employers buy and sell policies or administrative services that cover two or more individuals who are not members of the same immediate family. The individual market is the place where individuals and insurers buy and sell policies that cover an individual subscriber and her immediate family.

Both individuals and employers may purchase fully insured plans primarily from one of three types of private health insurers:

- Commercial health insurers: These companies are generally for-profit and organized as stock or mutual insurance companies. An example of a commercial health insurer is Aetna.
- Blue Cross and Blue Shield (BCBS): BCBS plans are nonprofit organizations. States regulate these plans, generally requiring them to have more of a community focus than commercial insurers. For example, they may have stricter requirements on excluding coverage of pre-existing conditions and on experience rating in order to make plans affordable to the sick. In some states (e.g., Connecticut, New Hampshire, Ohio), BCBS plans have converted to for-profit organizations and are now subject only to the state requirements for commercial insurers, but in other states (e.g., Arkansas, parts of California, New Jersey), BCBS plans remain nonprofits and continue to be subject to these requirements.

- Health maintenance organizations (HMOs): HMOs integrate health insurance with the provision of health care. An example of an HMO is Kaiser Permanente, in which Kaiser Health Plan has an exclusive relationship with the Permanente Medical Group and also owns hospitals, imaging centers, and other health care facilities. Health care services obtained outside of Kaiser's network of doctors, hospitals, and facilities are generally not covered by insurance. Most commercial insurers offer HMO products, but these plans generally do not integrate care delivery in the same way as a "true" HMO, because the insurer does not own facilities or contract exclusively with physicians.

For several reasons, large employers are more likely to bypass these options for health insurance and instead self-insure. While individuals and smaller employers pay insurers to take on the risk of illness or injury, self-insured employers take on this risk themselves. In other words, they are responsible for setting a premium that will cover the medical costs of their employees. Larger employers have the capacity to take on this risk because it is spread over many individuals. Therefore, the medical costs of a large group are more predictable from year to year than for an individual or small group, so a more accurate premium can be set each year.

But even if large employers have the capacity to take on risk, why would they want to? First, employers can save money on health insurance premiums by managing their own benefits and paying claims in-house (and anything that cannot be managed efficiently in-house can be purchased from a third-party insurer). Second, under the Employee Retirement Income Security Act of 1974 (ERISA), self-insured plans are exempt from many of the state regulations for fully insured plans, an important exemption for employers operating in multiple states. Designed to protect the assets of employees enrolled in private retirement plans, ERISA also sets rules for other employee benefit plans, including health insurance. While ERISA preempts most state laws regarding employee benefits, it does not preempt state laws for health insurance. Under the "deemer clause" (ERISA Section 514), however, states may not "deem" self-funded plans health insurance in order to subject them to state regulation. The deemer clause thus protects multi-state employers from facing inconsistent obligations in different states, so that they may offer employees working in different states the same package of health benefits.

Employment-based coverage is the most common type of private coverage and the most common type of health insurance, but not everyone has access to this coverage. Recall that in 2014, 66 percent of the population had private coverage, 55 percent had employment-based coverage, and 15 percent purchased insurance directly from an insurer (Smith & Medalia, 2015). Those without access may include workers in part-time or seasonal jobs, unemployed people, spouses and dependents of a worker without family coverage, and workers in firms that are too small to offer health insurance. Firms with fewer than 10 workers are the least likely to offer coverage; therefore, workers without employer-sponsored health insurance are most likely to be employed in small firms. Low-wage workers are also far less likely than higher-wage workers to have access to job-based coverage (Hoffman & Paradise, 2008).

Employees with access to coverage through their employer may still choose to purchase insurance on the individual market. There are benefits and costs to employment-based versus individual insurance. Employer and employee premium contributions to the employee's health insurance plan are exempt from federal and state income taxes, as well as Social Security and Medicare payroll taxes. Because of the tax treatment of health insurance benefits through an employer, and because of risk spreading across many individuals, employment-based insurance may be more generous than a policy on the individual market. But employment-based insurance may be unaffordable for some employees, or employers may not offer a plan option that the employee wants, for example because the plan excludes a certain provider or has out-of-pocket costs that are too high. Purchasing an employment-based plan also ties employees to their employers.

For just this reason, there are transitional options for those who lose access to employment-based insurance. Individuals might lose access when (1) they lose their jobs or move jobs; (2) they work fewer hours and lose eligibility for coverage; (3) a person reliant on a spouse's health coverage gets divorced or separated; (4) children age out of dependent coverage; or (5) a spouse who provides health insurance for a family dies or becomes eligible for Medicare. In these cases, workers or their [former] dependents may be eligible for the Consolidated Omnibus Budget Reconciliation Act (COBRA), a federal program applying to non-federal workplaces with 20 or more employees (some states have even more expansive policies). People eligible for the program may buy into their former plan for up to 18 or 36 months, depending on the reason for the loss of access. The employer, however, is not required to make any contribution to the premium, so plans purchased through COBRA may be very expensive. **Figure 2-1** illustrates the relationship among different types of private health insurance options in the United States.

PUBLIC HEALTH INSURANCE

Public health insurance is an agreement that the government will take on financial risk for health care costs, administer benefits, and pay claims, or contract these functions to a third party, for individuals and their families. The government may also administer benefits for public health insurance plans, or it may contract administration to a private third party. Six government health care programs—Medicare, Medicaid, the State Children's Health Insurance Program (SCHIP), TRICARE, the Veterans Health Administration (VHA), and the Indian Health Service (IHS) serve approximately one-third of Americans (Corrigan, Eden, & Smith, 2003).

Medicare

Title XVIII (18) of the Social Security Act, commonly known as Medicare, is a federally administered program that provides health insurance for the nation's aged and disabled. Modeled on the BCBS plans of the 1960s, Medicare benefits are divided into four parts. Part A covers hospital care; Part B covers physician, imaging, and laboratory services; Part C, also known as Medicare

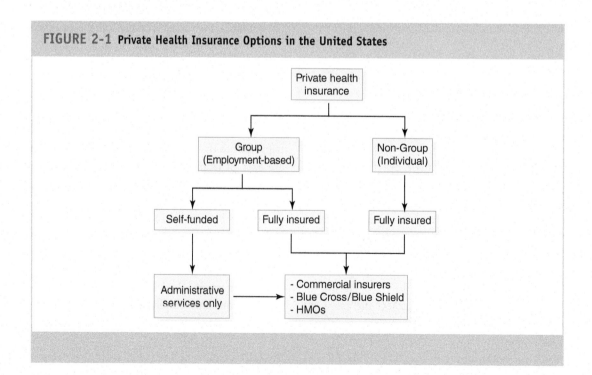

FIGURE 2-1 Private Health Insurance Options in the United States

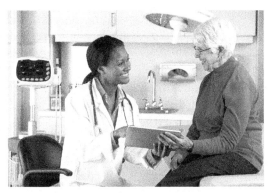

© Monkey Business Images/Shutterstock

Advantage, is a set of managed care options (e.g., HMO, preferred provider organization [PPO]) that are privately offered as an alternative to traditional Medicare (Parts A and B); and Part D covers outpatient prescription drugs. Traditional Medicare does not cover long-term care or assisted living services. It also does not pay for dental or vision care, or hearing exams and hearing aids.

Individuals may also purchase supplemental insurance called Medigap to help pay for out-of-pocket costs (such as deductibles, coinsurance, and copayments) and benefits not covered by Medicare. Medigap policies are offered through private health insurers and are not public health insurance. Medicare does not subsidize premiums for Medigap purchases, but some employers offer Medigap policies (Cubanski et al., 2015).

In general, most seniors qualify for Medicare. People who are age 65 and older qualify for Medicare Parts A and B if they are U.S. citizens or permanent legal residents with at least 5 years of continuous residence. Adults under age 65 with permanent disabilities are also eligible once they have received Social Security Disability Income (SSDI) payments for 24 months. People with end-stage renal disease (ESRD) or amyotrophic lateral sclerosis (ALS) are eligible for Medicare as well, as soon as they begin receiving SSDI payments. These individuals are not required to wait 24 months. People may enroll in Part C if they are entitled to Part A and are enrolled in Part B. People are eligible for Part D if they are enrolled in Parts A or B (Cubanski et al., 2015), though some Part C plans also integrate prescription drug coverage.

Part A, or inpatient hospital insurance, also covers short stays in a skilled nursing facility, some home health care, and hospice care. Enrollment in Part A is automatic for anyone who qualifies for Social Security on the basis of age or disability; only a very small proportion of beneficiaries who do not receive Social Security income must pay a premium to enroll. Part A is financed primarily through a 2.9 percent payroll tax—1.45 percent from the employer, and 1.45 percent from the employee. Higher-earning individuals are taxed 3.8 percent—1.45 percent from the employer, and 2.35 percent from the employee. These payroll taxes fund the Hospital Insurance (HI) Trust Fund, which pays Part A benefits (and Part C hospital benefits) (National Health Policy Forum, 2016).

Part B, the supplemental medical insurance (SMI) program, covers physician and laboratory services, durable medical equipment such as canes and walkers, and outpatient care. Those eligible must pay a premium to enroll in Part B, although these premiums are heavily subsidized by general tax revenue. Premiums finance only a quarter of Part B, while the remainder is funded primarily through general revenues (Cubanski & Neuman, 2016). There is a financial penalty for failing to enroll in Part B immediately upon eligibility, as much as 10 percent per year, in order to reduce adverse selection.

Part C, also called Medicare Advantage, is an alternative to Parts A and B. Over 30 percent of Medicare beneficiaries are enrolled in Part C (Jacobson, Casillas, Damico, & Neuman, 2016). Part C plans may offer additional benefits not covered by traditional Medicare. Like Part B, Part C plans are also financed in part by premiums, but these premiums are subsidized by general revenues for physician and laboratory care, and by the HI Trust Fund for inpatient hospital care.

Finally, Part D is the outpatient prescription drug benefit (drugs administered in a physician's office are covered under Part B). Those enrolled in traditional Medicare (Parts A and B) may also enroll in a private, stand-alone prescription drug plan (PDP), while those electing Part C benefits may enroll in an integrated Medicare Advantage Prescription Drug plan (MA-PD). Like Part C, Part D plans are private, and thus financed in part by premiums. General revenue covers just over three-quarters of the cost of Part D, while premiums and state funding cover the remainder (Cubanski & Neuman, 2016).

The federal government spent $539 billion (3 percent of Gross Domestic Product [GDP]) on Medicare in 2015 and provided health insurance coverage to approximately 55 million people: 46 million aged 65 years or older and 9 million people with permanent disabilities under age 65 (Box 2-1). When Medicare began on July 1, 1966, approximately 19 million people enrolled (Constantino & Angres, 2016; Cubanski et al., 2015). A majority of Medicare beneficiaries are female (55 percent), white (77 percent), and between the ages of 65 and 84 (71 percent). Most beneficiaries (74 percent) report being in "good" or "better" health, even though nearly half (45 percent) live with four or more chronic conditions, and one-third (34 percent) have one or more functional limitations in terms of activities of daily living (e.g., eating, bathing) that limit their ability function independently (Cubanski et al., 2015).

Most Medicare beneficiaries live on modest incomes. Nearly half of all Medicare beneficiaries (4 in 10) lived on an annual income of less than $20,000. Females, older beneficiaries (age 85 years

or older), black and Hispanic beneficiaries, and non-elderly beneficiaries with disabilities are more likely to be low income. Most Medicare beneficiaries (59 percent) with incomes over $20,000 rely upon either employer-provided health benefits to supplement Medicare or Medigap health insurance to fill gaps in covered benefits (Rowland, 2015).

Medicaid and the [State] Children's Health Insurance Program

Passed at the same time as Medicare, Title XIX of the Social Security Amendment of 1965 is otherwise known as the Medicaid program. Medicaid was designed to provide access to health care services for low-income persons and other "categorically needy"

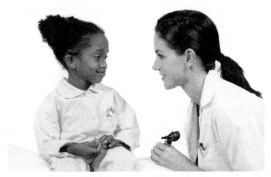
© wavebreakmedia/Shutterstock

BOX 2-1 Can Medicare Go Bankrupt?

Some policymakers claim that Medicare is running out of money and will eventually go bankrupt. To be clear, they are referring to the exhaustion of funds in the Part A Hospital Insurance (HI) Trust Fund, which pays for hospital benefits in traditional Medicare. While parts B, C, and D are funded mostly by premiums and general revenues, Part A is funded almost entirely by payroll taxes. The concern is that as the population ages, there will be too many Medicare beneficiaries and not enough workers contributing payroll taxes into the HI Trust Fund. In their 2016 annual report to Congress, the Medicare trustees projected that the HI Trust Fund would be depleted of assets by 2028.[1] But this situation is not bankruptcy, nor does it mean that hospital insurance for the elderly will cease to exist. Rather, it means that Medicare will cover most hospital benefits using income from sources other than HI Trust Fund assets, such as incoming payroll taxes. Ultimately, to ensure steady funding for hospital benefits, Congress must enact policy changes to slow cost growth and to raise revenue to strengthen the Trust Fund, for example by increasing the payroll tax.[2]

[1]Boards of Trustees of the Federal Hospital Insurance and the Federal Supplementary Medical Insurance Trust Funds. (2016, June 22). *Annual report*. Retrieved from https://www.cms.gov/Research-Statistics-Data-and-Systems/Statistics -Trends-and-Reports/ReportsTrustFunds/index.html?redirect=/reportstrustfunds/

[2]Van de Water, P.N. (2016, July 18). *Medicare is not "bankrupt": Health reform has improved program's financing.* Retrieved from http://www.cbpp.org/research/health/medicare-is-not-bankrupt

Data from: Boards of Trustees of the Federal Hospital Insurance and the Federal Supplementary Medical Insurance Trust Funds. 2016 Annual Report. Washington, D.C. June 22, 2016; Van de Water, Paul N. Medicare is not "Bankrupt." Center on Budget and Policy Priorities. July 18, 2016.

people—people who fall into some category of medical need based on illness or disability (Moore & Smith, 2005). Title XXI of the Social Security Act, known as the State Children's Health Insurance Program (SCHIP), or just CHIP, provides federal funds for states to expand eligibility to low-income children who otherwise would not qualify for Medicaid (Longest, 2010). Together, Medicaid and SCHIP are the largest health insurance programs in the United States. At the beginning of 2016, they provided coverage for 72 million Americans, including 35 million children, in all 50 states (The Henry J. Kaiser Family Foundation [KFF], 2016b).

States administer Medicaid and SCHIP, but in order to receive joint funding from the federal government (50 to 83 percent of the cost of the program, depending on state per capita income), benefits and eligibility thresholds must be at least as generous as the federal baseline. To receive federal funding, states *must* cover children ages 6 and over, up to 100 percent FPL ($11,880 for an individual or

$24,300 for a family of 4 in 2016); pregnant women and children under age 6 in households earning up to 133 percent of FPL; the elderly and those with disabilities who receive SSI benefits up to 75 percent FPL; very-low-income working parents eligible for welfare benefits; and some low-income seniors and other categories of disabled workers (KFF, 2011).

States may receive additional federal Medicaid funding to cover individuals above these thresholds. In particular, under the ACA, states have the option to expand Medicaid to all non-elderly individuals up to 138 percent FPL, and the federal government will cover nearly all of the costs of additional recipients. Even in states that have not expanded Medicaid, most have more generous eligibility requirements than the federal minimum for at least some groups, especially children. But across these non-expansion states, income and asset requirements vary considerably (**Figure 2-2**) (Gornick, Greenberg, Eggers, & Dobson, 1985; Morrisey, 2013).

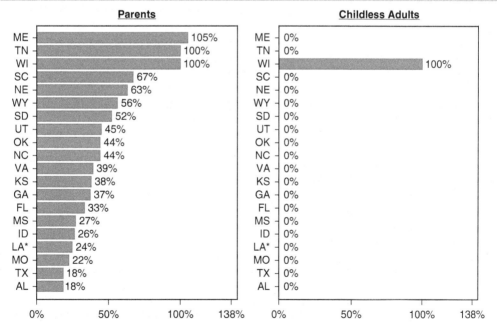

FIGURE 2-2 Variability in Eligibility Requirements Among States That Have Not Expanded Medicaid, January 2016

NOTE: Eligibility levels are based on 2016 federal poverty levels (FPLs) and are calculated based on a family of three for parents and an individual for childless adults. In 2016, the FPL was $20,160 for a family of three and $11,880 for an individual. Thresholds include the standard five percentage point of the federal poverty Level (FPL) disregard.
*Louisiana has adopted the Medicaid expansion, but it has not yet been implemented.

Similar to Medicare, Medicaid is called an "entitlement" program because anyone who meets eligibility requirements may enroll in Medicaid coverage. Individuals qualify for Medicaid only if they meet certain federal and state requirements pertaining to residency, immigration, and U.S. citizenship (Centers for Medicare and Medicaid Services [CMS], 2015b). Childless adults, or those over age 21 who are not disabled, pregnant, or elderly, are generally not eligible for Medicaid in the 19 states that have not adopted the health reform expansion, regardless of their poverty level, as of February 2016 (Center on Budget Policy and Priorities [CBPP], 2015; KFF, 2016a).

Although states have some flexibility in designing benefits for Medicaid recipients, every state Medicaid program must offer certain basic services to receive federal funding. These services include:

- Hospital inpatient and outpatient care
- Lab and X-ray services
- Physician services
- Skilled nursing facility care for individuals aged 21 years and older
- Home health care for persons eligible for skilled nursing services
- Rural health clinic services
- Pregnancy-related services, including pre-natal care and 60 days of postpartum care
- Pediatric and family nurse practitioner services
- Vaccines for children
- Family planning services and supplies

States may also receive federal funding to provide additional services such as physical therapy, vision care, and dental care, if they choose to do so (Longest, 2010). Coverage of nursing facility care and home health care is noteworthy, given that Medicare provides limited coverage of these services, and private insurance options are significantly less affordable. Medicaid, there-fore, is the primary payer for institutional and community-based long-term services and support (КГГ, 2013).

Some states do not comply with federal minimums for benefits and eligibility but still receive federal matching funds; these states have

an approved waiver under Section 1115 of the Social Security Act. Waivers may include provisions such as charging premiums, eliminating certain benefits to expand coverage, and mandating enrollment in managed care (Rudowitz & Musumeci, 2015).

Together, states and the federal government spent a combined $475 billion on Medicaid services in fiscal year (FY) 2014 (KFF, 2015). The federal government spent $350 billion (2 percent of GDP) (Constantino & Angres, 2016). States influence the total amount of spending on Medicaid because they have flexibility in determining who is eligible and what services they will cover, and because the federal government provides matching funds for the costs of services (CBPP, 2015). Most Medicaid spending (65 percent) is on acute care (e.g., physician services, inpatient and outpatient care, payments toward managed care plans). A significant portion (30 percent) of costs, however, is for long-term care services and supports. Administrative costs make up the remaining 5 percent of Medicaid spending (KFF, 2013).

Dual-eligible beneficiaries, low-income individuals who are enrolled in both Medicaid and Medicare, accounted for 38 percent of Medicaid spending, though they constitute just 15 percent of the Medicaid population. Most spending on dual-eligible beneficiaries is for long-term care services and supports. Children and non-elderly adults, including pregnant women, make up the majority of Medicaid enrollees (75 percent) but account for just one-third of Medicaid spending (KFF, 2013).

Tricare

Service members, their dependents, and retirees (and retirees' dependents) receive health insurance through TRICARE (formerly known as the Civilian Health and Medical Program of the Uniformed Services [CHAMPUS]). TRICARE was implemented in 1966 and provides health care benefits for all seven uniformed services—the Army, the Navy, the Marine Corps, the Air Force, the Coast Guard, the Commissioned Corps of the Public Health Service and the Commissioned Corps of the National Oceanic and Atmospheric

Administration, and the National Guard and Reserve (Committee on the Qualifications of Professionals Providing Mental Health Counseling Services Under TRICARE [TRI], 2010).

The "TRI" in TRICARE refers to its three main benefit options: an open-network option that covers most civilian providers (TRICARE Standard), a health maintenance organization option (TRICARE Prime), and a preferred provider option (TRICARE Extra). In 2002, a supplemental or "wrap-around" option much like Medigap was added for Medicare-eligible retirees (TRICARE for Life). Prior to TRICARE for Life, beneficiaries lost their TRICARE coverage when they reached age 65, and Medicare became their primary source of health coverage (TRI, 2010). TRICARE covers most medically necessary inpatient and outpatient care:

- Emergency and urgent care
- Medical and surgical procedures
- Home health care
- Hospice care
- Clinical preventive services
- Maternity care
- Pharmacy services
- Behavioral health care services

TRICARE generally does not cover services and supplies that are not medically or psychologically necessary for the diagnosis or treatment of an illness, injury, or treatment of pregnancy or well-child care. Nursing homes, long-term care, custodial care, and assisted living facility care are not covered under any circumstances (Defense Health Agency [DHA], 2016).

TRICARE served 9.5 million beneficiaries worldwide in FY 2014 (DHA, 2014). Only about 20 percent of beneficiaries are active-duty members of the armed forces or activated members of the National Guard or Reserve. Another quarter (26 percent) are family members of active duty or activated personnel; the remainder are retirees and their family members (TRI, 2010).

Veterans Health Administration

The Veterans Health Administration (VHA) was established in 1946 as a division within the Veterans

Administration (VA) to provide health coverage to U.S. veterans. The VHA is not an insurance plan, but rather a provider. VHA facilities provide comprehensive medical services, including inpatient and outpatient care, preventive care, mental health care, and health promotion and disease prevention services, among other services (United States Department of Veteran Affairs [VA], 2016b).

For medical conditions unrelated to military service, the VHA bills the veteran's insurer if he has private insurance, but not does not bill Medicare or Medicaid. For these non-service related conditions, some veterans are required to pay a copayment for services, though low-income veterans are generally exempt from cost-sharing. Service-related medical conditions are covered at no additional cost to the veteran or his insurer (VA, 2016a).

Generally, individuals who served in the active military service and were separated under any condition other than dishonorable qualify for health coverage through the VHA; veterans' families, however, are not eligible. Some current and former members of the Reserves or National Guard who were called to active duty and completed the full period may also qualify for coverage (VA, 2015). In 2014, the VHA provided care to more than 8.7 million veterans (VA, 2016c).

Indian Health Service

The Indian Health Service (IHS), an agency under the Department of Health and Human Services (HHS), provides health care services to over 2 million federally recognized American Indians and Alaskan Natives and their descendants (Department of Health and Human Services [HHS], 2015). Like the VHA, IHS is a provider, not an insurer. Unlike the VHA, however, IHS does not bill insurance for care; rather, the program pays IHS facilities and contracted providers directly. IHS users do not pay premiums, deductibles, or copayments for their care.

Due to limited funding, the IHS provides mostly primary care, including inpatient and outpatient care, ambulatory care, dental services, and pediatric care. Most IHS facilities are located on reservations; beneficiaries, therefore, typically live on or near federal reservations. Tribally operated health care facilities in Alaska, however, are located throughout the state (Boccuti, Swoope, & Artiga, 2014).

Other Government-Sponsored Health Insurance Programs

Some states and localities have their own health insurance or health provision programs for low-income and uninsured individuals. These health plans are known by different names depending on the state and have different eligibility and enrollment procedures (Summer, 1998; United States Census Bureau [USCB], 2016). Some programs require out-of-pocket payments (e.g., monthly premiums or copayments) from beneficiaries, although the amounts are typically low (Summer, 1998).

TRENDS IN HEALTH INSURANCE COVERAGE

For decades since the passage of Medicare and Medicaid, the uninsured rate at a given point in time remained relatively stable at around 15 percent of the population. After the ACA's major provisions went into effect in 2014, however, uninsurance began declining relatively rapidly; in 2015, 9 percent of the population was uninsured (**Figure 2**-3).

Beginning in the 1990s, enrollment in private health insurance among the non-elderly began to decline, more rapidly so just after the Great Recession (2007 to 2009) (Figure 2-3). Since the ACA and recovery from the recession, however, enrollment has risen again and is now at roughly 66 percent of the non-elderly population, compared to 71 percent in 1997 and 61 percent from 2010 to 2013. Meanwhile, enrollment in public insurance has steadily climbed from roughly 14 percent of the non-elderly population in 1997 to 25 percent in 2015. During this same time period, uninsurance among children declined dramatically, from 14 percent of children in 1997 to just 5 percent in 2015; most of this decrease was due to enrollment in public programs such as CHIP (Cohen, Makuc, Bernstein, Bilheimer, & Powell-Griner, 2009; Furman & Fiedler, 2014; Ward, Clarke, Nugent, & Schiller, 2016).

Most of the elderly have had coverage through Medicare since 1965. The share of beneficiaries enrolled in Part C plans has increased from 18 percent in 1999 to 31 percent in 2016 (Galewitz, 2011; Jacobson et al., 2016).

FIGURE 2-3 Trends in Insurance Enrollment for Adults Ages 18–64, 1997–2015

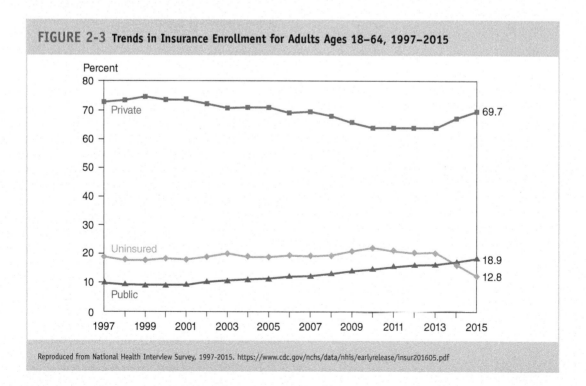

COMPARING PRIVATE AND PUBLIC COVERAGE

While many have strong opinions on whether private insurance is better than public insurance, it is important to understand the strengths and weaknesses of the two types.

Compared to public insurers, which generally offer a single benefits package at a fixed price, private insurers offer a wider variety of plans at different prices and benefits levels. Because private insurance companies compete for contracts with employers and individuals, they have developed numerous innovative tools and products with the goal of improving health and lowering costs, including pay-for-performance, disease management programs, and consumer-directed health plans (CMS, 2015a). Private insurance thus allows employers and individuals to select plans that are more tailored to their needs and preferences. The elderly, for example, may not care as much about the availability of obstetricians and pediatric providers, while younger adults may wish to have a variety of choice in pre- and post-natal care. The elderly, in contrast, may care much more about the inclusion of particular hospitals in the insurer's network or the availability of disease management programs, while the young may wish to pay lower premiums in exchange for more restricted networks and higher deductibles.

Because most private insurance in the United States is tied to employment, however, a major drawback compared to public insurance is that people lose their coverage when they leave their job or when a spouse leaves a job. This system leaves individuals vulnerable to losing insurance when they may need the most assistance—such as when a spouse dies or becomes unable to work, when a marriage dissolves, or when an employee must leave to take care of a sick parent. Further, job-based coverage leaves out the self-employed and the unemployed. Moreover, not all jobs offer insurance with dependent coverage, so some spouses and children are uninsured even when there is a worker in the family. Employer-based coverage also interferes with job mobility, called "job lock," which can result in employees taking or remaining in a job that is inappropriately matched to their skills and interests in order to maintain health insurance coverage.

The tax advantage to employment-based insurance also favors higher earners and results in the loss of billions of dollars of revenue. For example, suppose that Phil earns $50,000 per year, while Sandra earns $150,000 per year, but that both are offered health insurance at a premium of $10,000 per year. Sandra's income is taxed at a much higher rate than Phil's, perhaps 20 percent on average compared to Phil's 10 percent. Because employment-based insurance premiums are not taxed, Sandra saves 20 percent × $150,000 on taxes = $30,000 by purchasing the plan with pre-tax dollars, while Phil saves only 10 percent × $50,000 = $5,000. Not only does this tax treatment favor the wealthy, but it results in a $35,000 loss in revenue for the government. Because so many Americans have tax-free employment-based insurance, the estimated total revenue loss to the federal government is $248 billion dollars (Congressional Budget Office, 2013).

Further, the tax advantage also results in over-insurance. Phil and Sandra are now sitting on $35,000 of tax savings. One option is that they could spend this money, but the expenditures would be taxed. Another option is that they could put away the money for retirement in a tax-advantaged account, but they would not be able to spend it for decades. Yet another option is that they could contribute the money, tax-free, to pay for the premiums on an upgraded health plan, for example, a PPO with no deductible instead of an HMO that requires them to visit a primary care physician before seeing a specialist. Employment-based insurance thus encourages plans with benefits that are more generous than if those plans were to be purchased with taxed earnings.

Although employers usually contribute some share of the premium, employees may pay for health insurance in the form of lower wages, (or slower growing wages).But for some groups, wages may not adjust to accommodate the cost of insurance. Workers at minimum wage, for example, cannot by law accept wages that are below their current level. If the cost of health insurance is too high, then this group is at risk for unemployment. Likewise, sick and disabled employees and women of childbearing age cost more to insure, but employers cannot legally lower their wages to reflect this cost because of anti-discrimination statutes. Instead, employers may target these groups more subtly by hiring them less often and firing them more often (Summers, 1989).

Public insurance fills some of the gaps in the market for private insurance, providing coverage for some of the country's most vulnerable populations, including American Indians, the elderly, veterans, and the categorically needy (Iglehart, 1992). One of the biggest strengths of government-provided insurance is its size. With so many enrollees, the government has enormous influence over providers. In fact, Medicare does not negotiate with doctors and hospitals but rather sets administrative prices through the legislative process for Parts A and B. Providers must either accept the set prices or else lose a large volume of business.

With some exceptions (such as Medicare Parts C and D), however, the government does not offer those eligible for public insurance much choice in their plans, and universal benefits may not be universally appropriate. Individuals have different needs and preferences, and for some individuals, the government package of benefits may be inadequate, while for others, it may be too much (Summers, 1989).

One financing problem specific to Medicare is the high cost of health care coinciding with a declining ratio of workers to retirees. The aging baby boom population could potentially result in fewer contributors to the system while more beneficiaries simultaneously draw resources from it. Because Part A is financed through payroll taxes, insolvency of the HI Trust Fund is a threat if there are not enough workers to support the elderly (Moon & Davis, 1995).

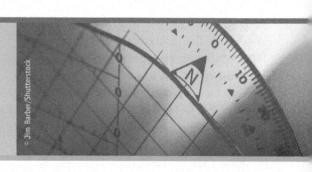

Summary

Although most adults (and their dependents) receive coverage through private, employer-based insurance, many special populations receive care through government-sponsored programs, including the elderly through Medicare, the categorically needy through Medicaid or through state or local programs, military service members through TRICARE, veterans through the VHA, and American Indians and Alaskan natives through the IHS. Some characterize the U.S. health insurance system as fragmented due to the many ways through which individuals may obtain coverage, the variability in benefits offered through health plans, and the variability in costs to the consumer. This "system" of coverage, consequently, means that some individuals "fall through the cracks," if they do not meet eligibility requirements for any of the government-sponsored programs or are not covered through their employer. Some individuals may also find they have more care than they need while others cannot access sufficient care to cover their needs at an affordable price. The health insurance system in the United States continues to evolve and improve, however, to reduce inequities and inefficiency through the passage of legislation, such as ERISA, Medicaid benefit expansions, and more recently, the Affordable Care Act.

References

Boccuti, C., Swoope, C., & Artiga, S. (2014). *The role of Medicare and the Indian Health Service for American Indians and Alaska natives: Health, access, and coverage.* Retrieved from http://kff.org/report-section/the-role-of-medicare-and-the-indian-health-service-for-american-indians-and-alaska-natives-health-access-and-coverage-report/

Center on Budget Policy and Priorities (CBPP). (2015, June). *Policy basics: Introduction to Medicaid.* Retrieved from http://www.cbpp.org/research/health/policy-basics-introduction-to-medicaid

Centers for Medicare and Medicaid Services (CMS). (2015a). *Linking quality to payment.* Retrieved from https://www.medicare.gov/hospitalcompare/linking-quality-to-payment.html

Centers for Medicare and Medicaid Services (CMS). (2015b). *Medicaid eligibility.* Retrieved from https://www.medicaid.gov/medicaid-chip-program-information/by-topics/eligibility/eligibility.html

Claxton, G., & Lundy, J. (2008, April). *How private health coverage works: A primer 2008 update.* The Henry J. Kaiser Family Foundation. Retrieved from https://kaiserfamilyfoundation.files.wordpress.com/2013/01/7766.pdf

Cohen, R. A., Makuc, D. M., Bernstein, A. B., Bilheimer, L. T., & Powell-Griner, E. (2009). Health insurance coverage trends, 1959–2007: Estimates from the National Health Interview Survey. *National Health Statistics Reports, 17,* 1–25.

Committee on the Qualifications of Professionals Providing Mental Health Counseling Services Under TRICARE, Board on the Health of Select Populations, Institute of Medicine. (2010). *Provision of mental health counseling services under TRICARE.* Washington, DC: National Academies Press. Retrieved from http://www.ncbi.nlm.nih.gov/books/NBK259179/

Congressional Budget Office. (2013). Options for reducing the deficit: 2013–2014. http://www.cbo.gov/sites/default/files/cbofiles/attachments/44715-OptionsForReducingDeficit-3.pdf

Corrigan, J., Eden, J., & Smith, B. (Eds.). (2003). Overview of the government health care programs. In *Leadership by example* (pp. 28–55). Washington, DC: The National Academies Press.

Constantino, M., & Angres, L. (2016, January). *The federal budget in 2015.* Retrieved from https://www.cbo.gov/publication/51110

Cubanski, J., & Neuman, T. (2016, July). *The facts on Medicare spending and financing.* The Henry J. Kaiser Family Foundation. Retrieved from http://kff.org/medicare/issue-brief/the-facts-on-medicare-spending-and-financing/

Cubanski, J., Swoope, C., Boccuti, C., Jacobson, G., Casillas, G., Griffin, S., & Neuman, T. (2015). *A Primer on Medicare: Key facts about the Medicare program and the people it covers.* The Henry J. Kaiser Family Foundation. Retrieved from http://kff.org/medicare/report/a-primer-on-medicare-key-facts-about-the-medicare-program-and-the-people-it-covers/

Defense Health Agency. (2014). *Evaluation of the TRICARE Program: Access, Cost, and Quality, FY 2014 Report to Congress.* Retrieved from http://www.health.mil/Military-Health-Topics/Access-Cost-Quality-and-Safety/Health-Care-Program-Evaluation/Annual-Evaluation-of-the-TRICARE-Program?type=Reports

Defense Health Agency. (2016, February). *TRICARE exclusions.* Retrieved from http://www.tricare.mil/CoveredServices/IsItCovered/Exclusions.aspx

Department of Health and Human Services. (2015). *Fiscal year 2016 Indian Health Service: Justification of estimates for appropriations committees.* Retrieved from https://www.ihs.gov/budgetformulation/includes/themes/newihstheme/documents/FY2016CongressionalJustification.pdf

Galewitz, P. (2011, September 15). Medicare advantage premiums falling 4% in 2012. *Kaiser Health News.* Retrieved from http://khn.org/news/medicare-advantage-premiums-falling-4-in-2012/

Gornick, M., Greenberg, J., Eggers, P., & Dobson, A. (1985). Twenty years of Medicare and Medicaid: Covered populations, use of benefits, and program expenditures. *Health Care Financing Review, Annual Suppl.,* 13–59.

Furman, J., & Fiedler, M. (2014, December 18). *2014 has seen the largest coverage gains on four decades, putting the uninsured rate at or near historic lows.* Retrieved from https://www.whitehouse.gov/blog/2014/12/18/2014-has-seen-largest-coverage-gains-four-decades-putting-uninsured-rate-or-near-his

The Henry J. Kaiser Family Foundation (KFF). (2011, April). *Federal core requirements and state options in Medicaid: Current policies and key issues.* Retrieved from http://kff.org/health-reform/fact-sheet/federal-core-requirements-and-state-options-in/

The Henry J. Kaiser Family Foundation (KFF). (2013). *Medicaid: A primer 2013.* Retrieved from https://kaiserfamilyfoundation.files.wordpress.com/2010/06/7334-05.pdf

The Henry J. Kaiser Family Foundation (KFF). (2015). *Total Medicaid spending.* Retrieved from http://kff.org/medicaid/state-indicator/total-medicaid-spending/

The Henry J. Kaiser Family Foundation (KFF). (2016a). *Current status of state Medicaid expansion decisions.* Retrieved from http://kff.org/health-reform/slide/current-status-of-the-medicaid-expansion-decision/

The Henry J. Kaiser Family Foundation (KFF). (2016b). *Total monthly Medicaid and CHIP enrollment.* Retrieved from http://kff.org/health-reform/state-indicator/total-monthly-medicaid-and-chip-enrollment/

Hoffman, C., & Paradise, J. (2008). Health insurance and access to health care in the United States. *Annals of the New York Academy of Sciences, 1136,* 149–160.

Iglehart, J. (1992). The American health care system. *New England Journal of Medicine, 326,* 962–967.

Jacobson, G., Casillas, G., Damico, A., & Neuman, T. (2016, May 11). *Medicare Advantage 2016 spotlight: Enrollment market update.* The Henry J. Kaiser Family Foundation. Retrieved from http://kff.org/medicare/issue-brief/medicare-advantage-2016-spotlight-enrollment-market-update/

Longest, B., Jr. (2010). Overview of Medicaid. In B. Longest Jr. (Ed.), *Health policymaking in the United States* (5th ed., pp. 233–244). Chicago, IL: Health Administration Press.

Moon, M., & Davis, K. (1995). Preserving and strengthening Medicare. *Health Affairs, 14,* 31–46.

Moore, J., & Smith, D. (2005). Legislating Medicaid: Considering Medicaid and its origins. *Health Care Financing Review, 27,* 45–52.

Morrisey, M. (2013). Health insurance in the United States. In G. Dionne (Ed.), *Handbook of Insurance* (pp. 957–995). New York, NY: Springer Science and Business Media.

National Health Policy Forum. (2016, January). *The basics: Medicare.* Retrieved from https://www.nhpf.org/library/the-basics/Basics_Medicare_01-04-16.pdf

Rowland, D. (2015). The Medicare and Medicaid partnership at age 50. *Generations: Journal of the American Society on Aging, 39,* 35–42.

Rudowitz, R., & Musumeci, M. (2015, 20 November). *The ACA and Medicaid expansion waivers.* The Henry J. Kaiser Family Foundation. Retrieved from http://kff.org/medicaid/issue-brief/the-aca-and-medicaid-expansion-waivers/

Smith, J., & Medalia, C. (2015). *Health insurance coverage in the United States: 2014.* Washington, DC: United States Census Bureau.

Summer, L. (1998). *State-subsidized health insurance programs for low-income residents: Program structure, administration, and costs.* Retrieved from http://www.commonwealthfund.org/usr_doc/Summer_statesubsidized.pdf

Summers, L. H. (1989). Some simple economics of mandated benefits. *The American Economic Review, 79,* 177–183.

United States Census Bureau. (2016, March). *Current Population Survey (CPS) Annual Social and Economic Supplement (CPS-ASEC): Types of health insurance.* Retrieved from http://www.census.gov/topics/health/health-insurance/guidance/cps-asec.html

United States Department of Veteran Affairs. (2015). *Veterans eligibility.* Retrieved from http://www.va.gov/HEALTHBENEFITS/apply/veterans.asp

United States Department of Veterans Affairs. (2016a). *Health benefits.* Retrieved from http://www.va.gov/HEALTHBENEFITS/index.asp

United States Department of Veteran Affairs. (2016b). *Medical benefits package.* http://www.va.gov/HEALTHBENEFITS/access/medical_benefits_package.asp

United States Department of Veteran Affairs. (2016c). *Veterans Health Administration.* Retrieved from http://www.va.gov/health/

Ward, B., Clarke, T., Nugent, C., & Schiller, J. (2016, May). *Early release of selected estimates based on data from the 2015 national health interview survey.* Retrieved from http://www.cdc.gov/nchs/data/nhis/earlyrelease/earlyrelease201605.pdf

CHAPTER 3

The Uninsured

Alexis Pozen, PhD

LEARNING OBJECTIVES

- Who are the uninsured, and why do they not have health insurance?
- What are the consequences of being uninsured?
- What programs and policies exist to assist the uninsured?

INTRODUCTION

In 2014, as part of the Affordable Care Act (ACA), almost all Americans were required to have health insurance. Yet years later, there are still people who remain chronically or periodically uninsured. This chapter will discuss characteristics of the uninsured, as well as programs and policies that address this population.

NUMBER OF UNINSURED

How many people are uninsured? The answer depends on how you ask the question: (1) Were you uninsured for the entire year last year? (2) Are you uninsured right now? and (3) Were you uninsured at any point during the year last year? The first question, about chronic uninsurance, yields an estimate that is lower than if you ask the second or third question, which are questions about periodic uninsurance. And comparing the second and third questions, the third (a "point-in-time" measure) yields a higher estimate than the second, because

even those with insurance *right now* may have been uninsured at some point during the year.

In fact, several major surveys of the U.S. population ask one or both types of questions. The Current Population Survey (CPS) (United States Census Bureau, 2015), a survey focusing on employment, has the most commonly cited estimate of the uninsured in part because it collects information from among the largest number of respondents. Before 2014 the CPS asked only about insurance status for the entire previous year, but now asks about coverage at the time of the interview. Surveys that estimate coverage based on all three questions include the National Health Interview Survey (NHIS), which measures population health and health care use; the Medical Expenditure Panel Survey (MEPS), a survey of health care use and spending; and the Survey of Income and Program Participation (SIPP), which is administered by the U.S. Census Bureau and focuses on income and employment. The American Community Survey (ACS), also administered by the Census Bureau and with an even larger number of participants than the CPS, collects information on demographics and socioeconomic indicators, but asks only whether respondents are currently insured.

Even comparing surveys that ask the same question (e.g., point-in-time), estimates of the uninsured may differ because of the different methods that surveys use. For instance, surveys may interview different participants. Prior to 2011 the Behavioral Risk Factor Surveillance System (BRFSS), which collects information on health behaviors and risk factors, surveyed people by calling their landline telephones. But not every household has a landline, especially younger and poorer households, so the survey could have been missing crucial information. After 2011, then, the survey added cell phone numbers, which increased the estimate of the uninsured. In comparison, the ACS conducts interviews by mail, in person, and by phone. It should not be surprising, then, that BRFSS estimates before 2011 were much lower than those of the ACS, and that estimates after 2011 were much more similar (Utah Department of Health, 2012).

Another reason that surveys asking the same question may generate different estimates of the uninsured is that surveys have different recall periods—how far back a participant must remember to answer the question. For example, before 2014 the CPS did not ask participants whether they were currently uninsured, only whether they had been uninsured for the entire year. But entire-year estimates so closely resembled other surveys' point-in-time estimates that analysts suspected that participants who were *currently* uninsured remembered themselves as having been *chronically* uninsured (U.S. Department of Health and Human Services, 2005). So beginning in 2014, the CPS made changes to its questions to improve accuracy. Participants asked to remember too far back may respond less accurately than those asked to remember more recent events. The CPS insurance question, for example, has a notoriously long recall period because the survey is administered in March, and respondents must remember their insurance status for the entire previous year—likely the cause of overestimates of entire-year uninsurance prior to the 2014 survey. MEPS, on the other hand, has a recall period of only about three to five months because participants are interviewed at several points during the year.

Estimates of the uninsured therefore vary because of differences in how the question is asked and because of differences in survey methods. These survey differences produce substantially different estimates. For example, the estimate for the number of people uninsured for the entire year in 2014 was 33.0 million (10 percent of the population) for the CPS and 26.3 million (8 percent of the population) for the NHIS, both large surveys with high response rates. In comparison, the estimate for the number of people uninsured at the time of the survey in 2014 was 36.7 million (12 percent of the population) for the ACS and 36.0 million (12 percent of the population) for the NHIS (Planalp, Au-Yeung, & Turner, 2015).

CHARACTERISTICS OF THE UNINSURED

Now that we understand that "the uninsured" is not a straightforward term (**Figure 3-1**), let us pick one survey, the CPS, and examine the characteristics of people who reported that they were uninsured *for the entire previous year* (Figure 3-1). As previously stated, 33.0 million people, or 10 percent of the population, were uninsured for the full year in 2014. The uninsured are almost all under 65, because most elderly people have Medicare; less than 1 percent of the elderly was uninsured. Over 4 million children (1 percent of the population) lacked health insurance in 2014 (U.S. Census Bureau, 2015).

Young adults are more likely to be uninsured than older adults. Although 18- to 34-year-olds constituted less than a quarter (24 percent) of the population, they constituted over one-third (38 percent) of the total uninsured population (U.S. Census Bureau, 2015). In fact, the uninsured in this age group have earned the name "young invincibles," so called because about a quarter believe that they are healthy enough to not need insurance, compared to 11 percent of the total population (The Henry J. Kaiser Family Foundation [KFF], 2013c). Perhaps because uninsurance is concentrated among younger people, the uninsured actually have *lower* rates of chronic conditions such as hypertension,

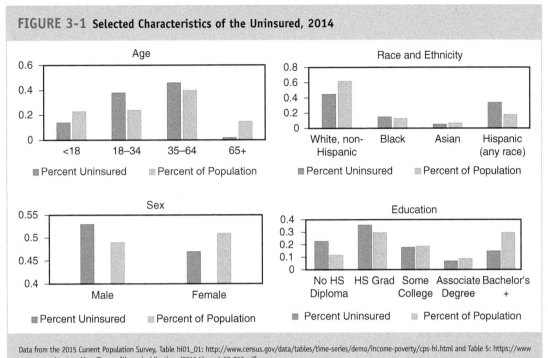

FIGURE 3-1 Selected Characteristics of the Uninsured, 2014

Data from the 2015 Current Population Survey, Table hi01_01: http://www.census.gov/data/tables/time-series/demo/income-poverty/cps-hi.html and Table 5: https://www.census.gov/content/dam/Census/library/publications/2015/demo/p60-253.pdf

heart disease, asthma, and diabetes, than the insured—45 percent compared to 55 percent (Davidoff & Kenney, 2005).

Males are more likely to be uninsured than females (53 percent compared to 47 percent), even though males make up less than half the population (U.S. Census Bureau, 2015). On one hand, this statistic seems odd because males are more likely to be part of the labor force, where most Americans obtain their insurance. For example, in a heterosexual couple where only one partner works, it is usually the male partner (Leppel, 2009). Not all jobs that offer insurance coverage also offer spousal coverage, so female partners of these workers would not necessarily be covered. Based on this information, then, we would expect more males to be insured. On the other hand, however, this statistic is not odd at all, because Medicaid does not cover healthy single men in some states.

The uninsured are more likely to be black and Hispanic. Although black people represent 13 percent of the population, they are 15 percent

of the uninsured; Hispanic people represent 18 percent of the population but 34 percent of the uninsured. Foreign-born people are also disproportionately uninsured, constituting 13 percent of the population but 27 percent of the uninsured. With limited employment opportunities and access to public programs, non-citizens are particularly at risk, constituting just 7 percent of the population but 21 percent of the uninsured (U.S. Census Bureau, 2015). In many states, even documented immigrants must wait to access Medicaid.

The vast majority (70 percent) of the uninsured population works. Over half (54 percent) work in full time jobs. Yet uninsurance is highly concentrated among the poor. People in households earning less than $25,000 constitute just 17 percent of the population but 28 percent of the uninsured, while those earning under $50,000 constitute over a third (38 percent) of the population but over half (57 percent) of the uninsured. And because earnings and education are so closely related, uninsurance is also concentrated among those with low levels of education. People with no high school degree or only a high school diploma represent 42 percent of the population but well over half (59 percent) of the uninsured (U.S. Census Bureau, 2015).

Finally, geography matters when it comes to health insurance, in part because states have varying requirements for private health insurers and public insurance eligibility, and in part because of the characteristics of people living in different regions of the country—for instance, the poor are concentrated in the South. As a result, people in the South are more likely to be uninsured, representing over a third (37 percent) of the population, but almost half (47 percent) of the uninsured. The states with the highest uninsured rates include Texas (19 percent), Alaska (17 percent), Florida (17 percent), and Georgia (16 percent), while the states with the lowest uninsured

rates include Massachusetts (3 percent), Vermont (5 percent), the District of Columbia (5 percent), and Hawaii (5 percent) (U.S. Census Bureau, 2015). Notably, Hawaii and Massachusetts both implemented health insurance expansions prior to the ACA—Hawaii enacted an employer mandate in 1974, and Massachusetts enacted comprehensive coverage expansion, including employer and individual mandates and Medicaid expansion, in 2006.

REASONS FOR UNINSURANCE

Although there are several reasons why people do not have health insurance, the most common reason is cost (**Figure 3-2**). Over half (60 percent) of adults under 65 reported that they did not have health insurance because they could not afford it. On the other hand, a fifth (20 percent) do not want health insurance. Fourteen

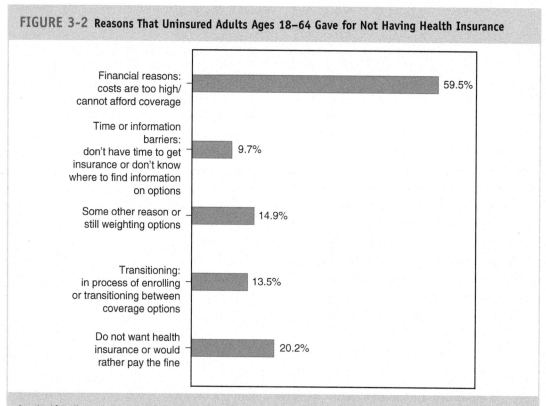

FIGURE 3-2 Reasons That Uninsured Adults Ages 18–64 Gave for Not Having Health Insurance

Financial reasons: costs are too high/cannot afford coverage — 59.5%

Time or information barriers: don't have time to get insurance or don't know where to find information on options — 9.7%

Some other reason or still weighting options — 14.9%

Transitioning: in process of enrolling or transitioning between coverage options — 13.5%

Do not want health insurance or would rather pay the fine — 20.2%

Reproduced from: Shartzer, A., Kenney G., Long, S., Hempstead, K., & Wissoker, D. (2014). Urban Institute Health Policy Center. Who-are-the-remaining-uninsured-as-of -june-2014. http://hrms.urban.org/briefs/who-are-the-remaining-uninsured-as-of-june-2014.pdf

percent do not have health insurance because they are transitioning between coverage options, for example because they were no longer eligible for Medicaid or had lost or moved jobs. And 10 percent reported that they did not have time to get insurance or did not know where to find information about options (Shartzer, Kenney, Long, Hempstead, & Wissoker, 2014). Note that some of the reasons for uninsurance are related. For example, people losing jobs may not be able to afford the cost of individual insurance, and people losing Medicaid eligibility because of higher pay may have an employment-based option. The so-called young invincibles who are thought to not have health coverage because they believe they are healthy may want coverage if the cost were lower; among the uninsured, younger people more often cite cost as the reason that they do not have health coverage (NHIS, 2014).

The ACA required everyone to have health insurance in 2014 and provided subsidies to purchase insurance. So why are there still uninsured people? First, the subsidies are only available for those earning 100 to 400 percent of the poverty level; those earning less were expected to obtain coverage through an expanded Medicaid program. But the Supreme Court ruled that states should not be required to expand Medicaid (NFIB v. Sebelius, 2012), and only 31 states and the District of Columbia have elected to expand their programs.

Second, while the ACA requires employers with 50 or more employees to offer coverage (or pay a penalty to finance coverage), these employers were largely already offering insurance (KFF, 2013d). Employees in small firms are more likely to be uninsured than those in large firms (U.S. Census Bureau, 2015).

Third, people may pay a penalty rather than comply with the individual mandate. The annual penalty for not having insurance is the higher of $695 per adult and $347.50 per child or 2.5 percent of household income. In contrast, the annual premium for an individual policy is an average of $2,800 per person in the individual market and $4,400 (employee contribution) in the group market (KFF, 2013a, 2013b). In 2015 7.5 million people, over one-fifth of the uninsured, elected to pay the penalty (Koskinen, 2015).

Finally, those most at risk for being uninsured are exempt from the individual mandate. For example, those living in states that did not expand Medicaid, but who would have qualified for Medicaid under the expansion, are exempt. People who are eligible to receive services from the Indian Health Services (IHS) are also exempt. Hardship exemptions include people who were homeless, experienced domestic abuse, became bankrupt, or were evicted from their homes. Finally, there are income-related exemptions for those who earn so little that they do not have to file a tax return or cannot afford even the lowest-priced plan. About 12 million people, roughly one-third of the uninsured, claimed an exemption from the individual mandate in 2015 (Koskinen, 2015).

CONSEQUENCES OF UNINSURANCE

Being uninsured affects health, health care, and financial security in numerous ways (**Figure 3-3**). The uninsured are not protected from catastrophic medical costs, which has profound consequences on the way that they engage with the medical care system.

Lack of Shared Risk or Negotiating Power

Insurance is meant to protect people against catastrophic, unpredictable out-of-pocket spending. But the uninsured have no protection against a catastrophe because they have no one else with whom to share risk. And should they decide (or be forced) to engage with the medical system, they will lack the benefit of an insurer's negotiating power for the price of hospital and physician services. Without an insurer to negotiate prices, consumers face the list price—the menu price reported by the hospital or physician. Ironically, even though the uninsured are poorer, the prices that they face are much higher. Uninsured consumers should know that they, too, may negotiate the list price, though they may not be able to get as far as an insurer, which negotiates on behalf of thousands of enrollees.

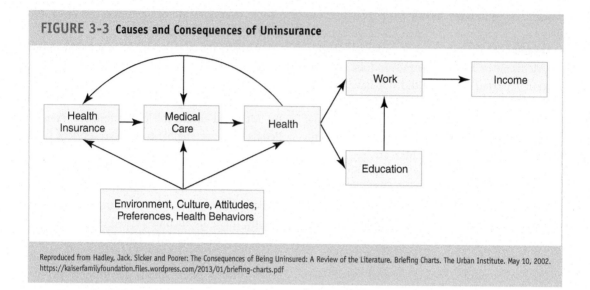

FIGURE 3-3 Causes and Consequences of Uninsurance

Because the uninsured enter the battle for medical care without any armor, they have less contact with the system compared with the insured. Over half of uninsured non-elderly adults do not have a usual source of medical care, compared with 10 percent of those publicly insured and 12 percent of those privately insured. The uninsured are also more likely to postpone care due to cost, go without needed care due to cost, and not be able to afford a prescription drug (Majerol, Newkirk, & Garfield, 2015).

In fact, then, it is the *insured* more so than the uninsured who accrue medical debt and report difficulty paying medical bills, because the uninsured do not have as much contact with the medical system. One-third (35 percent) of non-elderly adults reported accrual of medical debt or difficulty paying a medical bill in 2013, compared to half (51 percent) of those periodically uninsured and one-third (29) of those chronically uninsured. (Collins, Rasmussen, Doty, & Beutel, 2015).

Health Consequences of Uninsurance

Even among the uninsured who use the health care system, health outcomes are worse compared with those of the insured. Because health is a combination of social and environmental factors as well as medical care, one cannot attribute the entirety of health to the medical system. But even adjusting for the fact that the uninsured are poorer, less educated, and engage in riskier behaviors such as drinking and smoking, the uninsured die at higher rates than the insured (Baker et al., 2006; Card, Dobkin, & Maestas, 2009; McWilliams, Zaslavsky, Meara, & Ayanian, 2004).

Compared to the insured, the uninsured are more likely to go without influenza vaccinations, cholesterol testing, cancer screenings, and hypertension diagnosis (Card, Dobkin, & Maestas, 2004; Decker, 2005; McWilliams, Zaslavsky, Meara, & Ayanian, 2003). The uninsured see lower quality physicians and are treated at lower quality hospitals (Gardner & Vishwasrao, 2010). For the same type of hospital admission, they receive fewer services and are more likely to die (Card et al., 2004; Doyle, 2005). Evidence suggests that obtaining insurance at age 65 through Medicare is associated with improved health outcomes (Card et al., 2009; Decker, 2005).

Financial Consequences of Uninsurance

The causal link between uninsurance and financial distress is difficult to ascertain, because uninsurance can clearly cause financial distress, but financial distress can also cause uninsurance.

The authors of the Oregon study hypothesized that, on one hand, Medicaid might lead to increased employment and earnings, because improved health would reduce work absences and improve performance. On the other hand, however, Medicaid might reduce earnings because people would try to limit their earnings in order to maintain eligibility for Medicaid. In the experiment, the authors found no effect of Medicaid on employment or earnings (Baicker, Finkelstein, Song, & Taubman, 2014), though this finding could have been because the two effects cancelled each other.

In 2006 Massachusetts passed broad legislation expanding health insurance coverage, similar to the ACA, which one study found improved credit scores and reduced household debt and personal bankruptcy (Mazumder & Miller, 2015). As a caution to this interpretation, medical debt is usually just one part of the debt burden of those filing for personal bankruptcy (Dranove & Millenson, 2006), and as we have learned, it is the *insured*, not the *uninsured*, who accrue medical debt. It is not clear, then, how much the previously uninsured benefitted financially from the Massachusetts legislation. More comprehensive benefits for the *insured*, however, could have eased the burden of medical debt.

Whether financial benefits accrue to the previously insured or previously uninsured, however, there is strong evidence that coverage expansions ease financial strain. One survey estimated that after the ACA was implemented, the number of non-elderly adults that reported problems paying medical bills fell to levels similar to those in more robust economic times (Collins et al., 2015). Another study found that Medicare substantially eases financial strain related to medical costs (Barcellos & Jacobson, 2015).

Insurance is crucial to good health. As with financial distress, the causal link goes both ways. Poor health, for example, makes it difficult to hold a steady job that offers insurance. But uninsurance also causes poor health—the uninsured do not engage with the health system enough, and when they do, the intensity and quality of the services that they receive is insufficient. They die at higher rates than the insured, not just because they are disproportionately poor, less educated, and racial and ethnic minorities, but also because they receive worse medical care.

The financial consequences of uninsurance are less clear. Because the uninsured do not use the medical system as much as the insured, they—unintuitively—do not accrue medical debt at the same rate as the insured, though they may accrue other kinds of debt. Legislation such as Medicare, the Massachusetts health reform of 2006, and the ACA of 2010 eased the burden of medical debt and out-of-pocket spending on broad sets of the population.

What Steps Have Been Taken to Reduce Uninsurance?

States, cities, and the federal government have taken steps to address the uninsured. We have already discussed Medicare and Medicaid/SCHIP as policies that filled gaps in the private market for the elderly and the poor, respectively, and we will talk about the ACA at length. We have also examined some of the effects of the 2008 Oregon Medicaid expansion, including participants' increased use of health care services, improved self-reported health, and non-effects on employment and wages. This section will address other policies that have expanded insurance.

In 1974, Hawaii enacted the Prepaid Health Care Act, which required employers to offer health insurance to all employees who work over 20 hours per week. While evidence suggests that the mandate did increase coverage for some workers, others were shifted to part-time work where they were exempt from the mandate (but also safe from being laid off) (Buchmueller, DiNardo, & Valletta, 2011).

The previously mentioned Massachusetts health reform expanded health insurance coverage to its residents in 2006. Like the ACA, it implemented an individual mandate (requiring all residents to have health coverage), an employer pay-or-play mandate (requiring employers to offer health insurance coverage or pay a penalty to finance coverage), expanded Medicaid, and opened an online marketplace where insurers offered standardized, subsidized plans. Massachusetts currently has the lowest uninsured rate by far, a whopping 3 percent chronically uninsured. Like the Oregon plan, in Massachusetts health care utilization increased after reform, but unlike in

Oregon, preventable ER hospitalizations actually decreased (Miller, 2012). Some of this difference may be explained by the design of the policies—in Oregon, people voluntarily enrolled in coverage, while in Massachusetts, people were subject to a mandate (Taubman, Allen, Wright, Baicker, & Finkelstein, 2014). It is possible that participants in Oregon were more in need, more eager, or more capable of engaging in the health care system than the newly enrolled in Massachusetts. Despite this difference, the Massachusetts reform also improved self-reported health for the previously uninsured (Courtemanche & Zapata, 2014).

In 2006 San Francisco passed a pair of laws to expand health coverage to its residents and workers. Healthy San Francisco (HSF) is a health access program similar to insurance, although not generous enough to qualify as insurance. It is available to low- and middle-income adult San Francisco residents who do not qualify for public insurance and who have been uninsured for three months. For a small fee, participants in HSF may visit local physicians and public hospitals and clinics. The Health Care Security Ordinance (HCSO) is an employer mandate that requires employers to spend a fixed amount per employee per hour of work for for-profit firms over 19 employees and non-profit firms over 49 employees. A traditional mandate requires employers to pay a fixed amount per employee (in the form of insurance) regardless of hours worked, which makes low-wage employees relatively expensive and puts them at risk for layoffs. But as a result of the HCSO's design, low-wage workers by and large kept their jobs. In fact, evidence showed that employers instead passed on the cost of the HCSO to consumers (Colla, Dow, & Dube, 2011). For years after the mandate was enacted, diners at San Francisco restaurants might have found a line item at the bottom of their bill that said something like "Healthy SF Surcharge," sometimes with an additional explanation about how the restaurant provided health insurance for its staff.

TRENDS IN UNINSURANCE RATES

Health insurance as we know it in the United States began during the Great Depression. Even before the Depression, the advance of medical care had

made hospital and physician services too expensive for ordinary families. So when the stock market collapsed, medical providers looked to unions for a regular source of income. Providers and unions entered into mutually beneficial agreements that guaranteed medical care for the union workers and a prepaid income to the providers. But by the 1960s not everyone had access to such insurance, particularly those who did not work—children, the elderly, and the indigent. Medicare and Medicaid changed this situation, and the uninsurance rate dropped dramatically after these policies were passed in 1965 (**Figure 3-4**) (Furman & Fiedler, 2014).

But further coverage expansions until the ACA were small-scale, arguably with the exception of the 1997 State Children's Health Insurance Program (SCHIP), an extension of Medicaid. This program expands coverage to children whose parents' incomes are too high to qualify for Medicaid. Almost all children in the United States have health insurance coverage(Cohen, Martinez, & Zammitti, 2016).

The ACA, however, was anything but small scale. Estimates suggest that it expanded coverage to a net 16.9 million people. This number is quite large given that in 2013, before the ACA's major provisions took effect, there were an estimated 42.7 million uninsured (Carman, Eibner, & Paddock, 2015). In 2014, after major provisions were implemented, the full-year uninsurance rate was 10 percent of the population, among the lowest it has ever been in U.S. history (Cohen, Makuc, Bernstein, Bilheimer, & Powell-Griner, 2009; Furman & Fiedler 2014; U.S. Census Bureau, 2015).

WHAT IS UNDERINSURANCE?

Throughout this chapter, we have been discussing the problem of uninsurance. But as you may understand from personal experience, having insurance does not always make it perfectly easy to navigate the health care system. There is no accepted definition of underinsurance, but we can think of it as insurance that does not provide enough financial protection. We will develop a clearer definition for underinsurance in this section.

People who are *periodically* uninsured—not continuously insured throughout the year—are

FIGURE 3-4 Uninsurance Rate, 1963–2015

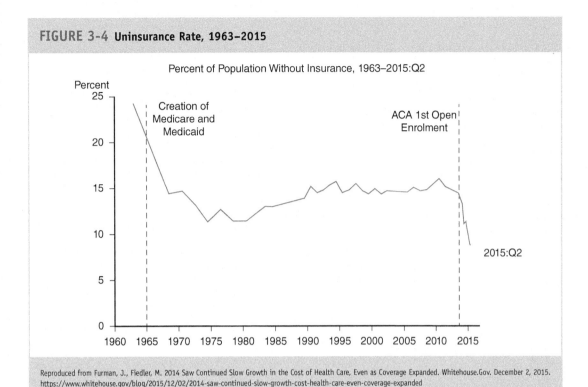

Percent of Population Without Insurance, 1963–2015:Q2

underinsured because they experience gaps in financial protection. Unstable earnings situations set people up for this type of periodic uninsurance; for example, those with incomes just at the threshold of Medicaid eligibility, or those with insecure employment. For example, consider Michael, a salesperson in Delaware, who has diabetes and an income that is low enough to qualify for Medicaid. He is offered a job that would allow him to earn a commission on his sales, but it does not come with health insurance. With the extra earnings, he might not qualify for Medicaid in a given month, and Delaware does not offer "continuous eligibility"—that is, he must prove eligibility for Medicaid each month. Given Michael's life-threatening condition, he does not want to take the job and risk becoming uninsured.

Relatedly, there are those who frequently *switch* insurance. This population is difficult to track because they appear to be continuously insured. But people who switch plans may also have to switch doctors, hospitals, or pharmacies, which is especially problematic for those with chronic conditions who rely on a team of providers that understand their medical history and care plan. Lapses in care as a result of switching plans and providers can be dangerous for frequent "switchers" (Ladapo & Chokshi, 2014). Therefore, "switchers" can also be underinsured.

There are also those who are continuously insured on the same plan, but for whom the out-of-pocket costs are too high to actually use the plan, such as costs amounting to 5 or 10 percent of income (Schoen, Doty, Collins, & Holmgren, 2005). Under the ACA, coverage for employees is deemed "affordable" if they must contribute no more than 9.5 percent of household income, though on average, employees pay only 4 percent of their income for single-person coverage (Collins, Radley, Schoen, & Beutel, 2014).

Another way to conceptualize how a plan might be unaffordable to an individual or a family is to recall that premiums are our expected medical costs. We do not expect to pay much more than our premium in any given year unless we get very sick or badly injured. If we do not get sick or injured, however, then we do not expect to pay large out-of-pocket sums. (There is one exception, which is high-deductible health insurance, but we will get to that. For now, let us focus on traditional plans). If at the end of the year, our deductibles, copayments, and coinsurance constitute a large proportion of our premium even though we have not gotten very sick, then our plan does not seem very generous. In 2013, out-of-pocket medical spending per capita was roughly $800 (Health Care Cost Institute [HCCI], 2015). Recall that in this year, the average premium for an individual policy was $2,800 per person per year in the individual market and $4,400 in the group market, and even more for a family policy (KFF, 2013a, 2013b). It appears from these data that underinsurance using the definition of "affordability" is not a big problem. But consider that the majority of people never visit the doctor, so that while for most, out-of-pocket spending is $0, but for a small minority, spending is very high. Distributed across the population, then, it would appear as if annual out-of-pocket spending per capita were reasonable—say, $800—but for some individuals, the cost is exorbitant.

Another way that plans can be unaffordable is by having very limited provider networks—the hospitals, physicians, imaging facilities, laboratories, and other health care facilities covered by insurance. Suppose that Deborah is a hotel manager who is on her feet all day. Her knee begins to bother her and she visits her physician, who tells her that she needs an MRI of her knee. There are no covered MRI facilities near her job, and if she misses a shift at work, then she might lose her job. The only way to get the MRI without missing work is to go to a facility that is not covered by insurance. A limited provider network, then, is another way that people can be underinsured. (And in fact, limited provider networks are what make it so difficult to "switch" insurance)

Further, while an insurer may include a wide array of providers in its network, the network may be insufficient in other ways. Providers may not accept new patients, may not accept patients with

public insurance, or may have long waiting times for new appointments or other inconveniences that make them difficult to use (no parking, not seeing patients on time, and so on).

Finally, the trend toward consumer-directed or high-deductible plans raises the question about whether these types of plans constitute sufficient insurance, or whether enrollees in these plans are underinsured. Because these plans require high up-front cost-sharing (a high deductible) before insurance coverage kicks in, they are also referred to as "catastrophic coverage." Under the ACA, they are treated separately from traditional health plans, and only young adults may use them to satisfy the individual mandate for coverage. The tradeoff for high up-front cost-sharing is a lower premium, which might appeal to young adults who do not expect to use the health care system regularly but want protection in case of a major hospitalization or medical emergency; evidence suggests that young workers disproportionately enroll in high-deductible health plans (Barry, Cullen, Galusha, Slade, & Busch, 2008; Greene, Hibbard, Dixon, & Tusler, 2006).

In some ways, this arrangement is underinsurance. Enrollees in these plans are expected to shop for several thousand dollars' worth of care based on price and quality, even though neither of those factors may be particularly transparent, even after receiving care. And because premiums are lower, these plans may be the only affordable option for some enrollees, as evidenced by the fact that they are only available to the relatively poor "young invincibles" in state health insurance marketplaces.

On the other hand, high-deductible health plans embody the true meaning of insurance; they protect enrollees against high, unpredictable medical costs (Arrow, 1963). Premiums can stay low in these plans because administrative costs for smaller claims do not consume so much of the premium. Instead, individuals pay their own costs for routine visits to the physician, for blood tests, and for daily medications, and only submit claims to the insurer for catastrophic medical expenses such as hospitalizations, emergencies, and specialty biologic drugs.

In sum, we can conceptualize underinsurance as several factors: (1) being periodically uninsured, (2) frequently switching insurance, and (3) having insurance that is unaffordable, whether because out-of-pocket costs (especially the deductible) are too high or the provider network is too narrow.

ALTERNATIVE SOURCES OF CARE AND PAYMENT FOR THE UNINSURED

If you are uninsured, then you should check healthcare.gov to see if you qualify for Medicaid or for subsidized private health insurance through the health insurance marketplace. As we have discussed in this chapter, health insurance is a critical component of good health. But being uninsured does not always mean going without care or paying the list price for care. First, if you are uninsured and need care at a hospital or physician's office, then you can negotiate the price; try doing so before you go in. Find out what a typical procedure, test, or service costs in your area by going to healthcarebluebook.com, or what a bundle of services costs by going to guroo.com. You may even want to use this website if you have insurance, for example if you have not met your deductible, to compare the price of a service offered by your provider to the typical price in your area. There are also professional medical billing negotiators.

Second, if you are uninsured and come to the emergency department of a hospital, then under the Emergency Medical Treatment and Labor Act (EMTALA), the hospital must stabilize or transfer you if you truly are experiencing a medical emergency. Consumers should understand, however, that EMTALA does not restrict providers from billing uninsured consumers for this service, only from turning them away from the hospital. Still, consumers may negotiate hospital bills, and most hospitals will check whether patients are eligible for Medicaid immediately upon admission.

Third, community health centers provide an array of services focused on primary care, but sometimes also including specialty care and

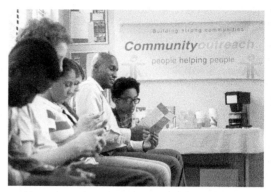

© Amble Design/Shutterstock

imaging and laboratory services, for fees that are often lower than at a traditional doctor's office. These fees may be on a sliding scale based on income, and some fees may be waived for those who cannot afford them. Health centers may also have special expertise in treating at-risk groups such as non-English speakers and the Lesbian, Gay, Bisexual, Transgender, and Queer/Questioning (LGBTQ) community. You can find a community health center at findahealthcenter.hrsa.gov.

Fourth, urgent care centers (walk-in clinics or retail clinics) are intended to treat conditions that are urgent but not life-threatening. Generally, there are primary care physicians on staff, and fees are usually lower than at a traditional doctor's office, although not as low as community health centers, whose focus is on the low-income and uninsured. Those with chronic conditions may find it difficult to see the same physician or nurse practitioner at every visit and to find an urgent care center with an in-house pharmacy.

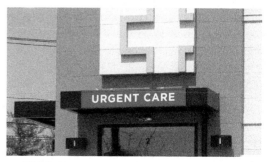

© raw206/Getty Images

Summary

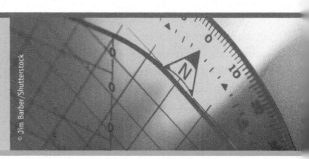

Despite the passage of the ACA, millions remain uninsured, periodically and chronically, throughout the year. Socioeconomic and political factors matter when it comes to insurance status. The uninsured are more likely to be black, Hispanic, less educated, Southern, and foreign-born. They are more likely to be young adults, and therefore, unintuitively, healthier. Because Medicaid has historically supported mothers and families, men are at greater risk for being uninsured.

Cost is the primary reason that people cite for being uninsured. While there are various secondary reasons—people have lost their jobs, or lost a family member on whom they were dependent for coverage, or they are exempt from the individual mandate—it is clear that most would purchase coverage if it were affordable.

While social and environmental factors may play a larger role in health than medical care, insurance is crucial to good health. The uninsured die at higher rates that cannot be explained by sociodemographic and environmental factors alone. They face out-of-pocket prices that are much higher than those of the insured, even though they are overwhelmingly poorer, and as a result they do not use as much medical care. When they do use care, they receive fewer services and experience worse outcomes. Giving people insurance improves their self-reported physical and mental well-being.

In 1965 Medicare and Medicaid were passed to address the problem of the uninsured. The dual policies were a success, drastically reducing the uninsured rate. Until the ACA, however, the uninsured rate remained steady at about 15 percent of the population, with only small-scale expansions

of coverage—perhaps with the exception of SCHIP in 1997. In 2010 the ACA was passed and expanded health insurance to millions.

But as we get closer to universal insurance, we must pay attention to the problem of underinsurance, which can be conceptualized as (1) being periodically insured, (2) frequently switching insurance, and (3) having insurance that is unaffordable because it has high out-of-pocket costs, especially a high deductible, or because it has a narrow provider network.

Finally, the uninsured should check healthcare.gov to see whether they are eligible for Medicaid or for subsidies to purchase a private health plan. But even the uninsured have options for low-cost care. Anyone may negotiate the price of their medical care, or even hire a professional negotiator. EMTALA is a federal protection for the uninsured experiencing a medical emergency. And community health centers and urgent care centers provide lower-cost alternatives to traditional care settings.

Achieving universal health insurance in a country where individual states are responsible for much of health insurance policy will require a coordinated effort. Many people are exempt from the individual mandate, and others have elected to pay the penalty. To get even these groups to participate, states must offer affordable health insurance plans.

References

Arrow, K. J. (1963). Uncertainty and the welfare economics of medical care. *The American Economic Review*, 53(5), 941–973.

Baicker, K., Finkelstein, A., Song, J., & Taubman, S. (2014). The impact of Medicaid on labor market activity and program participation: Evidence from the Oregon health insurance experiment. *The American Economic Review*, *104*(5), 322–328.

Baker, D. W., Sudano, J. J., Durazo-Arvizu, R., Feinglass, J., Witt, W. P., & Thompson, J. (2006). Health insurance coverage and the risk of decline in overall health and death among the near elderly, 1992–2002. *Medical Care*, *44*(3), 277–282.

Barcellos, S. H., & Jacobson, M. (2015). The effects of Medicare on medical expenditure risk and financial strain. *American Economic Journal: Economic Policy*, *7*(4), 41–70.

Barry, C. L., Cullen, M. R., Galusha, D., Slade, M. D., & Busch, S. H. (2008). Who chooses a consumer-directed health plan? *Health Affairs (Project Hope)*, *27*(6), 1671–1679.

Buchmueller, T. C., DiNardo, J., & Valletta, R. G. (2011). The effect of an employer health insurance mandate on health insurance coverage and the demand for labor: Evidence from Hawaii. *American Economic Journal: Economic Policy*, *3*(4), 25–51.

Card, D., Dobkin, C., & Maestas, N. (2004). *The impact of nearly universal insurance coverage on health care utilization and health: Evidence from Medicare*. Retrieved from http://www.nber.org/papers/w10365

Card, D., Dobkin, C., & Maestas, N. (2009). Does Medicare save lives? *The Quarterly Journal of Economics*, *124*(2), 597–636.

Carman, K., Eibner, C., & Paddock, S. (2015). Trends in health insurance enrollment, 2013–15. *Health Affairs*, *34*(6), 1044–1048.

Cohen, R. A., Makuc, D. M., Bernstein, A. B., Bilheimer, L. T., & Powell-Griner, E. (2009, July). Health insurance coverage trends, 1959-2007: Estimates from the National Health Interview Survey. *National Health Statistics Reports*, 17. Retrieved from https://www.cdc.gov/nchs/data/nhsr/nhsr017.pdf

Cohen, R., Martinez, M., & Zammitti, E. (2016). Health insurance coverage: Early release of estimates from the National Health Interview Survey, 2015. Retrieved from http://www.cdc.gov/nchs/data/nhis/earlyrelease/insur201605.pdf

Colla, C. H., Dow, W. H., & Dube, A. (2011). How do employers react to a pay-or- play mandate? Early evidence from San Francisco. *Forum Health Econ Policy*, *14*(2).

Collins, S. R., Radley, D. C., Schoen, C., & Beutel, S. (2014). National trends in the cost of employer health insurance coverage, 2003–2013. *Issue Brief*, *32*, 1–9.

Collins, S. R., Rasmussen, P. W., Doty, M. M., & Beutel, S. (2015). The rise in health care coverage and affordability since health reform took effect: Findings from the Commonwealth Fund biennial health insurance survey, 2014. *Issue Brief (Commonwealth Fund)*, *2*, 1.

Courtemanche, C. J., & Zapata, D. (2014). Does universal coverage improve health? The Massachusetts experience. *Journal of Policy Analysis and Management*, *33*(1), 36–69.

Davidoff, A., & Kenney, G. (2005). *Uninsured Americans with chronic health conditions: Key findings from the national health interview survey*. Washington, DC: The Urban Institute.

Decker, S. L. (2005). Medicare and the health of women with breast cancer. *The Journal of Human Resources*, *40*(4), 948–968.

Doyle, J. J., Jr. (2005). Health insurance, treatment and outcomes: Using auto accidents as health shocks. *Review of Economics and Statistics*, *87*(2), 256–270.

Dranove, D., & Millenson, M. L. (2006). Medical bankruptcy: Myth versus fact. *Health Affairs (Project Hope)*, *25*(2), 74–83.

Furman, J., & Fiedler, M. (2014, December 18). *2014 has seen the largest coverage gains on four decades, putting the uninsured rate at or near historic lows*. Retrieved from https://www.whitehouse.gov/blog/2014/12/18/2014-has-seen-largest-coverage-gains-four-decades-putting-uninsured-rate-or-near-his

Gardner, L., & Vishwasrao, S. (2010). Physician quality and health care for the poor and uninsured. *Inquiry*, *47*(1), 62–80.

Greene, J., Hibbard, J., Dixon, A., & Tusler, M. (2006). Which consumers are ready for consumer-directed health plans? *Journal of Consumer Policy: Consumer Issues in Law, Economics and Behavioral Sciences*, *29*(3), 247–262.

Health Care Cost Institute (HCCI). (2015, October). *2014 Health care cost and utilization report*. Retrieved from http://www.healthcostinstitute.org/2014-health-care-cost-and-utilization-report

The Henry J. Kaiser Family Foundation (KFF). (2013a). *Average monthly premiums per person in the individual market*. Retrieved from http://kff.org/other/state-indicator/individual-premiums/

The Henry J. Kaiser Family Foundation (KFF). (2013b). *Average single premium per enrolled employee for employer-based health insurance*. Retrieved from http://kff.org/other/state-indicator/single-coverage/

The Henry J. Kaiser Family Foundation (KFF). (2013c). *Kaiser health tracking poll: June 2013*. Retrieved from http://kff.org/health-reform/poll-finding/kaiser-health-tracking-poll-june-2013/

The Henry J. Kaiser Family Foundation (KFF). (2013d). *Percent of private sector establishments that offer health insurance to employees, by firm size*. Retrieved from http://kff.org/other/state-indicator/firms-offering-coverage-by-size/

Koskinen, J. A. (2015, July 17). *IRS commissioner Koskinen update to members of Congress on preliminary results from the 2015 filing season related to Affordable Care Act provisions*. Retrieved from https://www.irs.gov/pub/newsroom/irs_letter_aca_stats_010816.pdf

Ladapo, J., & Chokshi, D. (2014, November 18). *Continuity of care for chronic conditions: Threats, opportunities, and policy*. Retrieved from http://healthaffairs.org/blog/2014/11/18/continuity-of-care-for-chronic-conditions-threats-opportunities-and-policy-3/

Leppel, K. (2009). Labour force status and sexual orientation. *Economica*, *76*(301), 197–207.

Majerol, M., Newkirk, V., & Garfield, R. (2015). *The uninsured: A primer*. Retrieved from http://kff.org/uninsured/report/the

-uninsured-a-primer-key-facts-about-health-insurance-and-the-uninsured-in-the-era-of-health-reform/

Mazumder, B., & Miller, S. (2015). *The effects of the Massachusetts health reform on household financial distress.* Retrieved from https://www.chicagofed.org/publications/working-papers/2014/wp-01

McWilliams, J. M., Zaslavsky, A. M., Meara, E., & Ayanian, J. Z. (2003). Impact of Medicare coverage on basic clinical services for previously uninsured adults. *JAMA, 290*(6), 757–764.

McWilliams, J. M., Zaslavsky, A. M., Meara, E., & Ayanian, J. Z. (2004). Health insurance coverage and mortality among the near-elderly. *Health Affairs (Project Hope), 23*(4), 223–233.

Miller, S. (2012). Findings from Massachusetts's health reform: Lessons for other states. *Inquiry, 49*, 317–326.

National Federation of Independent Business et al. v. Sebelius, 132 S. Ct. 2566, 567 U.S. 1, 183 L. Ed. 2d 450 (2012).

National Health Interview Survey (NHIS). (2014). National Center for Health Statistics, Centers for Disease Control and Prevention. Retrieved from http://www.cdc.gov/nchs/nhis/

Planalp, C. Au-Yeung, C., & Turner, J. (2015, October). *Comparing federal government surveys that count the uninsured.* Robert Wood Johnson Foundation (RWJF). Retrieved from http://www.rwjf.org/en/library/research/2013/09/comparing-federal-government-surveys-that-count-the-uninsured.html

Schoen, C., Doty, M. M., Collins, S. R., & Holmgren, A. L. (2005). Insured but not protected: how many adults are underinsured? *Health affairs, 24*, W5.

Shartzer, A. Kenney, G. Long, S. Hempstead, K., & Wissoker, D. (2014). *Who are the remaining uninsured as of June 2014?* Retrieved from http://hrms.urban.org/briefs/who-are-the-remaining-uninsured-as-of-june-2014.pdf

Taubman, S. L., Allen, H. L., Wright, B. J., Baicker, K., & Finkelstein, A. N. (2014). Medicaid increases emergency-department use: Evidence from Oregon's health insurance experiment. *Science (New York, N.Y.), 343*(6168), 263–268.

United States Census Bureau. (2015). *Current population survey (CPS) health insurance: Data.* Retrieved from https://www.census.gov/cps/data/

United States Department of Health and Human Services. (2005, September). *Understanding estimates of the uninsured: Putting the differences in context.* Retrieved from https://aspe.hhs.gov/basic-report/understanding-estimates-uninsured-putting-differences-context-0

Utah Department of Health. (2012, June). *Utah health status update: Effect of improved survey methodology on BRFSS estimates.* Retrieved from http://health.utah.gov/opha/publications/hsu/1206_BRFSSCell.pdf

CHAPTER 4

The Affordable Care Act

Katie Keith, JD, MPH

LEARNING OBJECTIVES

- What were the goals of the Affordable Care Act?
- What gaps in the insurance market did the Affordable Care Act fill, and what gaps remain?
- What challenges arose in implementing the Affordable Care Act?

INTRODUCTION

Large-scale health reform efforts have long been elusive in the United States, where the expansion of benefits has, with few exceptions, been slow, hard-fought, and incremental. Reforms have generally targeted specific groups such as children, the elderly, and the poor. Prior to the Patient Protection and Affordable Care Act (ACA), 49.9 million Americans—about 16.3 percent of the population—were uninsured (Todd & Sommers, 2012). The ACA—or "Obamacare"—was the most significant expansion of health insurance coverage since Medicare and Medicaid in 1965 (Oberlander, 2010). Signed into law by President Barack Obama on March 23, 2010, the primary goal of the ACA was to expand health insurance coverage in the United States. Millions of people have gained coverage under the ACA, but the law has faced fierce political opposition and numerous legal challenges.

The ACA adopted three primary mechanisms to increase access to coverage: (1) rules for individuals, employers, and insurers to reduce barriers to private insurance markets; (2) state health insurance marketplaces or "exchanges" where consumers can compare coverage options and determine whether they are eligible for financial help; and (3) optional expansion of state Medicaid programs to cover more low-income adults. The law also made numerous changes in the delivery and quality of care, but its primary focus was on health insurance coverage. Figure 4-1 illustrates the major provisions of the ACA.

This chapter provides a brief history of the enactment of the ACA, discusses the main parts of the law, and summarizes how the law changes the way that consumers obtain health insurance coverage.

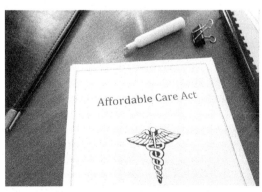

© zimmytws/Getty Images

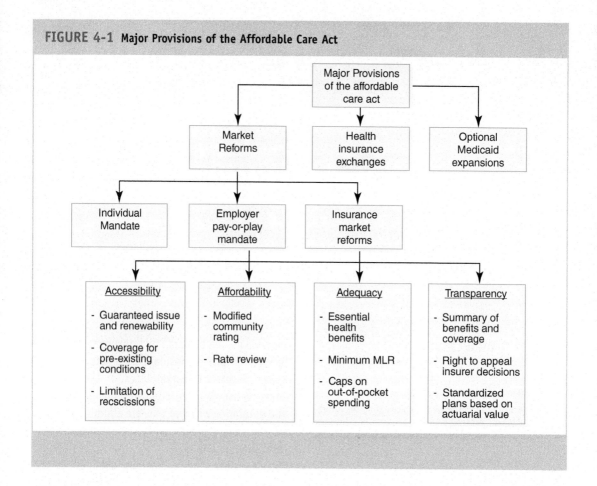

FIGURE 4-1 Major Provisions of the Affordable Care Act

HISTORY OF THE AFFORDABLE CARE ACT

The ACA was motivated by the high rate of uninsurance among non-elderly Americans, as well as underinsurance (insufficient benefits and unstable coverage), for which sick, low-income individuals were particularly at risk. At the time the ACA was passed, most Americans had health insurance through their employer, their spouse's employer, or through public programs like Medicare or Medicaid, but variations in state laws and insurance practices made it difficult to access coverage through the individual or small group markets. For example, insurers could deny coverage to sick or risky individuals (or small groups), or charge very high premiums for a policy.

Presidents and Congressional leaders since the Progressive era in the early twentieth century have made efforts at health insurance reform. But with some exceptions (such as Medicare and Medicaid), these efforts, rather than resulting in large-scale health insurance coverage increases, have instead been mostly incremental (Quadagno, 2005). The most recent failed health reform effort before the ACA, under President Bill Clinton, was criticized for being slow, secretive, and overly ambitious (Oberlander, 2007).

Health care was a topic of debate during the 2008 election, and President Obama cemented his commitment to health reform in a high-profile speech in February 2009 (Martin, 2009). In contrast with the Clinton reform efforts, the Obama Administration embraced a process that was speedy and transparent, and deferred to Congress on the details of the plan (Oberlander, 2010). Policymakers were also encouraged by successful health reform efforts in Massachusetts, where a law was passed in 2006 to expand insurance coverage through a state exchange, more generous Medicaid eligibility, and an individual mandate to purchase health insurance.

Responding to the president's call, the Democrat-controlled House and Senate each began working on health reform, which legislators and the public hotly debated throughout 2009 (Oberlander, 2010). By the fall, both chambers had passed a health reform bill, but the bills differed significantly. In most cases when the House and Senate disagree, a conference committee negotiates and drafts a compromise bill on which each chamber votes again. Senate Republicans vowed to delay voting on a compromise bill by employing a tactic called a filibuster, which can only be ended with a 60-vote "super-majority." But the death of Senator Ted Kennedy (a Democrat) in the fall of 2009 and the subsequent election of Senator Scott Brown (a Republican) as his replacement meant that the Senate no longer had the 60 votes it needed to break a filibuster and thus pass a compromise bill out of the Senate.

To salvage their efforts, the House abandoned the idea of a compromise bill and instead passed the Senate bill, which President Obama signed in March 2010. To incorporate House Democrats' concerns, Senate Democrats agreed to support a smaller bill called the Health Care and Education Reconciliation Act of 2010, which made budget-related amendments to the ACA and could not be delayed by filibuster. Together, these two bills constitute the largest expansion of health insurance coverage since Medicare and Medicaid in 1965.

The circumstances under which the ACA was passed puts into context some of the current controversy surrounding its implementation. Although President Obama and Congressional Democrats initially tried to gain bipartisan support, the final version of the bill was supported only by Democrats, which has given Republicans political fodder in their call for its repeal. In addition, the haste to pass the law meant that the final version included a number of inartful phrases and drafting errors (Pear, 2015). These errors have had considerable consequences. In 2015, for example, the Supreme Court debated whether a four-word phrase, "established by the State," should prevent individuals in states with federally established marketplaces from collecting health insurance subsidies, which would have left those individuals with few affordable options (King v. Burwell, 2015).

PROVISIONS OF THE AFFORDABLE CARE ACT

The ACA was not meant to restructure the U.S. health insurance system (for example, to a single-payer or voucher system), but rather to build upon the system that already existed, in order to minimize political opposition and disruption for those that were already satisfied with their plans. As such, the most significant changes were in expanding access to the individual and small group insurance markets, as well as Medicaid. These expansions were accomplished with (1) new responsibilities for individuals, employers, and insurers; (2) state health insurance exchanges; and (3) optional increased eligibility for Medicaid.

Individual Responsibilities

Most Americans are required to have health insurance under a provision known as the individual mandate, which is intended to encourage even the healthiest Americans to purchase insurance and spread the cost of premiums among a larger population. Coverage must meet certain minimum standards, known as minimum essential coverage. Those who do not comply with minimum essential coverage must pay a penalty when they file their federal taxes. The penalty is the greater of 2.5 percent of household income or $695 per adult ($347.50 per child) and is adjusted annually for inflation. The penalty is, however, capped at the cost of the average bronze plan (discussed in more detail below). This cap means that an individual will never be penalized more for lacking coverage than it costs to purchase health insurance.

Most comprehensive health insurance plans qualify as minimum essential coverage, including coverage through an employer (or spouse's employer), coverage on a parent's plan, Medicare,

Medicaid, the Children's Health Insurance Plan, most TRICARE plans, most student health plans, and private health insurance that meets marketplace standards. Note, however, that not everyone is subject to the individual mandate and thus not everyone who is uninsured must pay a penalty. Those exempt from the individual mandate include people from households with very low incomes or who cannot afford coverage; people who have suffered a hardship such as domestic violence, homelessness, or the death of a family member; people who are incarcerated; undocumented residents; members of federally recognized Indian tribes; those with religious objections; and people with short coverage gaps (fewer than three months) or who are members of a health care- sharing ministry.

Employer Responsibilities

Employers with 50 or more full-time employees are subject to an employer "pay-or-play" mandate, in which they have the option of offering health insurance ("playing") or paying a penalty ("paying"). Part-time employees (those averaging fewer than 30 hours per week) and seasonal employees are generally excluded from this mandate.

Employers are subject to penalties if at least one full-time employee receives a premium tax credit (subsidy) through the marketplace. Employees are entitled to receive these tax credits if (1) employers do not offer coverage; (2) employers offer coverage, but it is not "affordable" for the employee (meaning that the employee must contribute more than 9.5 percent of household income to the premium); or (3) employers offer coverage but it does not meet "minimum value" standards (meaning that the plan fails, on average, to cover at least 60 percent of health care costs). When employees claim a tax credit in these situations, employers must pay a penalty.

Insurer Responsibilities

Prior to the ACA, the rules for private health insurance varied by state, with few minimum federal standards. This meant that someone living in New York might have had dramatically different rights and protections than someone living in, say,

California or Texas. Provisions in the ACA established minimum national standards for accessibility, affordability, adequacy, and transparency of private health insurance coverage.

Accessibility

The ACA contains several provisions to protect those with pre-existing conditions—illness or injury that was present before coverage began. First, insurers may no longer exclude or limit coverage of pre-existing conditions. Second, prior to the ACA, insurers discovering a pre-existing health issue could legally rescind (cancel) coverage; under the ACA, however, rescissions of coverage are only allowed if consumers submit fraudulent insurance applications.

Third, insurers are subject to guaranteed issue, a requirement to offer coverage to anyone who applies, regardless of health status. Under federal law, guaranteed issue was already required in all states in the small group market, but the ACA extended this protection to the individual market as well. Prior to the ACA, only five states—Maine, Massachusetts, New Jersey, New York, and Vermont—required guaranteed issue in the individual market (The Henry J. Kaiser Family Foundation [KFF], 2012a). In any other state, insurers could refuse to sell someone a policy because that person already had, for example, diabetes or heart disease—or even just a family history of illness.

Finally, the ACA requires guaranteed renewability—insurers must offer to renew a policy each year to anyone who continues to pay premiums, regardless of health status. Prior to the ACA, if a consumer became sick or injured during the year, then an insurer could refuse to renew that consumer's policy the following year.

If insurers cannot deny coverage to sick enrollees, and consumers wait to obtain coverage until they are sick, then insurers face a serious adverse selection problem, with premiums that may be too low to cover sick enrollees who join the plan. To address this concern, the ACA established open enrollment, an established period of time during which consumers may purchase a policy for the following year. Once the open enrollment period ends, however, insurers can refuse to provide coverage unless a consumer qualifies for a special enrollment period. A special enrollment period is a limited period of time (generally 60 days) during which a consumer may enroll in health insurance outside of the open enrollment period. To qualify for a special enrollment period, a consumer must experience a "qualifying life event," such as the birth of a baby, marriage, the loss of a job, or the loss of existing coverage (Center on Budget and Policy Priorities, 2016). If a consumer does not take advantage of open or special enrollment periods, then they may be forced to remain uninsured until the next open enrollment period, even if they get sick or injured. The open enrollment period is therefore an incentive to purchase coverage even before consumers become sick or injured. Most employment-based plans and Medicare use this technique for the same reason.

The ACA also made it easier for young adults to stay enrolled in their parent's health insurance plan. Prior to health reform, dependent coverage in some states extended only to certain categories of young adults, such as students and unmarried children (National Conference of State Legislatures, 2016). The ACA required plans that offer dependent coverage to extend this coverage to all dependents until the age of 26. Because of this provision, 2.3 million young people gained health insurance through a parent's plan between 2010 and 2013 (Uberoi, Finegold, & Gee, 2016).

Affordability

Prior to the ACA, insurers commonly experience rated premiums (charged premiums based on previous year's costs) in the individual and small group markets, resulting in uneven access to coverage for the riskiest groups. In 2013, for instance, it was perfectly legal in 37 states to charge women more than men for the exact same coverage and to charge higher premiums to sicker individuals in 43 states and Washington, DC (KFF, 2012b).

To make coverage more affordable for these higher-cost groups, the ACA adopted a modified community rating system. Recall that community rating, unlike experience rating, sets premiums based on the average cost of all individuals in an area rather than just one individual or one group. The ACA allows increases to this premium based on only four factors: (1) family size, (2) geographic location, (3) age, and (4) tobacco use. Insurers cannot charge an older person more than 3 times as much as the youngest person or charge someone who uses tobacco more than 1.5 times as much as someone who does not use tobacco. Insurers may not use any factor other than these four cannot when risk-adjusting premiums for new plans in the individual and small group markets. These rating requirements are only minimum standards, meaning that states can adopt stricter rules. Some places—such as California and Washington, DC—have, for instance, prohibited surcharges for tobacco use, meaning that consumers that use tobacco are charged the same rate as those that do not (Giovanelli, Lucia, & Corlette, 2015).

Prior to the ACA, insurers in many states could raise premiums without justification and with little transparency for consumers. To address this issue, the ACA set national standards to review health insurance rate increases, such as requiring expert analysis to evaluate the rationale and assumptions made by insurers for raising rates. The federal government provided state departments of insurance with $250 million to support their rate review efforts (Center for Consumer Information and Insurance Oversight [CCIIO], n.d.b). In states that do not have an effective rate review program, the federal government will review rate increases.

Adequacy

Prior to the ACA, states were responsible for setting standards for coverage for fully insured (but not self-insured) plans. Coverage requirements varied widely among states, ranging from preventive health services, such as childhood immunizations and screening for colorectal cancer, to specialized benefits such as infertility treatment (National Conference of State Legislatures, 2015). The ACA sets minimum national standards, requiring plans in the individual and small group markets to include three components: (1) coverage of so-called essential health benefits, (2) limits on out-of-pocket costs, and (3) minimum actuarial value standards.

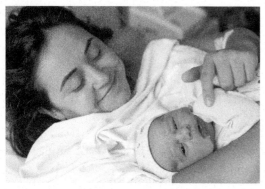

© Svetlana Solovjova/Shutterstock

In addition to state-mandated benefits, some insurers must also cover the following 10 categories of essential health benefits (EHB): ambulatory patient services; emergency services; hospitalization; maternity and newborn care; mental health and substance use disorder services, including behavioral health treatment; prescription drugs; rehabilitative and habilitative services and devices; laboratory services; preventive and wellness services and chronic disease management; and pediatric services, including oral and vision care. Some essential health benefits must be covered without cost-sharing; in particular, preventive services recommended by the U.S. Preventive Services Task Force with a high level of certainty as to the net benefit of the service.

Under the ACA, insurers are subject to a minimum medical loss ratio (MLR) requirement. The MLR is the percentage of the premium paid out in benefits. The minimum MLR is 85 percent in the large group market and 80 percent in the individual and small group markets, meaning that insurers must spend at least 85 (80) percent of premium dollars on medical care or quality improvement. If insurers fail to meet this threshold, then consumers receive a rebate directly from their insurance company.

The ACA caps annual and lifetime out-of-pocket spending (deductibles, copayments, and coinsurance) for essential health benefits. In 2014, the maximum out-of-pocket cost for individuals was $6,350 ($12,700 for families). By 2017, the maximum was $7,150 for individuals ($14,300 for families). This spending limit does not, however, include all potential out-of-pocket costs that a consumer might pay, such as monthly premium payments and costs associated with using an out-of-network provider (and of course, it does not cover indirect costs associated with using health care, such as transportation costs and lost work time).

Transparency

To make it easier for consumers to understand their health insurance plans, the ACA requires insurers (or employers) to provide enrollees with a summary of benefits and coverage (SBC). The SBC is a standardized form that summarizes the key features of a plan, including covered benefits, cost-sharing requirements, and coverage limits and exceptions. The SBC also includes examples to help consumers understand how much the plan would cover under common medical scenarios, such as a bone fracture or childbirth. This standardized document makes it easier for consumers to understand, compare, and evaluate their coverage options.

Plans on the exchanges must conform to one of four "precious metal" categories: bronze, silver, gold, or platinum (**Figure 4-2**). Within each of these categories, plans have the same actuarial value, meaning that they are estimated to cover the same proportion of total costs among enrollees, on average. Bronze plans are estimated to cover an average of 60 percent of costs among enrollees in that plan; silver plans 70 percent; gold plans 80 percent; and platinum plans 90 percent. The higher the actuarial value, the more generous the plan, which is usually reflected in a higher premium. Note, however, that actuarial value is only an *estimate* and that *actual* costs may vary by individual and by year. Some consumers—such as those under age 30 or facing a hardship—are eligible for a fifth type of plan known as catastrophic coverage, which has low monthly premiums and a high deductible.

The ACA also provides consumers with the right to appeal a decision made by their insurer, such as a claim denial, and requires insurers to follow standardized processes when resolving appeals. These standards apply to both the internal review process (an initial appeal to the insurer) and the external review process (a secondary appeal to an independent third party

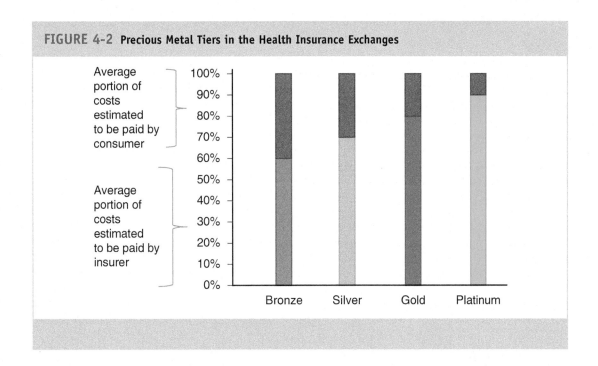

FIGURE 4-2 Precious Metal Tiers in the Health Insurance Exchanges

that can reverse or affirm the insurer's decision) (Andrews & Galewitz, 2010). These processes are the same in all 50 states and Washington, DC, but states may contract with different third-party external reviewers.

Must all plans comply with new insurer responsibilities? No, not all plans must comply with new insurer responsibilities. Two categories of plans are exempt from some types of regulations: self-funded plans and grandfathered plans (Table 4-1).

The first category of exempted plans is self-funded plans. Unlike fully insured plans, which are regulated by state insurance departments, self-insured plans are regulated at the federal level by the U.S. Department of Labor. In 1974, Congress enacted the Employee Retirement Income Security Act (ERISA) to regulate self-funded plans. Employers operating in multiple states, then, could offer uniform benefits to their employees across states, as ERISA generally pre-empted state laws and their various benefit mandates.

Crucial to the treatment of self-funded plans under the ACA, ERISA treats these plans not as insurance, but as administrative contracts between employers and insurers. In a self-funded plan, employers assume financial risk, while insurers administer claims. Under the ACA, then, insurance market reforms apply to insurance plans but not to administrative plans such as self-funded plans. Self-funded plans need not offer an essential health benefits package or meet the minimum medical loss ratio, nor are they subject to state review of premium increases. Some provisions, such as community rating and guaranteed issue and renewability, do not apply to self-funded plans, because insurers do not offer plans or set premiums for such a plan.

The second category of exempted plans is grandfathered plans, which are plans that were already in existence when the ACA was passed on March 23, 2010, and that have not undergone substantial changes to benefits or cost-sharing since then. "If you like your healthcare plan, you can keep your healthcare plan," President Obama repeated in selling the ACA to the public before it was passed. Grandfathered plans were built into the law to deliver the president's promise.

Grandfathered plans are exempt from a host of ACA regulations, including guaranteed issue and renewability and modified community rating. They need not offer essential health benefits. Grandfathered *group* plans may not

TABLE 4-1 Exemptions of Affordable Care Act Provisions

Provision	Grandfathered Plans[a]			New Plans- (Non-grandfathered)				
	Group Market[b]		Individual Market	Large-Group Market[c]		Small-Group Market[d]		Individual Market
	Fully Insured[e]	Self-Insured[f]		Fully Insured	Self-Insured	Fully Insured	Self-Insured	
Obtaining Coverage								
Guaranteed Issue	N.A.	N.A.	N.A.	✓	N.A.	✓	N.A.	✓
Nondiscrimination Based on Health Status	N.A.	N.A.	N.A.	✓	✓	✓	✓	✓
Extension on Dependent Coverage	✓	✓	✓	✓	✓	✓	✓	✓
Prohibition of Discrimination Based on Salary	N.A.	N.A.	N.A.	✓	✓	✓	N.A.	N.A.
Waiting Period Limitation	✓	✓	N.A.	✓	✓	✓	✓	N.A.
Keeping Coverage								
Guaranteed Renewability	N.A.	N.A.	N.A.	✓	N.A.	✓	N.A.	✓
Prohibition on Rescissions	✓	✓	✓	✓	✓	✓	✓	✓
Costs Associated with Coverage								
Rating Restrictions	N.A.	N.A.	N.A.	N.A.	N.A.	✓	N.A.	✓
Rate Review	N.A.	N.A.	N.A.	N.A.	N.A.	✓	N.A.	✓
Single Rick Pool	N.A.	N.A.	N.A.	N.A.	N.A.	✓	N.A.	✓
Covered Services								
Coverage of Essential Health Benefits	N.A.	N.A.	N.A.	N.A.	N.A.	✓	N.A.	✓

	C1	C2	C3	C4	C5	C6	C7
Coverage of Preventive Health Services Without Cost Sharing	N.A.	N.A.	N.A.	N.A.	√	√	√
Coverage of Preexisting Health Conditions	√	√	√	√	√	√	√
Cost-Sharing Limits							
Limits for Annual Out-of-Pocket Spending	N.A.	N.A.	N.A.	√	√	√	√
Minimum Actuarial Value Requirements	N.A.	N.A.	N.A.	N.A	N.A.	N.A.	N.A.
Prohibition on Lifetime Limits	√	√	√	√	√	√	√
Prohibition on Annual Limits	√	N.A.	√	√	√	√	√
Consumer Assistance and Other Patient Protections							
Summary of Benefits and Coverage	√	√	√	√	√	√	√
Medical Loss Ratio	√	√	N.A.	N.A.	N.A.	N.A.	N.A.
Appeals Process	N.A.	N.A.	√	√	√	√	√
Patient Protections	N.A.	N.A.	√	√	√	√	√
Nondiscrimination Regarding Clinical Trial Participation	N.A.	N.A.	√	√	√	√	√
Plan Requirements Related to Health Care Providers							
Nondiscrimination Regarding Health Care Providers	N.A.	N.A.	√	√	√	√	√
Reporting Requirements Regarding Quality of Care	N.A.	N.A.	√	√	√	√	√

exclude pre-existing conditions from coverage, but grandfathered *individual* plans may exclude such benefits. Grandfathered plans in both types of markets need not cover preventive services without cost-sharing, nor must they have a standardized internal or external appeals process.

Yet all plans, both self-insured and grandfathered, must comply with certain universal regulations. No plan may impose lifetime limits on coverage for essential health. Insurers may not rescind coverage for reasons other than fraud. Plans that offer dependent coverage must offer it to dependents up to age 26. Finally, all plans must offer enrollees a Summary of Benefits and Coverage document so that benefits and cost-sharing are clear.

Health Insurance Marketplaces

Prior to the ACA, consumers purchasing health insurance in the individual and small group markets could purchase a plan that excluded a pre-existing condition, but pay more for that condition anyway. They faced a confusing array of plans whose cost-sharing structures and provider networks were difficult to decipher; and in some areas, they may have only had one or two plans from which to choose. To address these issues, the ACA required that states establish health insurance marketplaces (also called exchanges) in every state. Exchanges are websites (and in some states, brick-and-mortar stores) where consumers can compare and purchase plans. There are two types of marketplaces in every state: the individual marketplace and the Small Business Health Options (SHOP) marketplace. In the individual marketplace, individual enrollees and their families can compare private plans, apply for premium and cost-sharing subsidies, determine eligibility for public coverage, and enroll in public coverage. In the SHOP marketplace, small employers aggregate their purchasing power to provide their employees with access to a wider range of plans at lower costs. Employees of these small businesses may then compare and purchase plans on the state SHOP marketplace website.

Plans offered through the exchanges are called qualified health plans (QHPs). A QHP is a plan that is ACA-compliant and approved by the state to be sold in the health insurance exchange. Some states have more restrictive standards, such as more generous benefit mandates and standards regarding an adequate provider network. Insurers must meet certain standards to offer a QHP, such as offering at least one silver plan and one gold plan and agreeing to set the same premium for QHPs sold inside and outside of the marketplace. Transparency in the marketplace is key; plans must conform to one of the "precious metal" tiers (or be a high-deductible plan for young people) so that consumers can more easily understand how much financial protection that the plan offers. For example, a "silver" Anthem plan in California is actuarially equivalent to (offers, on average, the same estimated financial protection as) a "silver" Empire plan in New York.

Enrollment in coverage through the individual or SHOP marketplaces is entirely voluntary, and, in most states, a robust private health insurance market continues to exist outside of the state exchanges. The individual exchange, however, may be the best option for low- and middle-income consumers because the government does not offer premium or cost-sharing subsidies outside of the exchanges.

States can choose to establish a state-based individual marketplace, a state-based SHOP marketplace, or neither. In states that declined to establish state-based individual marketplaces, federal regulators did so on their behalf. As of 2016, 16 states and Washington, DC, opted to establish state-based individual marketplaces (Figure 4-3) (KFF, 2016b). In states establishing their own exchanges, policymakers had significant flexibility regarding key decisions, such as financing and operations, and could adjust certain rules—such as extending open enrollment periods—to meet state needs or exceed minimum federal standards. In these states, marketplaces go by different names. For example, the marketplaces in California and the District of Columbia are called Covered California and DC Health Link, respectively.

In 27 states, the federal government operates the individual marketplace, and 7 states created a federal–state partnership. Three states—Arkansas, Mississippi, and Utah—established SHOP marketplaces, even though they ceded control of the individual market to the federal government; one state, New Mexico, established both a SHOP

FIGURE 4-3 State Health Insurance Marketplace Types, 2016

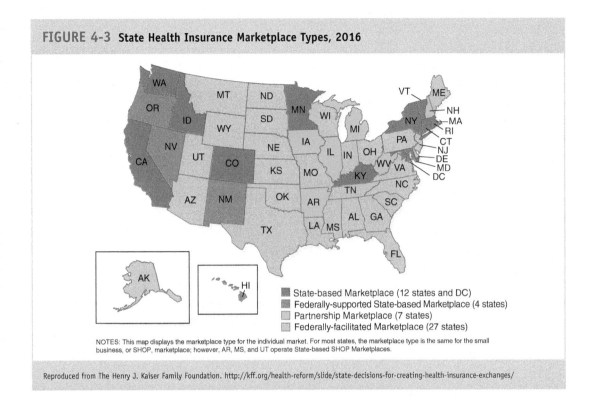

State-based Marketplace (12 states and DC)
Federally-supported State-based Marketplace (4 states)
Partnership Marketplace (7 states)
Federally-facilitated Marketplace (27 states)

NOTES: This map displays the marketplace type for the individual market. For most states, the marketplace type is the same for the small business, or SHOP, marketplace; however, AR, MS, and UT operate State-based SHOP Marketplaces.

Reproduced from The Henry J. Kaiser Family Foundation. http://kff.org/health-reform/slide/state-decisions-for-creating-health-insurance-exchanges/

marketplace and a federally supported state-based marketplace (KFF, 2016b).

Individual Health Insurance Marketplaces

Most Americans are eligible to purchase private health insurance through the individual marketplace in their state. The only people who are *not* eligible are those who are currently incarcerated or those who are not lawfully present in the United States. Although most people can purchase coverage through the marketplace, consumers must do so during annual open enrollment periods (or special enrollment opportunities), and not all will qualify for subsidies to reduce their monthly premiums or out-of-pocket costs. There are two types of subsidies available through the marketplace: premium tax credits and cost-sharing reductions (**Figure 4-4**).

A premium tax credit reduces the amount that consumers must pay in monthly premiums for

marketplace coverage (KFF, 2014). To be eligible for a premium tax credit, a consumer's annual household income must be between 100 and 400 percent of the federal poverty level (FPL), and she must not have access to public coverage or affordable coverage through an employer (or a spouse's employer).[1] The amount of the premium subsidy increases as household income declines. To claim a premium tax credit, individuals must file a federal income tax return, even if they are not usually required to do so.

Consider the following example: Lacy is 24 years old, lives in zip code 08062, and earned $23,760 (200 percent FPL) in 2016. She would like to purchase an individual policy. To do so, she will visit her state's marketplace, answer some demographic questions, and estimate her annual income for the following year. Using this information, the marketplace determines eligibility for premium tax credits, cost-sharing reductions, and Medicaid coverage. Lacy is eligible for a premium

[1] In states that have expanded their Medicaid program to cover low-income adults, premium tax credits are available to consumers whose income is between 138 and 400 percent FPL. The state's Medicaid program will cover those whose income is 138 percent FPL or less.

FIGURE 4-4 Subsidies on the Health Insurance Exchanges

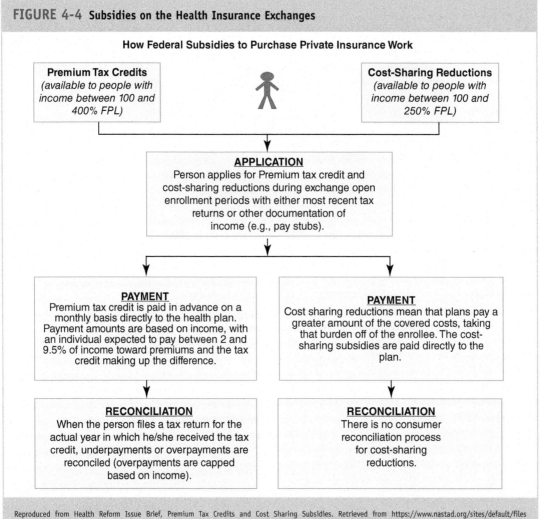

How Federal Subsidies to Purchase Private Insurance Work

Premium Tax Credits
(available to people with income between 100 and 400% FPL)

Cost-Sharing Reductions
(available to people with income between 100 and 250% FPL)

APPLICATION
Person applies for Premium tax credit and cost-sharing reductions during exchange open enrollment periods with either most recent tax returns or other documentation of income (e.g., pay stubs).

PAYMENT
Premium tax credit is paid in advance on a monthly basis directly to the health plan. Payment amounts are based on income, with an individual expected to pay between 2 and 9.5% of income toward premiums and the tax credit making up the difference.

PAYMENT
Cost sharing reductions mean that plans pay a greater amount of the covered costs, taking that burden off of the enrollee. The cost-sharing subsidies are paid directly to the plan.

RECONCILIATION
When the person files a tax return for the actual year in which he/she received the tax credit, underpayments or overpayments are reconciled (overpayments are capped based on income).

RECONCILIATION
There is no consumer reconciliation process for cost-sharing reductions.

tax credit of $296 per month, which she can apply toward any plan on the marketplace except for catastrophic coverage.

Once she selects her plan, Lacy must decide whether to take her premium tax credit in advance or wait until she files her taxes the following year. If she chooses to take the advance premium tax credit, then the federal government pays $296 per month directly to the insurer, and Lacy pays only her reduced portion of the premium. If Lacy's income is higher than estimated, then she may have to return some proportion of the subsidy when filing her federal taxes the following year, but if her income is lower than estimated, then she may receive a refundable credit.

Alternatively, Lacy may forgo advance premium credits. In this case, she will pay the full premium for whatever plan she chooses and receive a tax credit in the appropriate amount when she files her tax return the following year, estimated to be about $296.

The second type of marketplace subsidy is a cost-sharing reduction, which reduces out-of-pocket costs for health care services, like going to the doctor or filling a prescription (KFF, 2014). People are eligible for cost-sharing reductions if they are also eligible for a premium tax credit, have a household income of 100 to 250 percent FPL, and enroll in a silver plan. As with the premium tax credit, cost-sharing reductions increase as income declines. Unlike the premium tax credit, cost-sharing reductions can only be paid as an advance tax credit, directly to the insurer. However, consumers do not have to reconcile these payments at the end of the year and thus do not have to repay overpayments (but do not receive refunds for underpayments) because of income fluctuations. Cost-sharing reductions effectively raise the actuarial value of a plan because they increase, on average, the proportion of out-of-pocket costs from which enrollees are protected.

Once consumers know whether they are eligible for subsidies or Medicaid, they can review and compare their plan options (Figure 4-4). Selecting the right plan is critical for consumers, many of whom will be ineligible to switch to a different plan until the following year once the open enrollment period closes. For consumers with chronic diseases, switching plans from year-to-year means potentially facing a different network of providers who are unfamiliar with the patient's condition, drugs that may not be part of the new plan's formulary, and services that may be covered with higher cost-sharing.

Consumers will also have the option to purchase a stand-alone dental plan through the marketplace. After consumers select a plan, they may enroll in dental coverage through the marketplace and must pay the first month's premium directly to the insurer. They remain enrolled in this plan unless they fail to pay their premium or qualify for a special enrollment period that allows them to switch plans.

Consumers should return to the marketplace regularly to update income and demographic information to determine eligibility for subsidies and public coverage.

SHOP Marketplaces

Every state also has a SHOP marketplace designed to pool small businesses together, thereby increasing purchasing power to better negotiate with insurers for reasonable rates and benefits while also reducing administrative costs. To purchase coverage through the SHOP marketplace, employers must have at least 2 but no more than 50 full-time equivalent employees. Employers must also offer coverage to all full-time employees (those who average 30 or more hours per week) and meet minimum participation requirements set by the state, which require a certain percentage of employees—70 percent, in most states—to have health insurance (through either the employer or another source).

Unlike in the individual marketplace, which has a standard open enrollment period for all consumers, there is no open enrollment period in the SHOP marketplace, so employers may begin SHOP coverage at any time of the year. Although not required, small employers who enroll in SHOP coverage between November 15 and December 15 can waive the state's minimum participation requirement.

The shop marketplace may offer more options for coverage to employees of small businesses than prior to the ACA. Small employers generally offer only one or two plans to employees, if any, and rarely more (KFF, 2016a). But employers who participate in SHOP choose a "precious metal" level of coverage—such as bronze or silver—and employees may select any plan in that tier in their geographic area.

The Three-Legged Stool

The ACA's reforms are designed to complement each other and, indeed, depend upon one another. The "three-legged stool"—a piece of furniture that can remain steady on any surface, even one that is not level—also refers to a set of three provisions: guaranteed issue, the individual mandate, and subsidies to purchase insurance (**Figure 4-5**). Together, these reforms are the sturdy seat on which the exchanges sit; remove a "leg," however, and the exchanges topple over. For example, subsidies must accompany an individual mandate, or else low-income consumers could not afford to comply. Likewise, an individual mandate must accompany guaranteed issue, or insurers would face adverse selection severe enough to put them out of business. Insurers cannot offer coverage only to sick people; healthy people must also join the risk pool to balance the risk among enrollees. In fact, the individual mandate was critical to securing the support of insurers (Girion, 2009). Together, then, guaranteed issue, the individual mandate, and subsidies

FIGURE 4-5 Three-Legged Stool

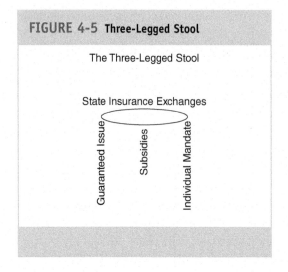

The Three-Legged Stool

keep the exchanges viable. The loss of any one of these interlocking reforms could destabilize state insurance exchanges.

Medicaid Expansion

Prior to the ACA, millions of low-income adults earned too much money to qualify for public coverage like Medicaid but too little to afford private coverage. Many states' Medicaid programs provided no coverage to adults without children and in states that did, such coverage was often limited (KFF, 2013). As a result, low-income, childless adults, especially poor, working males, were left without affordable coverage options.

As enacted, the ACA required all 50 states and the District of Columbia to expand eligibility for their Medicaid programs to individuals earning up to 138 percent FPL beginning in 2014. Additional enrollees would be 100 percent funded by the federal government through 2016, phased down to 90 percent by 2020.

In 2012, however, the Supreme Court ruled that this method of Medicaid expansion was too far-reaching and that expansion should be voluntary (*National Federation of Independent Business v. Sebelius, 2012*). As of March 2016, most states—31 and Washington, DC—had chosen to expand their Medicaid program (KFF, 2016c). Figure 4-6 maps state decisions to expand their Medicaid programs.

In states that do not expand their Medicaid programs, some low-income consumers with

FIGURE 4-6 State Decisions to Expand Medicaid, 2016

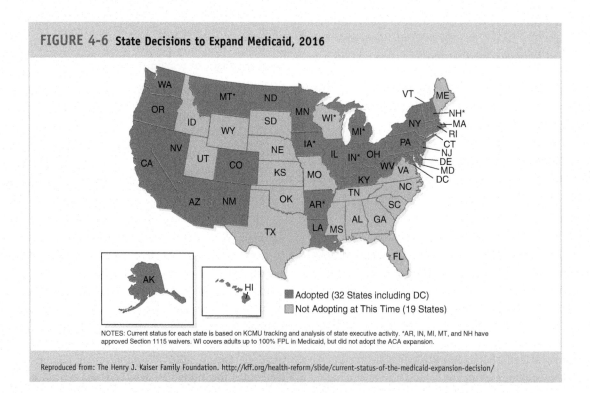

Adopted (32 States including DC)

Not Adopting at This Time (19 States)

NOTES: Current status for each state is based on KCMU tracking and analysis of state executive activity. *AR, IN, MI, MT, and NH have approved Section 1115 waivers. WI covers adults up to 100% FPL in Medicaid, but did not adopt the ACA expansion.

income below 100 percent FPL may fall into a "coverage gap" (**Figure 4-7**). Recall that to qualify for subsidies on the health insurance exchanges, consumers must earn between 100 percent and 400 percent FPL. Those earning below 100 FPL will therefore not qualify for any financial help. And if these very low-income adults also live in a state that did not expand Medicaid eligibility up to 138 percent FPL under the ACA, then they may not qualify for Medicaid either (for example, because they do not have children). These very poor adults may therefore lack access to any source of affordable insurance. Millions of individuals fall within this coverage gap and remain uninsured (Garfield & Damico, 2016).

Other Changes Under the Affordable Care Act

In addition to coverage expansions, the ACA also made changes to the health care delivery system. For the first time, Medicare is authorized to recognize accountable care organizations (ACOs), groups of providers—hospitals, physician organizations, and suppliers—responsible for coordinating care for a specified patient population and subject to quality standards. If an ACO saves money, then it may keep a percentage of cost savings, and some ACOs will even be responsible for paying a portion of losses—in exchange for a higher shared savings percentage. This introduction of ACOs has had a dramatic effect on the market, as private payers have followed Medicare's lead in recognizing their own ACOs, and providers have scrambled to form them. Because of the incentive to coordinate care (and also likely in response to the Great Recession of 2007 to 2009), providers responded to ACOs by engaging in a "merger frenzy" that has greatly consolidated hospitals and physicians across the United States (Dafny, 2014).

Among myriad other provisions, the ACA created the Center for Medicare and Medicaid Innovation to test new provider payment models to improve the value of payments for health care; created incentives for hospitals to reduce hospital-acquired infections; and established new institutes and agencies, such as the Patient-Centered Outcomes Research Institute. The law also created the Prevention and Public Health Fund, providing $5 billion over 10 years to invest in public health, wellness, and disease prevention. These funds have been used to help local officials prevent and respond to infectious disease outbreaks,

FIGURE 4-7 Coverage Gap for Low-Income Adults in States That Did Not Expand Medicaid

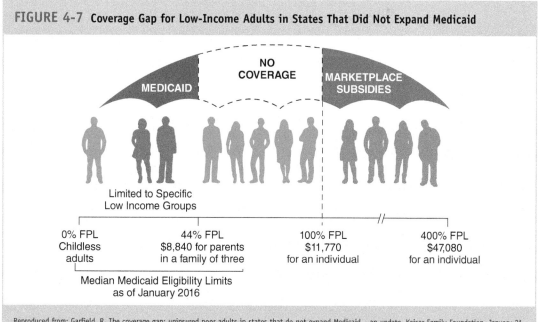

strengthen the primary care workforce, and fund community-based prevention programs (Haberkorn, 2012).

ENFORCEMENT

Different parts of the ACA are enforced by the federal government and the states, in accordance with the framework laid out by the Health Insurance Portability and Accountability Act of 1996 (HIPAA). Under HIPAA, states are presumed to be the primary enforcer of federal health insurance laws unless (1) a state reports that it is not enforcing federal law, or (2) the federal government determines that a state has failed to substantially enforce federal law (Pollitz, Tapay, Hadley, & Specht, 2000). This approach helps to ensure that states continue to be the primary regulators of private health insurance with the possibility of federal enforcement if needed. As we

have discussed, self-funded plans do not qualify as health insurance under ERISA, and so as per HIPAA, the federal government, rather than the states, enforces laws regarding self-funded contracts.

As of March 2016, five states—Alabama, Missouri, Oklahoma, Texas, and Wyoming—had declined to enforce or did not have the authority to enforce the ACA (CCIIO, n.d.a). In these states, the federal government—the Department of Health and Human Services (HHS)—enforces insurance market reforms and resolves consumer complaints. In the remaining states, state regulators—usually the state department of insurance—enforce the ACA. It is important to understand who is responsible for enforcing the law because consumers should know whom to contact if they need to file a complaint or otherwise report to a regulator.

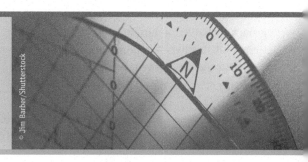

Summary

The ACA ushered in the most significant changes to the health care system since 1965. The law includes several mechanisms to increase access to health insurance, including new market reforms to improve the accessibility, affordability, adequacy, and transparency of private health insurance coverage; new health insurance marketplaces where low- and middle-income consumers can receive financial help with premiums and cost-sharing; and optional expansion of state Medicaid programs to low-income adults. These standards build upon the existing regulatory system for private health insurance, and the most extensive changes apply to coverage in the individual and small group markets.

Since the ACA went into effect in 2010, millions of Americans have enrolled in health insurance through the marketplaces, Medicaid, or a parent's plan, and the uninsured rate has reached historic lows. Despite this success, the law continues to face the threat of repeal in Congress, ongoing legal challenges, and resistance from state leaders. The continued controversy surrounding the ACA will result in state-by-state variability in how it is implemented and its success in further reducing the number of uninsured Americans.

References

Andrews, M., & Galewitz, P. (2010, July). New rules guarantee patients' right to appeal insurance claim denials. *Kaiser Health News*. Retrieved from http://khn.org/news/insurance-denials-2/

Center on Budget and Policy Priorities. (2016). *Guide to special enrollment period triggers and timing*. Retrieved from http://www.healthreformbeyondthebasics.org/wp-content/uploads/2015/06/SEP-Reference-Chart.pdf

Center for Consumer Information and Insurance Oversight (CCIIO). (n.d.a). *Compliance and enforcement*. Retrieved from https://www.cms.gov/cciio/programs-and-initiatives/health-insurance-market-reforms/compliance.html

Center for Consumer Information and Insurance Oversight (CCIIO). (n.d.b). *New resources to help states crack down on unreasonable health insurance premium hikes and to enhance health pricing transparency*. Retrieved from https://www.cms.gov/CCIIO/Resources/Regulations-and-Guidance/rates.html

Dafny, L. (2014). Hospital industry consolidation—still more to come? *New England Journal of Medicine, 370*, 198–199.

Garfield, R., & Damico, A. (2016). The coverage gap: Uninsured poor adults in states that do not expand Medicaid—An update. *Kaiser Commission on Medicaid and the Uninsured*. Retrieved from https://kaiserfamilyfoundation.files.wordpress.com/2016/01/8659-04-the-coverage-gap-uninsured-poor-adults-in-states-that-do-not-expand-medicaid.pdf

Giovanelli, J., Lucia, K., & Corlette, S. (2015). Implementing the Affordable Care Act: State action to reform the individual health insurance market. *Commonwealth Fund*. Retrieved from http://www.commonwealthfund.org/~/media/files/publications/issue-brief/2014/jul/1758_giovannelli_implementing_aca_state_reform_individual_market_rb.pdf

Girion, L. (2009, June 7). Private insurance companies push for individual mandate. *L.A. Times*. Retrieved from http://articles.latimes.com/2009/jun/07/business/fi-healthcare7

Haberkorn, J. (2012). The prevention and public health fund. *Health Affairs*. Retrieved from http://healthaffairs.org/healthpolicybriefs/brief_pdfs/healthpolicybrief_63.pdf

The Henry J. Kaiser Family Foundation (KFF). (2012a). *Health insurance market reforms: Guaranteed issue*. Retrieved from https://kaiserfamilyfoundation.files.wordpress.com/2013/01/8327.pdf

The Henry J. Kaiser Family Foundation (KFF). (2012b). *Health insurance market reforms: Rate restrictions*. Retrieved from https://kaiserfamilyfoundation.files.wordpress.com/2013/01/8328.pdf

The Henry J. Kaiser Family Foundation (KFF). (2013). *Medicaid: A primer*. Retrieved from https://kaiserfamilyfoundation.files.wordpress.com/2010/06/7334-05.pdf

The Henry J. Kaiser Family Foundation (KFF). (2014). *Explaining health care reform: Questions about health insurance subsidies*. Retrieved from http://files.kff.org/attachment/explaining-health-care-reform-questions-about-health-insurance-subsidies-issue-brief

The Henry J. Kaiser Family Foundation (KFF). (2016a). 2016 Employer health benefits survey. Retrieved from http://files.kff.org/attachment/Report-Employer-Health-Benefits-2016-Annual-Survey

The Henry J. Kaiser Family Foundation (KFF). (2016b). *Health insurance marketplace types, 2016*. Retrieved from http://kff.org/health-reform/state-indicator/state-health-insurance-marketplace-types/

The Henry J. Kaiser Family Foundation (KFF). (2016c). *Status of state action on the Medicaid expansion decision*. Retrieved from http://kff.org/health-reform/state-indicator/state-activity-around-expanding-medicaid-under-the-affordable-care-act/

King v. Burwell, 135 S. Ct. 475, 190 L. Ed. 2d 355, 576 U.S. (2014).

Martin, D. (2009, February 24). Obama calls for health-care reform in 2009. *CNN.com*. Retrieved from http://www.cnn.com/2009/POLITICS/02/24/obama.health.care/

National Conference of State Legislatures. (2015, December). *Mandated health insurance benefits and state laws*. Retrieved from http://www.ncsl.org/research/health/mandated-health-insurance-benefits-and-state-laws.aspx

National Conference of State Legislatures. (2016). *Dependent coverage and age for healthcare benefits*. Retrieved from http://www.ncsl.org/research/health/dependent-health-coverage-state-implementation.aspx#State_Actions

National Federation of Independent Business v. Sebelius, 132 S. Ct. 2566 (2012).

Oberlander, J. (2007). Learning from failure in health care reform. *New England Journal of Medicine, 357*, 1677–1679.

Oberlander, J. (2010). Long time coming: Why health reform finally passed. *Health Affairs, 29*(6), 1112–1116.

Pear, R. (2015, May 25). Four words that imperil health care law were all a mistake, writers now say. *New York Times*. Retrieved from http://www.nytimes.com/2015/05/26/us/politics/contested-words-in-affordable-care-act-may-have-been-left-by-mistake.html

Pollitz, K., Tapay, N., Hadley, E., & Specht, J. (2000). Early experience with "new federalism" in health insurance regulation. *Health Affairs (Project Hope), 19*(4), 7–22.

Quadagno, J. (2005). *One nation uninsured: Why the U.S. has no national health insurance*. New York, NY: Oxford University Press.

Todd, S. R., & Sommers, B. D. (2012). Overview of the uninsured in the United States: A summary of the 2012 current population survey report. *Office of the Assistant Secretary for Planning and Evaluation*. Issue brief. Retrieved from https://aspe.hhs.gov/basic-report/overview-uninsured-united-states-summary-2012-current-population-survey-report

Uberoi, N., Finegold, K., & Gee, E. (2016). Health insurance coverage and the affordable care act, 2010–2016. *Office of the Assistant Secretary for Planning and Evaluation*. Issue brief. Retrieved from https://aspe.hhs.gov/sites/default/files/pdf/187551/ACA2010-2016.pdf

CHAPTER 5

Covered Benefits

Katie Keith, JD, MPH

LEARNING OBJECTIVES

- What benefits and services are typically covered by health insurance?
- Who decides what is covered by health insurance?
- How do consumers know whether specific benefits are covered?

INTRODUCTION

Health insurance differs from other types of insurance in part because of its complexity. There are so many possible medical services and products that it is challenging for insurers to specify everything that a given policy might (or might not) cover. Clinical guidelines and state and federal requirements help to standardize coverage, but they, too, cannot address all possible types of care, nor can they always keep pace with technology and new evidence. Coverage differs from plan to plan because of variations in requirements across states, variations in interpretations of clinical guidelines, controversial evidence (and lack of evidence) about clinical services and products, and because plans offer different levels of benefits. Such complex variability in coverage makes health insurance notoriously difficult to navigate. This chapter discusses the ways that private health insurance covers certain services, medications, and providers, including the types of benefits that are typically covered, how insurers decide which benefits to cover, and what it means for consumers when benefits are not covered.

Consider the following example: Cara is a 25-year-old waitress who eats a nutritious diet and exercises regularly. Her job is exhausting, but lately she has been even more tired than usual. After a week of feeling this way, Cara collapses at work. At her mother's insistence, Cara goes to the hospital and receives a diagnosis of Hodgkin's lymphoma, a type of cancer in her lymphatic system. As Cara and her family consider their next steps, they realize that her health insurance—more of an afterthought until that point—will become very important. Fortunately, Cara has coverage through her mother's

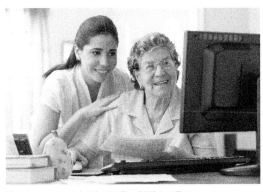

Blend Images - Jose Luis Pelaez Inc/Brand X Pictures/Getty

employer, but her family has many questions. Will she be able to pick her oncologist and get a second opinion if needed? Will she be able to afford chemotherapy if she needs it? Are there any limits to how much chemotherapy the plan will cover? Will the plan cover a risky procedure like a stem cell transplant? How much will she have to pay out-of-pocket for a hospital stay? We will revisit this example throughout the chapter.

TERMS OF COVERAGE

Health insurance is a contract: a private agreement between a health insurer (or employer) and a policyholder that the insurer will pay for certain specified medical expenses incurred by the policyholder.

Health insurance typically covers a portion of the bill when policyholders see a doctor, get surgery, and receive imaging and laboratory tests, but does not cover all out-of-pocket costs associated with obtaining care. Further, health insurance does not cover indirect costs, such as transportation costs or lost time at work or raising children, nor does it cover pain and suffering.

In designing a health insurance plan, insurers must balance comprehensiveness of coverage with affordability, in addition to complying with state and federal benefit mandates. The cost of coverage reflects a variety of factors. Costs increase when there are fewer coverage limitations (more services and products are covered), when cost-sharing requirements on consumers are lower (consumers are required to spend less out-of-pocket when obtaining services or products), and when the provider network is large (consumers have a wide choice of doctors and hospitals, and other health care facilities). Costs are also higher for plans with high administrative costs, which may reflect inefficiency and profits, but also actual administration: processing a large number of claims, investing in quality improvement programs, and managing population health. Costs are also higher for plans with riskier enrollees. Note that riskier enrollees tend to select plans (differentially enroll in plans) with more generous benefits, so more expensive plans may have higher premiums both because of their generous

benefits *and* because they attract enrollees who need to use these benefits.

Insurers list the terms, or rules, of an insurance contract in a document called the evidence of coverage (EOC) or certificate of coverage (COC), which provides comprehensive information about benefits, cost-sharing, coverage limitations, and other plan rules. A health insurance policy is the set of terms listed in the EOC or COC. Each plan has a different EOC or COC that is specific to the benefits that it covers and the rules that apply, and insurers look to the language in this document when determining whether a benefit is covered. The EOC or COC will also note the ways that the insurer limits coverage, including benefits that are covered only under certain conditions, such as when medically necessary, and benefits that are excluded from coverage altogether.

Insurers limit coverage of some treatments, procedures, or products to those that they deem medically necessary, or critical to a particular policyholder's health, based on clinical guidelines and the policyholder's condition. Insurers define medical necessity in advance, but must make individual determinations about whether a policyholder's case meets this definition. In Cara's case, for instance, the plan would likely conclude that chemotherapy, radiation therapy, and various lab tests are medically necessary to treating her cancer. The definition of medical necessity, however, varies by plan. If your provider and your insurer disagree about whether a particular service is medically necessary, then you can challenge the insurer's decision to deny coverage, first through the internal review process (an initial appeal to the insurer), and then through the external review process (a secondary appeal to an independent third-party that can reverse or affirm the insurer's decision).

Insurers also limit coverage by excluding some benefits from coverage under any circumstances, called coverage exclusions. Commonly excluded services include cosmetic surgery, dental services, long-term care, eye exams, home health care, and procedures that are considered experimental or investigational. Plans might also

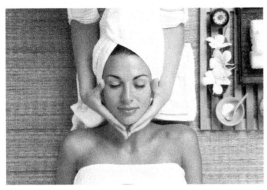

© Ersler Dmitry/Shutterstock

exclude coverage for some populations but not others; a common exclusion, for example, is limiting hearing aids to those under age 18. Cara's plan might exclude stem cell transplants but cover other types of transplants, such as heart or kidney transplants. If a service is explicitly excluded, then the plan typically will not cover it under any

circumstances, and the policyholder is unlikely to succeed in overturning the plan's decision through the appeals process.

If a benefit is *not* covered by insurance, then patients must pay for the care on their own if they wish to receive the service. The rate that patients face in this case may be much higher than if the service or product were covered, because insurers negotiate lower rates with providers. In some cases, a patient may have secondary insurance that will cover the service or supplemental insurance that will cover some of the out-of-pocket costs. Patients may also negotiate with their provider for a lower rate.

To improve the transparency of health insurance benefits, the Affordable Care Act (ACA) requires insurers and employers to provide individuals with a summary of benefits and coverage (SBC) (**Figure 5-1**). The SBC is a standardized form that summarizes the key features of a plan,

FIGURE 5-1 Excerpt from a Summary of Benefits and Coverage (SBC)

Coverage First Insurance: Basic PPO		Coverage Period: 1/1/2017–12/31/2017
Summary of Benefits and Coverage: What this Plan Covers and What it Costs		**Coverage for:** Individual and Family **Plan Type:** PPO

⚠ **This is only a summary.** If you want more detail about your coverage and costs, you can get the complete terms in the policy or plan document at www.jblearning.com/catalog/9781284113129/.

Important Questions	Answers	Why this Matters:
What is the overall deductible?	**$250** individual/ **$500** family. Does not apply to preventive and prenatal care, some laboratory tests, or prescription drugs.	You must pay the **deductible** before the plan begins to pay for covered services. Most, but not all, **deductibles** start over with each new coverage period, so you may need to pay your deductible again this year even if you paid it last year.
Are there other deductibles for specific services?	Yes. $100 individual/ $400 family for prescription drugs	You must meet a separate **deductible** for prescription drugs. See the chart on page 2 for additional information about the out-of-pocket costs of prescription drugs.
Is there an out-of-pocket limit on my expenses?	Yes. **$2,500** individual/ **$5,000** family.	The **out-of-pocket limit** is the maximum amount that you are required to pay in one coverage period (excluding your premium) before the plan covers 100% of costs.
What is not included in the out-of-pocket limit?	Premiums and services that are not covered by this plan are excluded from the out-of-pocket limit.	Even though these expenses may contribute toward your health spending, they do not count toward your **out-of-pocket limit**.
Is there an overall annual limit on what the plan pays?	No.	The chart beginning on the next page describes how the plan shares in the cost of covered services, but there is no limit in any coverage period or in your lifetime on how much the plan will contribute to these covered services.
Does this plan use a network of providers?	Yes. See http://bit.ly/2jrlMpN for a list of preferred providers.	You are responsible for lower out-of-pocket payments for preferred **providers** (also called in-network providers or participating providers) compared to non-preferred providers. See the chart starting on the next page to see how the plan pays different types of **providers**.
Do I need a referral to see a specialist?	No.	Because this plan is a PPO, you do not need a referral to see a **specialist**. However, the copayment for **specialist** visits is generally higher than for primary care provider (PCP) visits.
Are there services this plan doesn't cover?	Yes.	See page 4 for a list of services and supplies that this plan does not cover, as well as your policy or plan document for additional information about **excluded services**.

Questions: Visit us at www.jblearning.com/catalog/9781284113129/.
If you aren't clear about any of the bolded terms used in this form, see the Glossary. You can view the glossary in the back of this book or at www.healthcare.gov/glossary.

including covered benefits, cost-sharing requirements, and coverage limitations. The SBC is not as detailed as an EOC or COC—so a consumer may still need to review these documents—but it does explain how a plan covers key benefits.

While the focus of this chapter is on major medical insurance—comprehensive insurance that covers a wide range of medical benefits—consumers may also purchase plans that provide more limited coverage, generally to fill in gaps in major medical insurance policies. Such plans include critical illness insurance, which pays a lump sum in case of a pre-specified disease; disability income protection, which provides reimbursement in case the enrollee cannot work; accident-only insurance, which pays out-of-pocket costs and other related costs in case of an accidental injury; and fixed-benefit indemnity medical insurance, which pays the enrollee directly to assist with out-of-pocket payments for medical care. While these plans can offer considerable financial protection, none are considered comprehensive health insurance and thus do not satisfy the ACA's individual mandate. Rather, these types of plans are often purchased to supplement major medical insurance, similar to stand-alone dental plans or stand-alone vision plans.

COVERED BENEFITS

Insurers have broad discretion in designing their benefits, and coverage varies significantly from plan to plan. Common categories of covered services include physician services; hospitalizations for medical or surgical care (including room and board, nursing care, and inpatient pharmaceuticals); emergency services (including ambulance and emergency room care); mental health services; and lab and diagnostic tests (such as X-rays or MRIs). Some plans also include outpatient pharmaceuticals. To decide which services and products should be covered, insurers look to a variety of sources, including consumer demand, competition, scientific evidence and clinical guidelines, Medicare coverage decisions, and federal and state benefit mandates.

First, market conditions such as consumer demand and competition influence benefit design—which benefits are covered and under what conditions. Plans generally cover a comprehensive array of benefits because offering individual benefits piece by piece would lead to substantial adverse selection. Imagine a market in which you could purchase *just* cancer insurance, *just* diabetes insurance, or *just* insurance for heart disease. This market would attract only the highest-risk consumers, who have—or expect to have—these conditions. In contrast, a market that offers comprehensive benefits not only better protects consumers, but also ensures the stability of insurers by attracting lower-risk enrollees. Even before the ACA, then, almost all group health insurance plans were comprehensive plans, and covered services including hospitalizations, surgical procedures, and doctor visits (U.S. Department of Labor, 2011).

Second, competitive pressures drive benefit design. For example, self-funded employers have some flexibility in designing benefits for their employees, and can use a generous health insurance policy to recruit and retain talented employees. Further, competition can stimulate innovation in benefit design. As health care costs have risen, employers have developed new ways to limit spending, such as high-deductible health plans and employee wellness programs, which reward employees for participating in healthy activities or meeting other health goals.

Third, most insurers make decisions about what to cover based on clinical evidence. A chief medical officer (CMO), usually a physician leading a team of medical directors, is tasked with making these medical decisions. The medical team reviews protocols to ensure that coverage reflects the latest scientific evidence and clinical recommendations. Often, scientific evidence is controversial or non-existent, and clinical guidelines either do not exist or reflect this uncertainty. For example, it is not clear whether the benefits outweigh the risks for average-risk women in their 40s to get a mammogram every year, rather than every other year. So, while the U.S. Preventive Services Task Force recommends biennial screening (U.S. Preventive Services Task Force, 2016), the American Cancer Society recommends annual screening (Oeffinger et al., 2015), although both organizations have qualified their recommendations. As a result of this uncertainty, however, some plans cover screening every year for women in their forties, while other plans cover screening only every other year.

Fourth, many private health insurers model their coverage and reimbursement decisions after the Medicare program, the federal program that provides health benefits to older adults and people with disabilities. Many private insurers, for instance, refer to the Medicare fee structure when negotiating rates with providers. Although changes to the Medicare program often influence the benefits that private insurers offer and the prices that they pay (Clemens & Gottlieb, 2013), plans are not required to align their policies with Medicare.

Finally, federal and state laws dictate some of the benefits that must be covered. Benefit mandates are legal requirements that health insurance plans cover specific services or products provided by a specific type of provider, such as a hospital or a physician (Institute of Medicine, 2012). Some plans are exempt from mandates, depending on the type of plan. Self-funded plans, for instance, are primarily regulated under federal law and thus do not have to comply with state benefit mandates. Since self-funded plans are not considered insurance, they are exempt from some new federal mandates governing insurance under the ACA, such as the requirement to offer a package of essential health benefits. In contrast, fully insured plans are primarily regulated under state law and thus must comply with state benefit mandates, as well as new federal mandates under the ACA (except for grandfathered plans, which are exempt from some new regulations).

Benefit mandates are an important determinant of coverage, but are themselves determined by the medical needs and preferences of the population targeted by the mandate. State legislatures began adopting benefit mandates as early as 1949 as a way to fill gaps in coverage. By the 1980s, insurers were subject to various state laws requiring them to cover newborn children of insured parents, treatment for alcoholism, and

psychologist services (Jost, 2009). Today, all states have at least some mandates, but requirements vary considerably and range from requiring coverage for preventive health services, such as immunizations and cancer screening, to specialty care likely to be used by fewer individuals, such as the chemotherapy that Cara will likely need (National Conference of State Legislatures, 2015). Benefit mandates often generate debate about the balance between comprehensiveness and the affordability of coverage; the more generously benefits are covered, the more consumers will have to pay for them.

Prior to the ACA, federal law included some benefit mandates, but they applied only to plans choosing to cover certain services. For instance, plans covering mastectomy, maternity care, and mental health services were also required to cover, respectively, breast reconstructive surgery, a hospital stay of at least 48 hours following childbirth, and mental health benefits at parity with (the same level of cost-sharing as) medical or surgical benefits (Kofman & Pollitz, 2006).

The ACA adopted more extensive federal benefit mandates. Under the law, all new plans must cover preexisting medical conditions, certain preventive services, and—for plans with dependent coverage—dependent children up to age 26. Large employers must also cover hospitalizations and physician services to avoid paying a penalty. And the law imposes its most extensive mandates on new plans in the individual and small group markets, which must cover at least 10 categories of essential health benefits (EHB) (**Box 5-1**).

BENEFIT DESIGN

Even if two plans cover the same benefits, they may still differ in other aspects of benefit design. For example, while one policy might require a $30 copayment for a doctor's visit, another might cover the same visit without cost-sharing (no copayment). New plans must offer some preventive services, like routine immunizations, without cost-sharing. While zero cost-sharing incentivizes the use of these services because it makes them appear "free," in fact policyholders must pay for "free" services in

BOX 5-1 Essential Health Benefits*

Ambulatory (outpatient) care

Emergency services

Inpatient hospitalization

Pregnancy, maternity, and newborn care, before and after birth

Mental health and substance abuse services

Prescription drugs

Rehabilitative and habilitative services and devices

Laboratory services

Preventive and wellness services and chronic disease management

Pediatric services, including oral and vision care

*Coverage of essential health benefits required only for fully insured plans in the individual and small group markets.

Reproduced from: Healthcare.gov; https://www.healthcare.gov/coverage/what-marketplace-plans-cover/

their premiums. (Have you ever heard the expression, "there is no such thing as a free lunch?" Well, there is no such thing as a free checkup, either). In other cases, cost-sharing can be used to discourage the use of certain services or products, with many plans imposing the highest cost-sharing for specialty brand-name drugs and out-of-network care, for which plans face the highest prices.

Benefits may also differ with regard to utilization management. Utilization management is a broad set of tools that plans use to influence a policyholder's use of covered benefits. Two primary utilization management tools include referral and prior authorization. A referral is when a physician (usually a primary care physician) directs a patient to another physician (usually a specialist). Prior authorization is required approval before policyholders receive a covered benefit. So for example, while some plans require a referral for specialty care, other plans allow patients to self-refer. And while some plans require prior authorization for only the most expensive or experimental care, other plans require it for more routine specialty care and imaging services. If the policyholder fails to obtain a referral or prior authorization when it is necessary, then the plan may decline to cover the service. In Cara's case, chemotherapy,

radiation, or a stem cell transplant would all likely require prior authorization by the plan before they are covered, as they are all very expensive services.

Other utilization management tools are intended to improve health while reducing wasteful spending. Disease management programs, for example, help patients coordinate care among multiple providers and keep patients on a medication regimen. Discharge planning services assist patients with care that they will need at home after a surgery or other hospitalization.

In summary, coverage of health benefits and services varies by plan, insurer, and state, and plans have adopted new benefit design features in response to market conditions and state and federal regulations. Given the complexity of private health insurance and its contractual nature, it is important for consumers to understand key design features—such as coverage exclusions, cost-sharing, and utilization management—before selecting and enrolling in a plan.

COVERAGE OF PRESCRIPTION DRUGS

Like medical coverage, prescription drug coverage also varies by plan. There are, however, far fewer mandates and guidelines related to prescription drug coverage, so there is even more variability this type of coverage.

A key tool for insurers to drive policyholders to low cost drugs is a formulary, a list of medications covered by the plan. Common categories of covered prescription drugs include medications to treat asthma, high blood pressure, diabetes, cholesterol, and depression, as well as pain medications, antacids, and antibiotics. A tiered formulary is one that charges lower cost-sharing for generic drugs and discounted branded drugs, and higher cost-sharing for undiscounted branded drugs, or drugs for which there are no competitors. For example, in a classic four-tier formulary, the first tier contains the lowest copayment for generic drugs; the second tier contains a higher copayment for *preferred* (discounted) branded drugs; the third tier contains an even higher copayment for *non-preferred* (undiscounted, or less heavily discounted) branded drugs; and the fourth tier contains a very high copayment, or sometimes coinsurance, for the most expensive drugs, such as biologics, which generally must be administered in a physician's office. The price of some drugs has become so high that fifth and even sixth tiers are not uncommon.

Another strategy that insurers use to contain drug costs is to limit the number of drugs covered in each drug class (drugs with the same chemical mechanism, generally used to treat the same disease) to obtain volume discounts. Insurers may also choose whether the formulary will be an open formulary or a closed formulary. In a closed formulary, drugs not listed will not be covered; in an open formulary, drugs not listed may be covered, but at a higher copayment, analogously to a medical plan with out-of-network benefits.

We expect to find expensive drugs in high tiers, but in adverse tiering, insurers place all drugs used to treat a high-cost condition (such as angina, bipolar disorder, or multiple sclerosis) into the same high tier. The ACA generally prohibits this practice. In Florida, for instance, insurers placed all HIV/AIDS medications—including generic drugs—at the highest formulary tier, prompting a federal complaint of discrimination

and a settlement with Florida insurance regulators (Thomas, 2014). Insurers have also been engaging in adverse tiering for several classes of cancer medications, including those that Cara will likely need to treat her Hodgkin's lymphoma (AvalereHealth, 2014).

Pharmacy and therapeutics (P&T) committees guide insurers' pharmaceutical benefit policies., Comprising physicians, pharmacists, and other health professionals, these committees are responsible for developing and updating formularies, as well as access to medication policies such as prior authorization, step therapy (when a patient must try other medications before "stepping up" to a more expensive drug), and exceptions protocols (when a patient requests coverage of a non-formulary medication). Because P&T committees meet regularly to review evidence about new and currently covered drugs, formularies may change from one year to the next, or even in the middle of a coverage year.

Most health insurers do not administer pharmaceutical benefits themselves, but rather contract with a pharmacy benefit manager (PBM), a third party that manages formularies and access to medication policies (with the guidance of a P&T committee), processes and pays pharmaceutical claims, and contracts with local pharmacies and online wholesalers and manufacturers. The role of PBMs has become complex; some may even take on risk for the primary medical insurer and thus become an insurer-within-an-insurer. PBMs use their specific expertise and large volume of contracts to negotiate volume discounts with drug manufacturers and pharmacies, and increasingly, pharmacies have been acquiring PBMs.

No plan will cover every medication, so it is important for consumers to understand how certain drugs will be covered before enrolling in a plan. Most plans make their formulary available online, and a plan's SBC must include a link to the formulary. The SBC will also provide information about cost-sharing on each level of a tiered formulary. Publicly accessible information allows consumers to see whether their medication is listed on the formulary, on which tier, and whether they will have to comply with other policies before receiving the medication, such as prior approval or step therapy.

Many consumers also purchase over-the-counter drugs (OTC drugs) without a prescription. Common OTC drugs include aspirin, allergy medication, heartburn treatment, and some forms of birth control. Most plans, however, do not cover the purchase of OTC drugs, which results in a tradeoff for patients: on one hand, there is not the hassle or the copayment associated with visiting a doctor for a prescription; on the other hand, consumers must pay for the drug out-of-pocket. This cost may be burdensome for consumers who need the drug for a chronic condition. Policyholders may consider asking their doctor to prescribe an OTC drug so it will be covered by the plan. Alternatively, some employers offer a health care flexible spending arrangement (FSA) or health reimbursement arrangement (HRA), through which employees may purchase drugs with pre-tax dollars.

COVERAGE OF MEDICAL PROVIDERS

Limited provider networks are another tool that insurers use to limit costs (**Figure 5-2**). Different plans will cover different doctors, hospitals, nurse practitioners, clinics, and specialty care centers. The threat of exclusion from a provider network allows the insurer to negotiate lower prices for care. Further, restricting access to certain providers discourages the enrollment of high-risk individuals. For instance, if a plan does not have a pediatric oncologist in its network, then what are the options for a family whose child was just diagnosed with cancer?

Most, but not all, plans contract with provider networks to pass on a discounted price to consumers. But plans manage these networks in very different ways. To become part of a preferred provider organization (PPO), for example, providers agree to contract with the plan at a discounted rate and use certain evidence-based quality protocols. Policyholders may use out-of-network providers, but the plan's

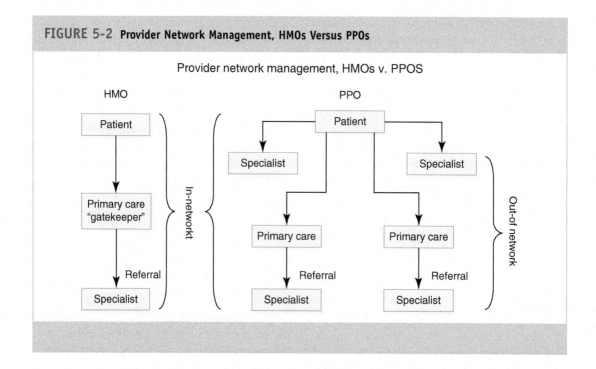

FIGURE 5-2 Provider Network Management, HMOs Versus PPOs

Provider network management, HMOs v. PPOS

cost-sharing is structured in a way that incentivizes use of in-network providers. Health maintenance organizations (HMOs), in contrast, generally have smaller provider networks, and out-of-network benefits are less common. Some HMOs even enter into exclusive contracts with a provider group, such that the HMO covers care for only providers in that group. Kaiser Permanente is an example of such an exclusive relationship between an insurer (Kaiser Health Plan) and a physician group (Permanente Medical Group). The plan also owns its own hospitals, which Kaiser members must use. If Cara is enrolled in an HMO plan, then her provider options may be much more limited than under a PPO plan.

Given the differences among plans and the implications for receipt of care, it is important for consumers to understand their plan's provider network. Most plans make their provider directories available online, and a plan's SBC must include a link to the provider directory. Consumers may use the directory to see whether their doctor is part of the plan's network and to view the other providers covered under the plan. Note, however, that contracted providers change frequently and directories are not always accurate, so you should contact your doctor's office to confirm that they are in-network. The SBC will also provide information about whether out-of-network providers are covered and, if so, the difference in cost-sharing compared to in-network care.

Most states have set some standards to regulate the scope of provider networks (**Figure 5-3**). These network adequacy standards vary significantly by state and type of

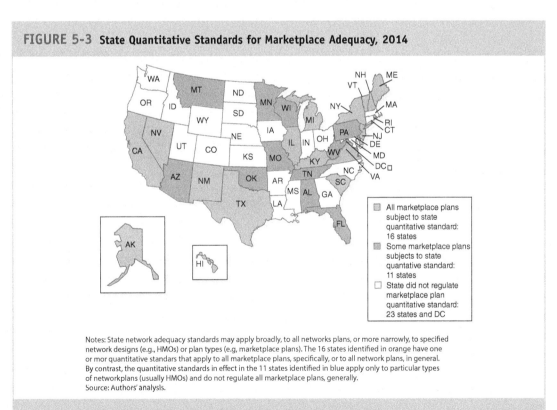

FIGURE 5-3 State Quantitative Standards for Marketplace Adequacy, 2014

- All marketplace plans subject to state quantitative standard: 16 states
- Some marketplace plans subjects to state quantative standard: 11 states
- State did not regulate marketplace plan quantitative standard: 23 states and DC

Notes: State network adequacy standards may apply broadly, to all networks plans, or more narrowly, to specified network designs (e.g., HMOs) or plan types (e.g, marketplace plans). The 16 states identified in orange have one or mor quantitative standars that apply to all marketplace plans, specifically, or to all network plans, in general. By contrast, the quantitative standards in effect in the 11 states identified in blue apply only to particular types of networkplans (usually HMOs) and do not regulate all marketplace plans, generally.
Source: Authors' analysis.

Reproduced from: Giovanelli J, Lucia KW, Corlette S. Implementing the Affordable Care Act: State regulations of marketplace plan provider networks. *The Commonwealth Fund*. May 2015. http://www.commonwealthfund.org/~/media/files/publications/issue-brief/2015/may/1814_giovannelli_implementing _aca_state_reg_provider_networks_rb_v2.pdf plan but may be qualitative (by requiring plans to have, for instance, a sufficient number and type of in-network providers) or quantitative (by requiring plans to have, for instance, at least two in-network primary care physicians within 10 miles for 90 percent of enrollees). In some cases, network adequacy standards apply only to HMO plans or to plans that use a certain network design. Under the ACA, plans sold in state marketplaces must meet additional federal qualitative and quantitative standards for network adequacy. For example, enrollees must be able to secure an appointment within a reasonable time frame without having to travel an unreasonable distance. Networks must also be sufficiently large to cover the number of enrollees in the plan (Giovanelli, Lucia, & Corlette, 2015).

Network adequacy standards were a response to plans as they experimented with more limited network designs, such as narrow networks (severely restricting the available providers to negotiate price discounts with the providers willing to join), tiered networks (networks in which consumers pay less for providers with steeper discounts), and high-performance networks (tiered networks in which consumers pay less for providers noted for high-quality or high-value care). Collectively, these strategies are referred to as value-based networks. Because provider network restrictions influence so many aspects of care, including cost-sharing, access to specialists, convenience, and continuity of care, it is critical for consumers to understand how to find out which providers are in their network, and how much it will cost out-of-pocket to see an in-network or out-of-network provider.

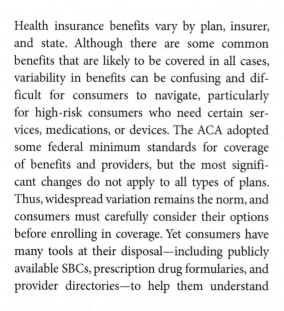

Summary

© Jim Barber/Shutterstock

Health insurance benefits vary by plan, insurer, and state. Although there are some common benefits that are likely to be covered in all cases, variability in benefits can be confusing and difficult for consumers to navigate, particularly for high-risk consumers who need certain services, medications, or devices. The ACA adopted some federal minimum standards for coverage of benefits and providers, but the most significant changes do not apply to all types of plans. Thus, widespread variation remains the norm, and consumers must carefully consider their options before enrolling in coverage. Yet consumers have many tools at their disposal—including publicly available SBCs, prescription drug formularies, and provider directories—to help them understand

various coverage options and select a plan that is appropriate for their health care needs and budget.

References

AvalereHealth. (2014). *An analysis of exchange plan benefits for certain medicines.* Retrieved from http://www.phrma .org/sites/default/files/20140521_FINAL%20PhRMA _High%20Coinsurance%20and%20Tier%20Placement _Avalere%5B7a%5D_0.pdf

Clemens, J., & Gottlieb, J. D. (2013). *In the shadow of a giant: Medicare's influence on private physician payments.* Cambridge, MA: National Bureau of Economic Research. Retrieved from http://www.nber.org/papers/w19503.pdf

Giovanelli, J., Lucia, K., & Corlette, S. (2015). *Implementing the Affordable Care Act: State regulation of marketplace plan provider networks.* Commonwealth Fund. Retrieved from http://www.commonwealthfund.org/publications /issue-briefs/2015/may/state-regulation-of-marketplace -plan-provider-networks

Jost, T. (2009). *The regulation of private health insurance*. Retrieved from https://www.nasi.org/usr_doc/The_Regulation_of_Private_Health_Insurance.pdf

Kofman, M., & Pollitz, K. (2006). Health insurance regulation by states and the federal government: A review of current approaches and proposals for change. *Journal of Insurance Regulation*, 24(4), 77.

National Conference of State Legislatures. (2015, December). *Mandated health insurance benefits and state laws*. Retrieved from http://www.ncsl.org/research/health/mandated-health-insurance-benefits-and-state-laws.aspx

Oeffinger, K. C., Fontham, E. T. H., Etzioni, R., Herzig, A., Michaelson, J. S., Shih, Y. C., … American Cancer Society. (2015). Breast cancer screening for women at average risk: 2015 guideline update from the American Cancer Society. *JAMA*, 314(15), 1599–1614.

Thomas, K. (2014, November 7). Cigna agrees to reduce H.I.V. drug costs for some Florida patients. *New York Times*. Retrieved from http://www.nytimes.com/2014/11/08/business/cigna-to-reduce-hiv-drug-costs-for-some-florida-patients.html?_r=0

U.S. Department of Labor. (2011). *Selected medical benefits: A report from the Department of Labor to the Department of Health and Human Services*. Retrieved from http://www.bls.gov/ncs/ebs/sp/selmedbensreport.pdf

U.S. Preventive Services Task Force. (2016, January). Breast cancer: Screening. Retrieved from https://www.uspreventiveservicestaskforce.org/Page/Document/UpdateSummaryFinal/breast-cancer-screening1

CHAPTER 6

Consumer Financial Responsibility for Health Care

Erin Hemlin, MA

LEARNING OBJECTIVES

- What factors contribute to health insurance premiums?
- Why is there a tradeoff between monthly premiums and out-of-pocket spending?
- What role does provider network design play in out-of-pocket spending for health care services?

INTRODUCTION

Health insurance protects consumers from financial strain due to medical costs, but paying a monthly health care premium does not mean that the insurer will pay 100 percent of costs; rather, it guarantees enrollees access to the insurer's network of providers. In many cases, consumers must share in the costs of their care by paying deductibles, copayments, and coinsurance (**Figure 6-1**). This chapter will discuss consumer financial responsibility for insurance and medical care.

PREMIUMS

Though health insurance in the United States is expensive, most public and private premiums are subsidized in some way. The monthly premium is the price of belonging to an insurance plan. Similar to a gym membership or cable subscription, the consumer pays a fixed amount every month to maintain coverage, regardless of whether she uses any services. Premiums in any insurance plan,

public or private, are based on the riskiness of the insured group (how likely people in the group are to get sick or injured, and how severely so), as well the generosity of the benefits. The total cost of the premium is the actuarially fair premium (which reflects these costs) plus the loading charge (to cover administrative expenses and profits). Employment-based private premiums are subsidized by a large tax advantage, whereas public premiums are subsidized by general revenues.

Premiums for Employment-Based Insurance

Risk-spreading (sharing the risk of high medical costs over more people) makes employment-based insurance more affordable, but risk-spreading is not a subsidy, it is just economical. Employer-sponsored insurance (and for that matter, Medicare, Medicaid, and any insurance other than insurance on the individual market) is a form of group insurance, in which more than one individual enters a shared contract and pays a monthly premium to an insurance provider (or employer), who pools this money to cover the costs of medical care for the group. A small group is an unpredictable group whose costs must be buffered by high premiums; similarly, an unhealthy or high-risk group must be buffered by high premiums. Therefore, the larger and healthier the group, the lower the premiums.

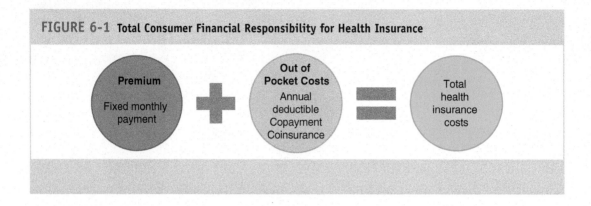

FIGURE 6-1 Total Consumer Financial Responsibility for Health Insurance

The federal government provides subsidies to employer-sponsored insurance plans by exempting employer and employee premiums from taxation. Premiums are deducted tax-free directly from an employee's paycheck, and tax-free from an employer's payroll. Suppose that you earned $5,000 and had to pay $500 in taxes. Then you could purchase an insurance policy that costs $4,500. But now suppose that your earnings were tax-exempt; then you could purchase an insurance policy that costs $5,000. You can see from this simple example that the federal subsidy of health insurance encourages more generous policies than if premium contributions were taxed.

Some people also think that employers who contribute to employee health insurance are "paying" for this benefit, but in fact it is usually the employee who is paying in the form of lower, or slower growing, wages (Currie & Madrian, 1999). Employees generally accept this tradeoff because health insurance through a job compared to the individual market has so many benefits. For example, sharing risk makes it cheaper to purchase a more generous policy, and the policy is subsidized through the tax advantage. In fact, health insurance is a key recruitment and retention tool for firms. There are, however, drawbacks to obtaining health insurance through an employer—it ties insurance to employment and limits the employee's options to those that the employer offers. Some employees may not be able to afford the insurance that their employer offers.

Premiums for Insurance in the Individual Market

Prior to the ACA, sick and high-risk individuals without access to group insurance through an employer or the government had limited options for affordable coverage. Although premiums were actually lower on average in the individual market than in the small and large group markets (Clemans-Cope & Karpman, 2015), this difference reflected lower enrollee risk and less generous coverage. Because enrollees in the individual market do not share financial risk, insurers generally excluded coverage for pre-existing conditions, and sometimes denied coverage altogether for individuals with such a condition. Further, while employees paid for health insurance with tax-free dollars, encouraging generous benefits, individual market enrollees paid for insurance as they would any other taxable good.

Under the ACA, however, pre-existing conditions may not be excluded from coverage. While this protection generally increases premiums, the ACA offers financial assistance for premiums and cost-sharing for plans purchased in the state health care marketplaces. Further, premiums in the marketplaces are calculated based on the average risk in the community (they are community rated), rather than the risk of each individual (experience rated). While this protection increases premiums for those who have lower than average risk (healthier individuals), it decreases premiums for those with higher than average risk (sicker individuals).

Premiums for Medicaid

States may not charge premiums to Medicaid enrollees who qualify for the program with incomes below 150 percent of the federal poverty level (FPL). For enrollees earning 150 percent FPL or more, or for enrollees qualifying for the program because of an illness or disability, states have some flexibility in charging a premium, and most do for at least one of these groups (Brooks, Miskell, Artiga, Cornachione, & Gates, 2016). Premiums do not cover the entire estimated cost of care for the enrollee, but are subsidized by state and federal taxes.

Premiums for Medicare

Medicare beneficiaries have a default option of traditional, fee-for-service (FFS) Medicare (Parts A and B), but may choose to forgo this option for Medicare Advantage (Part C), offered through the private market. In FFS Medicare, most beneficiaries will not owe any additional premium for Part A (hospital insurance), because a portion of their paycheck has been deducted to cover this expense. The baseline monthly premium for Part B benefits is $121.80; enrollees pay more if they earn more or if they delay enrollment in Part B (enrollment in Part A is automatic). There is a penalty for late enrollment in order to reduce adverse selection. Premiums in Parts C and Part D depend on the plan. Because general revenues heavily subsidize premiums in the Medicare program, beneficiaries' premiums are not as high as in the private market, even in Parts C and D, which use private plans (The Henry J. Kaiser Family Foundation [KFF], 2015). Dual eligibles (Medicare enrollees also eligible for Medicaid) receive assistance paying their premiums.

COST-SHARING

In many cases, consumers must pay out-of-pocket to use their health insurance, even if they have been paying their monthly premium (**Figure 6-2**). Out-of-pocket costs are payments that the consumer makes for medical services or products, and include copayments, a fixed dollar amount per service, such as a doctor's visit, or product, such as a 30-day supply of a prescription; coinsurance, a percentage of the price of a service or product; and an annual deductible, a fixed dollar amount that the consumer must meet before the insurer begins to pay for services. Out-of-pocket costs are also referred to as consumer cost-sharing because they represent the costs in which the consumer must participate in order to receive care (analogously, the insurer's portion of the bill is referred to as insurer cost-sharing).

Consumers can generally expect to trade off premiums with out-of-pocket costs. Plans with lower premiums tend to have higher out-of-pocket costs, while plans with higher premiums generally have lower out-of-pocket costs. For example, all silver plans on the health exchanges must have an actuarial value of 70 percent, meaning that they must cover, on average, 70 percent of health care costs among enrollees in that plan. But there is room for variation within silver plans, and consumers may pay lower premiums in return for higher cost-sharing or vice versa. For example, one silver plan might have a $3,000 deductible with a $10 copayment for doctor's visits, while another plan has a $2,000 deductible, but a $50 copayment for doctor's visits. Depending on the individuals enrolled, both plans could have an actuarial value of 70 percent, making them technically comparable, but the costs to the consumer could vary substantially under each plan based on the care that they need.

Cost-Sharing in Medicaid

Cost-sharing is permitted for most services in the Medicaid program, but it is generally limited to only a few dollars per service, and cannot be imposed for emergency care, family planning services, or preventive care for children. Most states do impose cost-sharing on some services, such as non-preventive physician visits, inpatient care, and prescription drugs (Brooks et al., 2016). Like cost-sharing in the private market, copayments and deductibles in Medicaid are intended to reduce moral hazard. But although the level of cost-sharing in Medicaid is low compared to the private market, it may still be high enough to make care unaffordable for many beneficiaries, who have been shown to delay or avoid necessary care (Ku, 2003).

FIGURE 6-2 Cost-Sharing Illustration

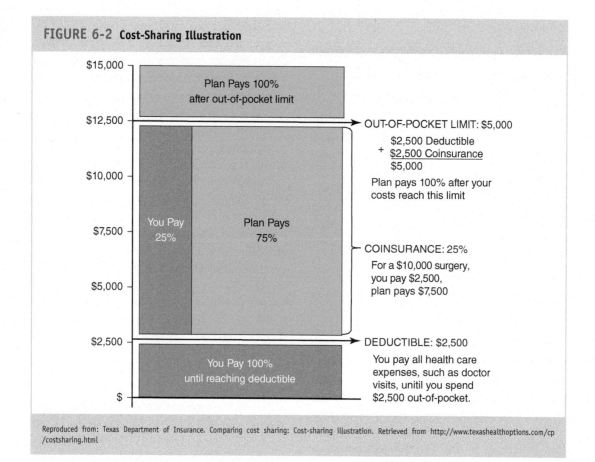

Cost-Sharing in Medicare

The federal government sets the FFS Medicare cost-sharing structure, while private insurers set varying structures in Parts C (Medicare Advantage) and D (prescription drugs). In the FFS program, beneficiaries are responsible for an annual $1,288 deductible in Part A (the hospital benefit), with no additional cost-sharing for the first 60 days, a $322 copayment per day for days 61 through 90, and a $644 copayment per day for each day after 90 days. In Part B of the FFS program, the annual deductible is $166, with 20 percent cost-sharing for some services and no cost-sharing for other preventive services. Dual eligibles receive assistance with cost-sharing. Unlike typical employment-based plans, there is no annual limit on how much Medicare beneficiaries may owe out-of-pocket.

In-Network Versus Out-of-Network Providers

Out-of-pocket costs also vary depending on whether consumers visit a provider that is a member of a plan's network. A provider network (also called in-network providers) is a group of physicians, hospitals, clinics, laboratories, and imaging and testing facilities that have agreed to accept a discounted negotiated price from a private insurer or an administered price from a public insurer. Plans incentivize patients to visit in-network providers over out-of-network (non-network) providers (those that have not agreed to accept the insurer's discounted price). Network providers thus receive patient volume in exchange for accepting lower prices.

Patients using in-network providers are generally responsible for a lower portion of the bill than patients using out-of-network providers. Some plans may not offer out-of-network benefits, in which case care is entirely the patient's financial responsibility, and costs incurred will not count toward fulfillment of a deductible or an out-of-pocket maximum. Health maintenance organizations (HMOs) keep premiums low by restricting provider networks and limiting out-of-network benefits, while preferred provider organizations (PPOs) tend to have wider networks and more generous out-of-network benefits. PPO enrollees who visit preferred providers (in-network providers for a PPO) incur lower out-of-pocket payments, while those who visit nonpreferred providers (out-of-network providers for a PPO) incur higher out-of-pocket payments. Point-of-service (POS) plans usually have some out-of-network benefits but are more restrictive than PPO plans. Exclusive provider organizations (EPOs), like HMOs, have restrictive networks and limited out-of-network benefits but differ from HMOs in that they usually do not require referrals for specialty care.

Even when patients visit an in-network provider, they may receive an out-of-network bill. For example, your in-network primary care physician orders a blood test from an out-of-network laboratory. Or you have a medical emergency, and an [in-network] ambulance takes you to an out-of-network hospital. Or you undergo surgery at an in-network facility with an in-network surgeon, but the anesthesiologist, who negotiates separately with your plan, is out-of-network. When you unexpectedly receive care from an out-of-network provider, the bill from that provider is called a surprise medical bill. Consumers have the right to negotiate surprise medical bills with the out-of-network provider and their insurance company, and may seek help from a patient advocate in order to avoid exorbitant costs. In some states, such as New York, patients who visit in-network providers are not responsible for surprise medical bills.

Care Setting and Intensity

The intensity of the care setting also drives consumers' out-of-pocket costs. For example, suppose that your stomach hurts and you are concerned that you have appendicitis. During normal business hours, if an appointment were available, you might be able to see your primary care provider (PCP). But if an appointment were not available, then you might instead go to a retail clinic, a clinic located within a pharmacy or grocery store that provides preventive care and limited care for conditions that might otherwise be treated in a doctor's office, and generally has hours that extend beyond those of a normal doctor's office. If the nurse practitioner or physician assistant at the retail clinic suspected that you might indeed have appendicitis based on a physical exam, then they might send you to a nearby urgent care center for an X-ray to confirm the diagnosis. Urgent care centers are free-standing clinics that treat pressing, but not life-threatening, conditions and also generally have extended hours. (Both retail clinics and urgent care centers are referred to as walk-in clinics because you do not need an appointment to visit these clinics.) If you were really doubled over in pain and the providers at the retail clinic suspected that you were in an emergent, life-threatening situation, then they would send you to the emergency room instead of the urgent care center.

The out-of-pocket costs of each of these options will be quite different, depending on the plan. Generally, the less intensive the setting, the lower the out-of-pocket cost to the consumer. A PCP's office or retail clinic is generally less expensive than an urgent care center or emergency room, though the insurer generally waives the copayment if the enrollee is admitted to the hospital.

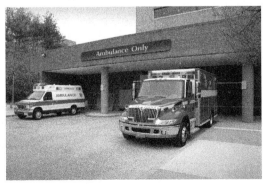
© Christian Delbert/Shutterstock

Although a PCP is the cheapest out-of-pocket option, there are tradeoffs to using less intensive care settings. PCPs offer preventive care and care for minor illnesses and injuries, as well as ongoing care for chronic conditions. They provide referrals and prescriptions when necessary. A PCP that you visit regularly may recognize patterns that are cause for concern. Yet most PCP offices have limited hours and thus may not be available when an urgent or emergent problem arises. Retail clinics, on the other hand, are usually open later in the evening and on weekends. Compared to about 5,000 acute care hospitals (American Hospital Association, 2015), there are 6,400 urgent care centers (Barnet, 2015) and 1,914 retail clinics, with retail clinics growing rapidly (Accenture, 2015). Walk-in clinics generally accept payment from most major commercial insurers, as well as Medicaid and Medicare.

In practice, using the most appropriate setting may be difficult for a number of reasons. First, if individuals do not live near an urgent center or retail clinic, then an emergency room may be the only option for urgent care after hours. Second, some people are unaware of cheaper alternatives such as retail clinics and urgent care centers. Third, plan restrictions may lead individuals to seek care in an inappropriately intensive setting. Suppose in our appendicitis example that a plan's provider network excludes nearby PCPs whose hours extend beyond normal business hours. Then enrollees from that plan might seek care from a nearby emergency room. Finally, both underinsured and uninsured individuals may delay care for a non-urgent problem until it has become an urgent (or emergent) problem. These individuals may end up in settings, such as emergency rooms, that are more intensive than necessary had their problem been sufficiently covered by insurance.

PRESCRIPTION DRUGS

Consumers must also factor in costs of any medications they need when comparing health insurance plans. Prescription drug costs are determined by a drug formulary, which is a list of prescription drugs covered by the plan. Some plans

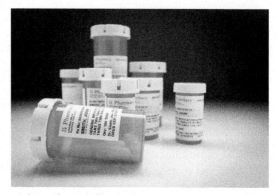

© Andy Dean Photography/Shutterstock

use a closed formulary, in which drugs not listed are not covered, while others use an open formulary, in which drugs not listed may be covered but with higher cost-sharing.

A tiered formulary lists drugs by levels of consumer cost-sharing **Figure 6-3**. Drugs at higher levels—or tiers—have higher cost-sharing. There are typically four to five tiers, but sometimes up to six or seven (Figure 6-3). A simple four-tier formulary might include generic drugs in the first tier; preferred brand-name drugs (brand-name drugs for which the insurer obtains a discount) in the second tier; non-preferred brand-name drugs (brand-name drugs that are less discounted or not discounted); and specialty drugs and biologics in the fourth tier. A six-tier formulary might make these categories even more granular: preferred generics in the first tier; non-preferred generics in the second tier; preferred brand-name drugs in the third tier; non-preferred brand-name drugs in the fourth tier; preferred specialty in the fifth tier; and non-preferred specialty in the sixth tier.

The purpose of the drug formulary is to steer consumers to the least expensive drug option. Most plans charge a copayment for each prescription fill (for example, a 30-day supply of a medication), and this copayment increases with each tier in the formulary. For drugs on the highest tiers, and for off-formulary drugs (for plans with open formularies), plans may charge coinsurance. For example, a plan with a four-tier open formulary might charge a $10 copayment for medications in the first tier, $30 for medications in the second, $50 for medications in the third, 20 percent

FIGURE 6-3 Tiered Formulary with Four Tiers

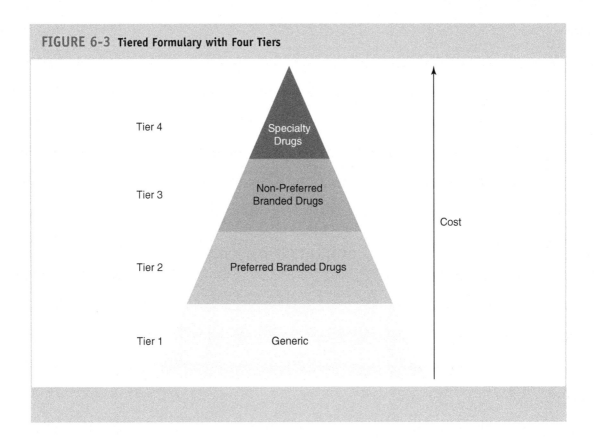

coinsurance for medications in the fourth, and 50 percent coinsurance plus a $500 deductible for non-formulary medications.

Medicare beneficiaries in the traditional program or in Part C may obtain insurance for outpatient prescription drugs through a private Medicare Part D plan. Like any private plan, the premium for a Part D drug plan depends on the generosity of the benefits and the estimated risk of enrollees in the plan. Medicare subsidizes the Part D premium but requires enrollees with higher incomes (over $85,000) to pay a larger proportion of the premium. Cost-sharing varies among Part D plans, but by law, all must be at least as generous as the so-called standard plan, which covers prescription drugs (with beneficiary cost-sharing) up until the costs of the drugs add up to a few thousand dollars. At that point, the beneficiary enters a coverage gap known as the doughnut hole and must pay for 100 percent of their drugs until catastrophic coverage kicks in. The ACA gradually closes the doughnut hole

through 2020, and Medicare will subsidize costs in the doughnut hole in the interim.

Consumers with chronic conditions who take medications regularly should look up a plan's drug formulary before enrolling to ensure that the out-of-pocket costs for their medications will be affordable. Drug formularies are set every year by the insurer but are subject to change during the year. For example, an insurer may remove a medication from its formulary if new evidence emerges that its risks outweigh its benefits, or it may add a medication that has recently been approved by the Food and Drug Administration (FDA).

HIGH-DEDUCTIBLE HEALTH PLANS

High-deductible health plans (HDHPs) or consumer-directed health plans are, as their name suggests, plans that impose a high deductible on consumers, sometimes thousands of dollars, usually in exchange for a lower premium (**Figure 6-4**). The rationale behind HDHPs is twofold. First, every insurance claim costs money to process, a

FIGURE 6-4 High-Deductible Plans Versus Traditional Plans

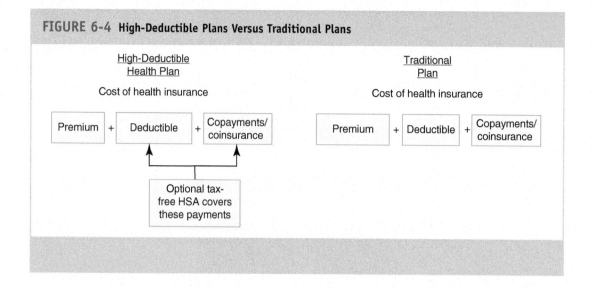

cost that is added to the premium in the form of a loading charge. For smaller claims, such as doctor visits, outpatient prescription drug fills, and blood tests, the loading charge constitutes a large percentage of the total cost of the claim, but for larger claims, such as inpatient surgery, the loading charge constitutes a small percentage of the total cost. If consumers pay directly out-of-pocket for lower-cost visits and tests, then they bypass the insurer and do not incur a loading charge. The administrative costs involved in claims processing are reserved only for higher-cost care. Second, when consumers must use their own funds, rather than the insurer's, to pay for care, they are encouraged to consider the value of that care; in this way, HDHPs are intended to curb moral hazard.

Enrollment in HDHPs has grown quickly. In 2009 HDHPs covered just 8 percent of workers, but by 2015, they covered 24 percent (Islam, 2015). Under the ACA, these plans have been a key component of the state health insurance marketplaces to appeal to younger enrollees.

A person enrolled in an HDHP is also entitled to enroll in a health savings account (HSA), an account owned *by the enrollee* into which she (and her employer) may contribute tax-free dollars to spend on out-of-pocket costs, including deductibles, copayments, and coinsurance. If the enrollee changes jobs, then she may keep the

HSA and the funds in it. An employer may set up an HSA, but individuals who do not work and are enrolled in an HDHP are still entitled to an HSA and may set one up with a trustee, such as an insurer or a bank. Yet among the non-elderly with private insurance, 37 percent are enrolled in an HDHP, but only 13 percent have an HSA (Cohen & Martinez, 2012).

There are other accounts that may be paired with an HDHP, including a health reimbursement arrangement (HRA), an account owned by the *employer* in which the employer contributes funds for pre-determined medical expenses, such as cost-sharing; and a flexible spending account (FSA), which is also owned by the employer, but is "flexible" in that the employee funds it for most qualified medical expenses. Only an HSA, however, may be set up without an employer and is "portable," in that the employee owns it and may thus take it from job to job or into and out of employment.

In theory, HDHPs encourage consumers compare the price and quality of options available to them. Yet price and quality data are not always readily available or easy to decipher. In practice, HDHPs appeal to consumers who do not expect to use much health care, and thus will not need to spend their deductible. So while costs in HDHPs appear to be lower, some of this difference is because enrollees in HDHPs are healthier to begin with (Barry, Cullen, Galusha, Slade, & Busch, 2008; Greene, Hibbard, Dixon, & Tusler, 2006; Tollen, Ross, & Poor, 2004).

NARROW NETWORKS AND TIERED NETWORKS

We have discussed how insurers use provider networks to contain costs by paying discounted prices to in-network physicians; in-network physicians, in turn, are willing to accept these discounts in exchange for patient volume. Taking network design one step further, insurers have introduced two alternative network designs: narrow networks and tiered networks. Narrow networks are a more extreme version of a typical provider network; in a narrow network, an insurer contracts with a much more restricted group of providers than in a typical network. Because there are fewer providers per enrollee, the insurer can promise each provider a greater volume of patients and in turn negotiate an even steeper discount. For enrollees, narrow networks offer lower premiums and out-of-pocket costs as a tradeoff for restricted provider choice.

Tiered networks are less restrictive than narrow networks, offering lower patient cost-sharing for providers with steeper discounts or for high-value providers, much in the same way a tiered formulary incentivizes patients to use low-cost drugs. High-performance networks, a type of tiered network, direct patients to high-quality or high-value providers, rather than just low-cost providers.

Yet tiered networks may have limited efficacy in some markets. For example, in rural areas where there is less competition among providers for patients, providers have less incentive to accept a discounted rate for their services in exchange for higher volume. Similarly, hospitals have monopolies in some markets (they are the only hospital in the area) and thus may not wish to join a narrow network in which their prices are steeply discounted (Summer, 2015).

It is important for consumers to understand how their provider network is structured. In comparing plans, consumers should evaluate the cost-sharing rules for in-network versus out-of-network providers, and for providers in each tier of a tiered network. It is the shared responsibility of the insurer to make this information transparent and easily accessible, and the consumer to obtain this information before seeking care.

REFERENCE PRICING (REVERSE DEDUCTIBLE)

Reference pricing (reverse deductible) is a cost-sharing structure in which the *insurer* pays the initial cost-sharing for a service or product, and the consumer is responsible for any remaining cost.

As an example of how reference pricing works, an employer or insurer might determine from assessing area claims that the appropriate price for a colonoscopy is $1,200 and set a reference price at that amount. Enrollees would then be able to get a colonoscopy at any facility priced $1,200 or less without any additional cost-sharing (sorry, no keeping the difference if you go to a cheaper facility). Enrollees may visit more expensive facilities but must pay the difference out-of-pocket.

Like many cost-saving tools, reference pricing has advantages and disadvantages. On one hand, it incentivizes high-cost providers to lower costs so that they may be listed as facilities that offer services at or below the reference price; on the other hand, low-cost providers may have the opposite incentive—that is, to raise their price to the reference price, because insurers will pay it and because consumers do not get to keep any of the savings from visiting a lower-cost facility. Reference pricing works best for services where there is little variation in clinical quality, because higher-quality providers are not paid more for their services under a reference pricing scheme; rather, all providers are paid the same fixed price (Fronstin & Roebuck, 2014). As with provider network structure, the success of reference pricing depends on patients' understanding of their choices under such an arrangement, and the participation of geographically convenient, high-quality providers.

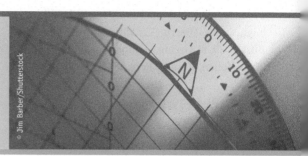

Summary

Health insurance is intended to protect consumers from catastrophic financial losses from illness or injury. Consumers share in the cost of their care through some combination of enrollment fees (premiums) and out-of-pocket costs (deductibles, copayments, and coinsurance). As costs have risen, insurers have looked to both providers and consumers to contain spending. Plans direct consumers to discounted providers, generic medications, and less intensive care settings. In addition, there has been a trend toward increasing consumer cost-sharing and limiting provider networks. Yet without transparent information on price and quality, it will be difficult for consumers to "comparison shop" for providers and make informed decisions about the value of their care. Consumers must have access to this information in order for these cost-containment tools to be effective.

References

Accenture. (2015). *U.S. retail health clinics expected to nearly double by 2017 according to Accenture analysis.* Retrieved from https://www.accenture.com/t20150827T034830__w__/us-en/_acnmedia/Accenture/Conversion-Assets/DotCom/Documents/Global/PDF/Digital_2/Accenture-Retail-Health-Clinics-POV.pdf

American Hospital Association. (2015). Number of community hospitals, 1994–2014. In *Chartbook: Trends affecting hospitals and health systems* (Ch. 2). Retrieved from http://www.aha.org/research/reports/tw/chartbook/index.shtml

Barnet, S. (2015, June 23). 20 things to know about urgent care 2015. *Beckers Hospital Review.* http://www.beckershospitalreview.com/lists/20-things-to-know-about-urgent-care-2015.html

Barry, C. L., Cullen, M. R., Galusha, D., Slade, M. D., & Busch, S. H. (2008, December/November). Who chooses a consumer-directed health plan? *Health Affairs, 27*(6), 1671–1679.

Brooks, T., Miskell, S., Artiga, S., Cornachione, E., & Gates, A. (2016). *Medicaid and CHIP eligibility, enrollment, renewal, and cost-sharing policies as of January 2016: Findings from a 50-state survey.* Retrieved from http://kff.org/medicaid/report/medicaid-and-chip-eligibility-enrollment-renewal-and-cost-sharing-policies-as-of-january-2016-findings-from-a-50-state-survey/

Clemans-Cope, L., & Karpman, M. (2015, October). *Changes in claims, premiums, and medical loss ratios across and within states' individual markets between 2010 and 2014.* Retrieved from http://www.rwjf.org/en/library/research/2015/10/where-might-premiums-be-heading-.html

Cohen, R. A., & Martinez, M. E. (2012). Health insurance coverage, early release of estimates from the national health interview survey, 2011. *National Center for Health Statistics.* Retrieved from http://www.cdc.gov/nchs/data/nhis/earlyrelease/insur201206.pdf

Currie, J., & Madrian, B. (1999). Health, health insurance and the labor market, ch. 50, p. 3309–3416 in, vol. 3, part C, Elsevier. In O. Ashenfelter & D. Card (Eds.), *Handbook of Labor Economics* (Vol. 3, pp. 3309–3416). Oxford, United Kingdom & Amsterdam, The Netherlands: Elsevier.

Fronstin, P., & Roebuck, M. C. (2014). Reference pricing for health care services: A new twist on the defined benefit contribution concept in employment-based health benefits. *Employment Benefit Research Institute* (Vol. 398). Retrieved from https://www.ebri.org/pdf/briefspdf/ebri_ib_398_apr14.refprcng.pdf

Greene, J., Hibbard, J. H., Dixon, A., & Tusler, M. (2006, September). Which consumers are ready for consumer-directed health plans? *Journal of Consumer Policy, 29*(3), 247–262.

The Henry J. Kaiser Family Foundation. (2015, July 24). *The facts on Medicare spending.* Retrieved from http://kff.org/medicare/fact-sheet/medicare-spending-and-financing-fact-sheet/

Islam, I. (2015, October 7). Trouble ahead for high deductible plans? *Health Affairs Blog.* Retrieved from http://healthaffairs.org/blog/2015/10/07/trouble-ahead-for-high-deductible-health-plans/

Ku, L. (2003). *Charging the poor more for health care: Cost-sharing in Medicaid.* Center on Budget and Policy Priorities. Retrieved from http://www.cbpp.org/archiveSite/5-7-03health.pdf

Summer, L. (2015). Health plan features: Implications of narrow networks and the trade-off between price and choice. AcademyHealth Research Insights.

Tollen, M., Ross, M., & Poor, S. (2004, August). Risk segmentation related to offering of a consumer-directed health plan: A case study of Humana Inc. *Health Services Research, 39*(4), 1167–1188.

CHAPTER 7

Consumer Protections

Deanna Meyler, PhD

LEARNING OBJECTIVES

- What rights do patients have?
- What U.S. laws have guided patient care?
- How can patients help themselves?

INTRODUCTION

We go to the doctor when we don't feel well and the hope is that our doctor will help us feel better. In the background of a doctor visit, and all health care contacts, there are many federal and state laws, as well as national association and local hospital policies, guiding the interaction. As patients, we have many rights in this process that are often not discussed when we visit a doctor. These laws and policies attempt to protect us from harm such as fraud or mistreatment, but also from confusion and unwarranted discomfort. This chapter explores patient rights and responsibilities when accessing health care, patient resources, and financial assistance.

PATIENT RIGHTS

Patient rights are the basic protections a patient has when accessing medical care. Accessing medical care can include, but is not limited to, doctor appointments, hospital visits, and any other time spent with a health care institution such as a recovery center, billing office, or insurance agency.

History of Patient Rights in the United States

Patients are protected under many types of laws. Malpractice laws, for example, protect patients from harm as a result of professional negligence. Privacy laws protect patients from mishandling of their medical information. As early as 1973, groups have been concerned with listing all of these rights so that patients know and understand them.

American Hospital Association

In 1973 the American Hospital Association (AHA) outlined the first patient bill of rights, incorporating patient opinions and institutional policies about informed consent and patient autonomy. Their 12 principles (Paasche-Orlow, Jacob, Hochhauser, & Parker, 2009) were the following:

1. The right to considerate and respectful care
2. The right to obtain current and understandable information
3. The right to make decisions about the plan of care and to refuse recommended treatment
4. The right to have an advance directive
5. The right to privacy
6. The right to confidential communications and records

7. The right to review medical records and to have them explained
8. The right to indicated medical care, including transfer to another facility
9. The right to be informed of business relationships that influence care
10. The right to refuse participation in research
11. The right to reasonable continuity of care
12. The right to be informed of charges, as well as policies for patient care and responsibilities, and resources for resolving conflicts

The AHA intended for these principles to be treated as guidelines for patients rather than as key provisions for legislation, yet many of these guidelines have been key parts of subsequent legislation.

Health Insurance Portability and Accountability Act

In 1996, Congress passed the Health Insurance Portability and Accountability Act (HIPAA). The law is so named because it makes it easier to change jobs by limiting exclusions of pre-existing conditions, but it is better known for its privacy protections. HIPAA requires "covered entities," including health plans and providers to keep your information private. Such information includes medical records, associated demographic information including where you live and work, and billing information. In general, providers and insurers can only use this information for limited purposes, such as to coordinate your care and to bill insurance, and for some public health and law enforcement uses, but they cannot report information to your employer or to marketers or advertisers, nor can they share this information with your family and friends without your permission (Civic Impulse, 2016b). The U.S. Department of Health and Human Services (HHS) helps patients who feel their HIPAA rights have been violated and offers forms and local contact information for reporting violations (Civic Impulse, 2016b). See Box 7-1 for an example of a patient privacy notice.

BOX 7-1   Example of a Notice to Protect the Privacy of Patient Medical Information

Your Information. Your Rights. Our Responsibilities.

This notice describes how medical information about you may be used and disclosed and how you can get access to this information. **Please review it carefully.**

Your Rights

You have the right to:

- Get a copy of your paper or electronic medical record
- Correct your paper or electronic medical record
- Request confidential communication
- Ask us to limit the information we share
- Get a list of those with whom we've shared your information
- Get a copy of this privacy notice
- Choose someone to act for you
- File a complaint if you believe your privacy rights have been violated

Your Choices

You have some choices in the way that we use and share information as we:

- Tell family and friends about your condition
- Provide disaster relief
- Include you in a hospital directory
- Provide mental health care

- Market our services and sell your information
- Raise funds

Our Uses and Disclosures

We may use and share your information as we:

- Treat you
- Run our organization
- Bill for your services
- Help with public health and safety issues
- Do research
- Comply with the law
- Respond to organ and tissue donation requests
- Work with a medical examiner or funeral director
- Address workers' compensation, law enforcement, and other government requests
- Respond to lawsuits and legal actions

Your Rights

When it comes to your health information, you have certain rights. This section explains your rights and some of our responsibilities to help you.

Get an electronic or paper copy of your medical record

- You can ask to see or get an electronic or paper copy of your medical record and other health information we have about you. Ask us how to do this.
- We will provide a copy or a summary of your health information, usually within 30 days of your request. We may charge a reasonable, cost-based fee.

Ask us to correct your medical record

- You can ask us to correct health information about you that you think is incorrect or incomplete. Ask us how to do this.
- We may say "no" to your request, but we'll tell you why in writing within 60 days.

Request confidential communications

- You can ask us to contact you in a specific way (for example, home or office phone) or to send mail to a different address.
- We will say "yes" to all reasonable requests.

Ask us to limit what we use or share

- You can ask us not to use or share certain health information for treatment, payment, or our operations. We are not required to agree to your request, and we may say "no" if it would affect your care.
- If you pay for a service or health care item out-of-pocket in full, you can ask us not to share that information for the purpose of payment or our operations with your health insurer. We will say "yes" unless a law requires us to share that information.

Get a list of those with whom we've shared information

- You can ask for a list (accounting) of the times we've shared your health information for six years prior to the date you ask, who we shared it with, and why.
- We will include all the disclosures except for those about treatment, payment, and health care operations, and certain other disclosures (such as any you asked us to make). We'll provide one accounting a year for free but will charge a reasonable, cost-based fee if you ask for another one within 12 months.

Get a copy of this privacy notice

You can ask for a paper copy of this notice at any time, even if you have agreed to receive the notice electronically. We will provide you with a paper copy promptly.

(Continues)

BOX 7-1 Example of a Notice to Protect the Privacy of Patient Medical Information   (*Continued*)

Choose someone to act for you

- If you have given someone medical power of attorney or if someone is your legal guardian, that person can exercise your rights and make choices about your health information.
- We will make sure the person has this authority and can act for you before we take any action.

File a complaint if you feel your rights are violated

- You can complain if you feel we have violated your rights by contacting us using the information on page 1.
- You can file a complaint with the U.S. Department of Health and Human Services Office for Civil Rights by sending a letter to 200 Independence Avenue, S.W., Washington, D.C. 20201, calling 1-877-696-6775, or visiting **www.hhs.gov/ocr/privacy/hipaa/complaints/.**
- We will not retaliate against you for filing a complaint.

Your Choices

For certain health information, you can tell us your choices about what we share. If you have a clear preference for how we share your information in the situations described below, talk to us. Tell us what you want us to do, and we will follow your instructions.

In these cases, you have both the right and choice to tell us to:

- Share information with your family, close friends, or others involved in your care
- Share information in a disaster relief situation
- Include your information in a hospital directory

If you are not able to tell us your preference, for example if you are unconscious, we may go ahead and share your information if we believe it is in your best interest. We may also share your information when needed to lessen a serious and imminent threat to health or safety.

In these cases we never share your information unless you give us written permission:

- Marketing purposes
- Sale of your information
- Most sharing of psychotherapy notes

In the case of fundraising:

- We may contact you for fundraising efforts, but you can tell us not to contact you again.

Our Uses and Disclosures

How do we typically use or share your health information?

We typically use or share your health information in the following ways.

Treat you

We can use your health information and share it with other professionals who are treating you.

Example: A doctor treating you for an injury asks another doctor about your overall health condition.

Run our organization

We can use and share your health information to run our practice, improve your care, and contact you when necessary.

Example: We use health information about you to manage your treatment and services.

Bill for your services

We can use and share your health information to bill and get payment from health plans or other entities.

Example: We give information about you to your health insurance plan so it will pay for your services.

How else can we use or share your health information?

We are allowed or required to share your information in other ways—usually in ways that contribute to the public good, such as public health and research. We have to meet many conditions in the law before we can share your information for these purposes. For more information see: www.hhs.gov/ocr/privacy/hipaa/understanding/consumers/index.html.

Help with public health and safety issues

We can share health information about you for certain situations such as:

- Preventing disease
- Helping with product recalls
- Reporting adverse reactions to medications
- Reporting suspected abuse, neglect, or domestic violence
- Preventing or reducing a serious threat to anyone's health or safety

Do research

We can use or share your information for health research.

Comply with the law

We will share information about you if state or federal laws require it, including with the Department of Health and Human Services if it wants to see that we're complying with federal privacy law.

Respond to organ and tissue donation requests

We can share health information about you with organ procurement organizations.

Work with a medical examiner or funeral director

We can share health information with a coroner, medical examiner, or funeral director when an individual dies.

Address workers' compensation, law enforcement, and other government requests

We can use or share health information about you:

- For workers' compensation claims
- For law enforcement purposes or with a law enforcement official
- With health oversight agencies for activities authorized by law
- For special government functions such as military, national security, and presidential protective services

Respond to lawsuits and legal actions

We can share health information about you in response to a court or administrative order, or in response to a subpoena.

Our Responsibilities

- We are required by law to maintain the privacy and security of your protected health information.
- We will let you know promptly if a breach occurs that may have compromised the privacy or security of your information.
- We must follow the duties and privacy practices described in this notice and give you a copy of it.
- We will not use or share your information other than as described here unless you tell us we can in writing. If you tell us we can, you may change your mind at any time. Let us know in writing if you change your mind.

For more information, see: www.hhs.gov/ocr/privacy/hipaa/understanding/consumers/noticepp.html.

Changes to the Terms of This Notice

We can change the terms of this notice, and the changes will apply to all information we have about you. The new notice will be available upon request, in our office, and on our website.

Other Instructions for Notice

- Insert Effective Date of this Notice

(Continues)

BOX 7-1 Example of a Notice to Protect the Privacy of Patient Medical Information *(Continued)*

- Insert name or title of the privacy official (or other privacy contact) and his/her email address and phone number.
- Insert any special notes that apply to your entity's practices such as "we never market or sell personal information."
- The Privacy Rule requires you to describe any state or other laws that require greater limits on disclosures. For example, "We will never share any substance abuse treatment records without your written permission." Insert this type of information here. If no laws with greater limits apply to your entity, no information needs to be added.
- If your entity provides patients with access to their health information via the Blue Button protocol, you may want to insert a reference to it here.
- If your entity is part of an OHCA (organized health care arrangement) that has agreed to a joint notice, use this space to inform your patients of how you share information within the OHCA (such as for treatment, payment, and operations related to the OHCA). Also, describe the other entities covered by this notice and their service locations. For example, "This notice applies to Grace Community Hospitals and Emergency Services Incorporated which operate the emergency services within all Grace hospitals in the greater Dayton area."

Reproduced from: http://www.hhs.gov/hipaa/for-professionals/privacy/guidance/model-notices-privacy-practices/

Patient's Bill of Rights

In 1997, President Bill Clinton appointed the U.S. Advisory Commission on Consumer Protection and Quality in the Health Care Industry to draft a patient bill of rights. The Commission's recommendations have become the standard adopted by many payers and providers (Commission, 1998). The principles of the Patient's Bill of Rights echo those of the AHA:

1. The right to information disclosure
2. The right to a choice of providers and plans
3. The right to access emergency services
4. The right to participation in treatment decisions
5. The right to respect and nondiscrimination
6. The right to confidentiality of health information
7. The right to complaints and appeals
8. The encouragement of consumer responsibilities, including the responsibility for health and treatment decisions

The Patient's Bill of Rights was not a piece of legislation but rather policy guidance that was voluntarily adopted by some covered entities and used as a framework by states that passed a state-level patients' bill of rights into law.

Bipartisan Patient Protection Act

Some legislators were determined to protect patient rights at the federal level. In 2001, Senator John McCain sponsored the Bipartisan Patient Protection Act, which would have strengthened consumer protections in managed care plans by amending two other pieces of legislation: the Public Health Service Act, which allows the government to regulate public health, and the Employee Retirement Income Security Act, which sets minimum standards for health insurance provided by private industry (Civic Impulse, 2016a, 2016d). But despite wide public support, the House and Senate could not agree on a version of the bill (Moore, 2001). Physician groups were suspicious of the bill, fearing that it would expose them to new malpractice litigation and interfere with their autonomous practice (Kaiser Health News, 2009).

The Affordable Care Act

In 2010, the ACA was signed into law. Part of this landmark legislation included the first federal patient bill of rights. Some of these protections will not apply to those in grandfathered health insurance plans. The protections include the following (Families USA, 2011):

1. The right to coverage despite pre-existing medical conditions
2. The right to choose any doctor in your plan's network
3. The right to speedy emergency care even in out-of-network facilities
4. The right to limit your out-of-pocket liability for out-of-network services
5. The prohibition of rescissions (cancellations) of coverage, except in the case of fraud
6. The prohibition of annual and lifetime limits on coverage for essential benefits
7. The right to certain preventive services without a copayment
8. The right to appeal a health plan decision
9. The right to dependent coverage for young adults up to age 26, for families with qualifying plans

Rights are enforced at many levels. State insurance commissioners regulate health insurers. The federal government regulates self-insured employers. Employers must demonstrate compliance through paperwork (Engle-Hambright & Davies, Inc., 2014). Consumers may file complaints with the state or the federal government. Employees may file a whistleblower complaint against an employer not complying with the ACA with the United States Department of Labor, Occupational Safety and Health Administration. These complaints are not anonymous, but the employer may not legally retaliate since the passage of the Whistleblower Protection Act (Civic Impulse, 2016c).

Rights at the State Level

States have the option to implement their own state-level patients' bill of rights. Yet in 2009 over half of the states have not done so (Paasche-Orlow et al., 2009). In part, the lack of action at the state level is because there had been several attempts at the federal level (described previously) to enact patients' rights legislation. However, when states do enact legislation, it can be supplemental to rights provided at the federal level. For example, New York offers numerous rights that are unique from the ACA.

PATIENT RESPONSIBILITIES

In addition to being protected with certain rights, patients have responsibilities and obligations to fulfill within the health care system. Here we outline these responsibilities within the U.S. health care system and also provide some recommended methods for patients to advocate for their own health.

Personal Responsibility for Health

As patients, we are expected to take responsibility for our own health. The Clinton Commission guidelines (described previously) included responsibilities such as exercising and refraining from smoking; maintaining a healthy diet; being involved in health care decisions; disclosing relevant information and communicating preferences; and avoiding knowingly spreading disease (Commission, 1998). Doctors have the responsibility to help patients understand treatment options and must provide understandable information that meets patient education levels and language needs, but health is much more than medical care and health insurance. Those who wish to be healthy must take responsibility, to the extent possible, to engage in a healthy lifestyle (Commission, 1998).

Financial Responsibilities

In the United States, patients are expected to pay for services rendered depending on the structure of their insurance plan. In many health insurance plans, patients are expected to pay a copay at the time of service. The cost of health care can be high, even with health insurance, and unaffordable for low-income households. Patients with language barriers and low socioeconomic status have more difficulty managing medical bills. Medical bills are rarely accompanied with options for patients to lower costs.

However, patients have some options to lower their medical bills.

Patient Advocates

Most hospitals have patient advocates or patient representatives. These employees are available to patients at any point during their care. They can help patients make sure they are receiving the right care, get a ride home after a procedure, or understand a bill. When patients have complaints, they are often referred to a patient advocate. Because the onus of responsibility is on the patient to understand their medical bill, the patient advocate can be an information resource for understanding the bill and options to reduce the cost and pay the bill (Gilkey & Earp, 2009).

Payment Plan

Many hospitals are willing to set up a payment plan with patients. If a determined amount is paid within each predetermined span of time, usually a month, bills will not be sent to collection agencies. Payment plans can be interest-free (Lee, 2014).

Haggle

Although it may sound unusual, patients can haggle to lower their charges. For example, sometimes a hospital will agree to a lower cost if a patient can pay all remaining charges immediately (Lee, 2014). Patients can research their charges and compare costs for the same care from other doctors and hospitals. If costs are higher than what other providers charge, this information can be brought to the attention of the hospital and sometimes the hospital will match the lower cost. There is no obligation for a hospital to lower the cost, but if lowering a well-researched cost will improve the chances that the patient can pay the bill, they may consider doing so (Lee, 2014).

Charitable Programs

Many hospitals, especially nonprofit hospitals, have charitable programs that can help with medical costs. These programs may not be visible, and so patients must research and inquire about availability. Patient advocates can assist with locating appropriate charitable programs. Most programs are based on income (Chazin, Friedenzohn, Martinez-Vidal, & Somers, 2010).

Crowdfunding

Some patients have turned to online crowdfunding opportunities, such as Kickstarter or YouCaring, to raise money for medical bills. Others who know large medical bills are forthcoming will begin asking for donations before beginning care through sites such as GiveForward.

Bankruptcy

Unfortunately, after following all options already listed, costs can still be too high for many patients. In fact, a major cause of personal bankruptcy in the United States is medical bills (Himmelstein, Thorne, Warren, & Woolhandler, 2009). Declaring bankruptcy is an option of last resort for patients to resolve medical bills.

Advocating for Your Own Health

Despite the policies and protections that are now in place for patients, it is still largely the responsibility of patients to advocate for their own health. Table 7-1 gives several resources to help patients advocate for themselves. Patients decide when they need to see a doctor and doctors advise and provide the care they think will be best for the patient. Ultimately, it is the responsibility of patients to seek and receive the best care and

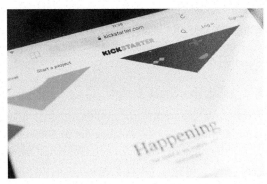

© spaxiax/Shutterstock

TABLE 7-1 **Selected Resources for Patient Advocacy**

Organization	Website
Agency for Healthcare Research and Quality—Patient Safety Organization Program	https://pso.ahrq.gov/listed
CenterWatch	http://www.centerwatch.com/
Community Health Advocates	http://www.communityhealthadvocates.org
FAIR Health Consumer Cost Lookup	http://fairhealthconsumer.org
Federal Trade Commission	https://www.identitytheft.gov/
Health Advocates for Older People	http://www.hafop.org
Health and Human Services: HIPAA	http://www.hhs.gov/hipaa/filing-a-complaint/index.html
Healthcare Bluebook	https://www.healthcarebluebook.com
Healthcare.gov	https://www.healthcare.gov/health-care-law-protections/
Medical Identity Fraud Alliance	http://medidfraud.org
National Patient Safety Foundation	http://www.npsf.org/
Occupational Safety and Health Administration	https://www.osha.gov/whistleblower/WBComplaint.html
Patient Advocate Foundation	http://www.patientadvocate.org

treatment. Social disadvantages such as language barriers and low education will shape and determine which options patients advocate for and access. However, patients can advocate for themselves in this process:

- Patients can be informed about their symptoms before seeing a doctor. They can keep a journal of symptoms to know the duration and intensity while also noting any additional observations that seem unrelated. This kind of information helps doctors with a diagnosis.
- Patients can research symptoms, diseases, conditions, and health care providers on the Internet or at the local library.
- Patients can bring questions to their doctor appointments. Writing down questions ahead of time and bringing them to appointments reduces the chance a question will be forgotten.
- Patients can get a second and even third opinion from a health care provider. If

there is any concern that the diagnosis or treatment is not right, patients can visit a new health care provider and share information from the prior visit. Depending on the health insurance policy, the cost of a second opinion is often covered.

- Patients can explore alternative approaches such as diet and exercise, acupuncture, and chiropractic adjustments. Complementary and alternative medicine approaches are not usually covered by insurance, but, depending on the diagnosis, could be more accessible and beneficial.
- Patients can continue to do research. Once diagnosed, patients can explore additional therapies and options their doctor may not be able to access. This is common among cancer patients and other complex diseases. With multiple studies of new treatments in progress, patients can approach doctors involved with the studies to potentially gain access to a new drug or approach as a study participant.

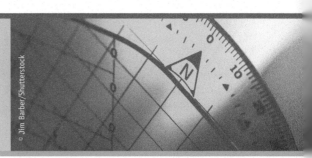

Summary

The American Hospital Association drafted the first U.S. patient bill of rights in 1973, but it was not until 2010 that a federal, enforceable Patients' Bill of Rights was passed into law. Some states go beyond these federal regulations and provide even more protections for patients in their state.

Despite these protections, patients bear many responsibilities for their health and for advocating for their health care needs. They are responsible for speaking openly with doctors to receive appropriate care and implement agreed upon treatments. They are also responsible for their own health outside of the doctor's office. Social and environmental factors can affect the ability of individuals to practice healthy lifestyles and to self-advocate for medical treatment.

References

Chazin, S., Friedenzohn, I., Martinez-Vidal, E., & Somers, S. A. (2010, August). *The future of U.S. charity care programs: Implications of health reform*. Retrieved from http://www.chcs.org/media/The_Future_of_Charity_Care_Programs.pdf

Civic Impulse. (2016a). H.R.2—93rd Congress: Employee Retirement Income Security Act of 1974. Retrieved from https://www.govtrack.us/congress/bills/93/hr2

Civic Impulse. (2016b). H.R.3103—104th Congress: Health Insurance Portability and Accountability Act of 1996. Retrieved from https://www.govtrack.us/congress/bills/104/hr3103

Civic Impulse. (2016c). S.20—101st Congress: Whistleblower Protection Act of 1989. Retrieved from https://www.govtrack.us/congress/bills/101/s20

Civic Impulse. (2016d). S.1052—107th Congress: Bipartisan Patient Protection Act of 2001. Retrieved from https://www.govtrack.us/congress/bills/107/s1052

Commission on Consumer Protection and Quality in the Health Care Industry. (1998). *Quality first: Better health care for all Americans*. Retrieved from http://archive.ahrq.gov/hcqual/

Engle-Hambright & Davies, Inc. (2014). *Affordable Care Act (ACA) violations—Penalties and excise taxes*. Retrieved from http://www.ehd-ins.com/assets/2014/10/2014Oct-HCRACAViolations.pdf

Families USA. (2011, April). *The Affordable Care Act: Patients' Bill of Rights and Other Protections*. Retrieved from http://familiesusa.org/product/affordable-care-act-patients-bill-rights-and-other-protections

Gilkey, M. B., & Earp, J. A. L. (2009). Defining patient advocacy in the post-quality chasm era. *North Carolina Medical Journal, 70*(2), 120–124.

Himmelstein, D., Thorne, D., Warren, E., & Woolhandler, S. (2009). Medical bankruptcy in the United States, 2007: Results of a national study. *American Journal of Medicine, 122*(8), 741–746. doi: 10.1016/j.amjmed.2009.04.012

Kaiser Health News. (2009, June). AMA "alarmed" over increased liability for physicians under Patients' Rights Bill. Retrieved from http://khn.org/morning-breakout/dr00004453/

Lee, J. (2014). *Slash your medical bills: 7 ways to haggle*. Retrieved from http://billadvocates.com/save-money/slash-medical-bills-7-ways-haggle/

Moore, D. W. (2001, July). Public supports patient's bill of rights. *Gallup*. Retrieved from http://www.gallup.com/poll/4588/public-supports-patients-bill-rights.aspx

Paasche-Orlow, M. K., Jacob, D. M., Hochhauser, M., & Parker, R. (2009). National survey of patients' bill of rights statutes. *Journal of General Internal Medicine, 24*(4), 489–494.

CHAPTER 8

Payment Mechanisms

Alexis Pozen, PhD and John A. Gravina, MPH

LEARNING OBJECTIVES

- What are common mechanisms of payment from insurers to providers?
- What are the tradeoffs associated with each payment mechanism, and for what types of care does each payment mechanism work best?
- What is the purpose of risk adjustment to insurers and providers?

INTRODUCTION

How insurers pay for care is profoundly important to balancing health care costs, quality, and accessibility for consumers. Insurers pay providers in a variety of ways. Public payers, such as Medicare and Medicaid, generally reimburse providers at rates set by government regulators. Private payers, on the other hand, negotiate with providers for the price of services and supplies. Prices for both types of payers can be set per office visit, per day in the hospital, or per service rendered. While the price of a service is important, what the price *covers* is equally important. Payment mechanisms influence the amount and intensity of care provided, as well as the types of services available to enrollees.

COMMON PAYMENT MECHANISMS

In this section, we will define and compare the most common payment mechanisms, including

fee-for-service, capitation, salary, per diem, and per admission. Bundled payment (also known as episode-of-care or case rate) is newer and not as common, but worth including in this list because of its increasing importance in several public and private initiatives to improve the value of care. No single payment mechanism works best in every circumstance; rather, each has its relative advantages and disadvantages.

Fee-for-Service

Fee-for-service (FFS) reimburses providers for each procedure or service rendered. For example, if you see your primary care physician for a flu shot, then under fee-for-service, your insurance pays separate reimbursements for the consultation and the immunization. Fees are paid according to a fee schedule, a list of prices for each service that is either negotiated (private payers) or administered (public payers).

Capitation

Capitation is a flat dollar payment per patient per month (sometimes per year). A capitation can be thought of as a treatment "budget." Patients (usually HMO enrollees) sign up with a physician (or physician group), and the HMO makes a monthly payment for that patient, usually at the beginning of the month. The group then pools the money from all of the patients and spends it on those who need care. Groups that stay within their budget may keep the remainder and invest it into their practice; those who go over the budget must make up the deficit with their own funds.

Salary

A salary is a fixed dollar amount per year. Physicians earning a salary are generally employees of, or exclusively contracted with, a medical group.

Per Diem

A per diem (per day) payment is a fixed dollar amount per day (e.g., in the hospital or other health care facility) regardless of the intensity of services provided that day.

Per Admission

A payment per admission is a fixed payment to the hospital or health care facility based on the diagnosis at admission, and similarly to a per diem, does not vary with the intensity of the services provided for that admission.

Bundled Payment (Episode-of-Care Payment)

In a bundled payment arrangement, insurers pay a fixed amount for the entire continuum of care. For example, a bundled payment for a knee surgery might include payment for all of the pre-surgical tests, the surgery itself, and any follow-up care. Instead of paying for an individual service or hospital day, the unit of service is the entire episode of care, and so this arrangement is also referred to as episode-of-care payment (or case rate, because it covers the entire medical case).

COMPARISON OF PAYMENT MECHANISMS

All payment mechanisms come with tradeoffs, and no single mechanism works best in every situation. For example, FFS payment puts relatively little financial risk on providers, while capitation is more financially risky. FFS is a type of retrospective payment, meaning that reimbursement varies with the cost of the patient, while capitation is a type of prospective payment, meaning that reimbursement does not vary with the cost of the patient. Under FFS, then, providers will be compensated more for treating costly patients, but under capitation, providers must cover these patients with funds from their monthly budget. On the other hand, if capitated physicians provide care at a lower cost, then they can increase their profits. Providers can also increase revenue by registering more patients. FFS, then, incentivizes a higher volume and intensity of care compared to capitation, while capitation incentivizes efficient but potentially inadequate care for a less risky patient population.

These two payment types represent relative extremes of retrospective and prospective payment, but there are other payment types in between. Hospitals paid per diem, for example, receive higher reimbursement if patients stay in the hospital for longer, but not if care is costlier per day. Therefore, per diem creates an incentive to prolong a patient's stay while providing only low-intensity, low-cost services. Providers paid bundled payments receive no additional payment for a costlier surgery, but nor are they incentivized to keep their patients out of surgery to begin with, because they receive the bundle only if their patients end up on the operating table. Somewhere between prospective and retrospective, these payment mechanisms require providers to be responsible for some, but not all, of the financial risk of treating their patients.

Figure 8-1 illustrates the relative levels of risk to the provider versus the payer for each type of payment mechanism discussed here. Because retrospective payment mechanisms pay providers more for sicker patients, they are associated with less risk to the provider (more risk to the payer); and because prospective payment mechanisms do not pay more for sicker patients, they are associated with more provider risk (less payer risk).

Because of the various advantages and disadvantages of payment mechanisms, there is no "best" payment mechanism; rather, some work better for different types of care than others. Bundled payments, for example, work best for well-defined episodes, such as surgeries or acute medical conditions. They do not work as well for chronic conditions, where there is no clear beginning or end. Further, there is less compelling need for bundled payment for episodes that do not have much variability in price,

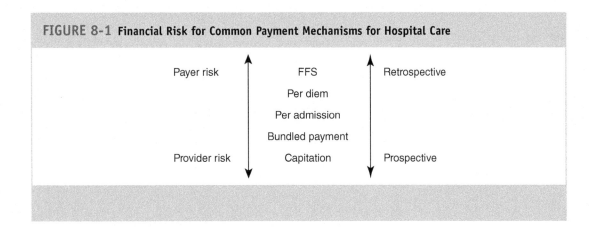

FIGURE 8-1 Financial Risk for Common Payment Mechanisms for Hospital Care

as bundled payment is meant to address this problem (Miller, 2009).

And while FFS is widely disdained for the incentive it provides to increase the quantity and intensity of services (Epstein, Begg, & McNeil, 1986), doing away with it entirely seems unwise. One study found that Americans receive only half of recommended preventive care (McGlynn et al., 2003). It is difficult to make the argument that primary care physicians should take on more financial risk for services that are underprovided. On the other hand, there is clearly waste in the system due to duplication of services and overprovision of high-intensity services. Capitation may help control costs, but it also incentivizes provision of fewer services and cream-skimming (targeting low-risk or otherwise profitable patients, also known as cherry-picking), so it works best for practices that are skilled at managing a budget for chronically ill patients. Figure 8-1 shows an approximation of the levels of risk for the different payment mechanisms discussed here.

HISTORY OF PAYMENT

It may seem strange that we have so many ways to pay providers, but some history will put these mechanisms into context. The earliest reimbursement innovations began in the Medicare program but have extended to other public and private payers. Unlike these other payers, however, reimbursement policies in traditional (FFS) Medicare are standard across the country, so as health care costs rose with new medical advances and expanded coverage, policymakers turned to Medicare to test new ways

to pay providers that could be implemented uniformly. Because many of these mechanisms proved successful in limiting cost growth, private payers followed suit. Even today, private insurers look to the Medicare program for guidance in decisions regarding reimbursement and coverage.

Payment reform began in hospitals, because hospital care accounted for, and still accounts for, the largest proportion of health care spending—32 percent in 2014 (Centers for Medicare and Medicaid Services [CMS], 2015). Changes in physician payments were slower, in part because physicians were always well organized as a profession, and in part because their fees represented a smaller proportion of total health care spending (Starr, 1982; CMS, 2015). As outpatient care grew in importance, however, managed care organizations experimented with new ways to reimburse physicians.

Medicare Cost-Plus Era: 1960s and 1970s

Early health insurance plans provided protection primarily for hospital expenses. Indemnity plans, in which consumers paid providers directly for services and then submitted the bill for reimbursement, were more common, and reimbursed at per diem rates. Less commonly, workers enrolled in prepaid group plans that paid a monthly capitation in exchange for hospital care.

As medical technology rapidly progressed throughout the 1950s and 1960s, however, the American Hospital Association encouraged the growth of service benefit plans, which reimbursed providers directly. While indemnity plans required patients to pay out-of-pocket for expensive hospital services and wait for reim- bursement, service benefit plans protected patients from this financial burden. Service bene- fit plans, however, did not become the norm until the managed care era of the late 1980s and 1990s, because during the middle of the century, limiting hospital spending became a more urgent problem than limiting consumer spending.

To protect vulnerable populations from high out-of-pocket costs, Congress passed Medicare and Medicaid, but these programs in turn fueled cost growth (Catlin & Cowan, 2015) (**Figure 8-2**). Expanded coverage increased the demand for care, and this demand was unhindered by Medi- care's payment policy toward hospitals. To secure wide access to services for beneficiaries, Medicare initially paid hospitals FFS based on the costs incurred plus 2 percent, called a "cost-plus" fee schedule. This system encourages the provision of high intensity services and long stays in the hospi- tal. One study estimated that the passage of Medi- care was associated with a 37 percent increase in inflation-adjusted hospital expenditures from 1965 to 1970 (Finkelstein, 2007).

In response to such generous Medicare reim- bursement, hospitals flooded the market. Although people were not necessarily getting sicker, the cost-plus system incentivized administrators to fill an increasing supply of beds. New medical interventions helped to fill the empty beds by giving hospitals reasons to admit patients and keep them for longer periods of time (Gruber & Owings, 1996). This phenomenon, known as supplier-induced demand, is consumer use of health care services beyond the volume and inten- sity that she would prefer if she had full informa- tion on the costs and benefits, that occurs because of influence from providers.

Voluntary and Mandatory Cost Containment: 1970s and 1980s

To address rapid health care spending growth, policymakers implemented various cost- containment efforts, aimed especially at hospitals. Not all of these efforts were successful. Part of an economy-wide program to limit inflation, President Nixon's Economic Stabilization Program (ESP) of the 1970s applied price and wage controls to hospitals.

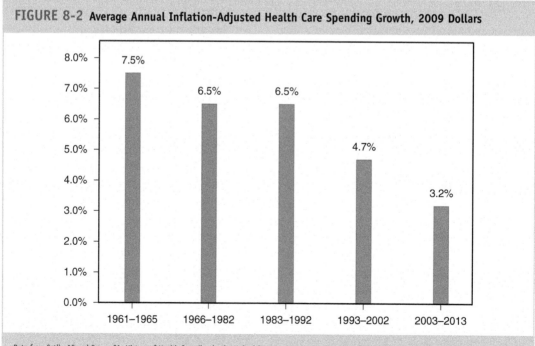

FIGURE 8-2 **Average Annual Inflation-Adjusted Health Care Spending Growth, 2009 Dollars**

Data from Catlin AC and Cowan CA. History of Health Spending in the United States, 1960-2013. 2015 (Data from U.S. National Health Expenditures)

While this program was temporarily successful in suppressing inflation, it did so at the expense of hospital profits and, in particular, wages. And when the program ended, inflation again increased (Gold, Chu, Felt, Harrington, & Lake, 1993).

President Carter inherited the problem of hospital costs from his predecessor. As Congress tried to pass legislation to replace the ESP, hospitals mounted their own campaign to voluntarily control costs to fend off any mandatory controls. The bills that were introduced would have capped revenues, set floors for occupancy (implicitly constraining how many hospitals could be built), and limited overall expenditures, but were never passed (H.R. 6575/S. 1391, 1977; H.R. 2626/S. 570, 1979). Evidence suggests that the threat of mandatory controls made voluntary efforts successful but, as with ESP, only temporarily (Gold et al., 1993).

In 1964, New York became the first state to establish a certificate-of-need (CON) program, which imposed regulations on construction of new hospitals and other health care facilities in the state. Other states soon followed, and in 1974 the federal government required states to implement CON laws to receive funding for certain federal programs, though this condition was repealed in 1987. CON programs require developers to apply for a certificate from the state for any projects that cost above a certain amount to build. Some CON programs are more restrictive than others; for example, some have lower dollar thresholds requiring an application to the state, or apply to a wide variety of facilities in addition to hospitals, such as physician offices, ambulatory surgery facilities, and nursing homes. Today, 36 programs remain (Mitchell & Koopman, 2014). There is limited evidence about the effectiveness of CON laws in reducing cost growth (Conover & Sloan 1998; Grabowski, Ohsfeldt, & Morrisey, 2003). In states that have a particularly cumbersome CON process, facilities that are successful in obtaining a certificate may actually have an incentive to provide costly care to recoup their initial investment.

Another state-led initiative aimed at reducing hospital costs is all-payer rate setting. Beginning in the 1970s states began to set their own prices for hospital services, overriding Medicare and privately negotiated fees. By 1980 over half of states had such a policy. In some states, all-payer programs were voluntary for hospitals, and in most, they did not cover all payers, despite the name. Because states had flexibility in setting fees, all-payer programs were effective in reducing hospital spending growth (Gold et al., 1993). Today, only Maryland still has an all-payer policy, including an exemption from Medicare and Medicaid rates.

Medicare Prospective Payment System, 1983

Medicare began to shift away from the cost-plus system in 1983, when it adopted the Prospective Payment System (PPS) for inpatient hospital care, which was implemented gradually over several years. Instead of paying hospitals for every cost incurred, under the PPS, Medicare pays hospitals per admission, grouped by diagnosis, regardless of the length of stay.

PPS signified a fundamental shift in provider reimbursement policy. After PPS, Medicare experimented with prospective payment for other types of providers. Further, private payers used PPS as the basis for their own changes in hospital reimbursement.

PPS was undoubtedly successful in stemming hospital cost growth (Bamezai, Zwanzigier, Melnick, & Mann, 1999). In the cost-plus era, hospitals did not have to consider strategies to limit costs, only to increase revenue—more admissions, longer lengths of stay, and limitless tests and procedures. Under PPS, however, hospitals receive a flat rate per admission, so stays in the hospital cannot be so long or so costly. Sicker patients are a liability. Indeed, shortly after the PPS was first implemented, the average length of stay at PPS facilities dropped (Gold et al., 1993), though it is difficult to know whether hospitals were admitting healthier patients or reducing the intensity of admissions or treatment (Ellis & McGuire, 1996).

Managed Care, 1980s and 1990s

In 1973, Nixon signed the bipartisan HMO Act, which provided funding to establish and expand HMOs, and preempted state laws prohibiting them. It also required employers offering health insurance to offer at least one HMO. But because Congress passed the Employee Retirement and Income Security Act (ERISA) just one year later, making it easier for employers to leave their insurance plans and self-insure, HMOs were not widely available at first. Health care cost growth during the 1970s and 1980s, however, made these plans increasingly attractive for employers, and by the mid-1990s, growth in offer rates of HMOs far outpaced growth in offer rates of traditional indemnity plans (American Hospital Association [AHA], 2016).

HMOs were the first managed care organizations (MCOs). Other MCOs that followed include preferred provider organizations (PPOs), point-of-service organizations (POSs), and exclusive provider organizations (EPOs). MCOs have experimented with different payment mechanisms for both hospital and physician services, often looking to Medicare for guidance. What distinguishes MCOs from Medicare (and from indemnity plans), however, is that while Medicare contracts with most providers willing to accept its fees, HMOs selectively contract with providers, engaging them in price and quality competition.

The obstacles to obtaining care in MCOs and the concern that they withheld necessary care resulted in a public backlash (Blendon et al., 1998). While this backlash did not end managed care altogether, by the late 1990s most Americans had left their HMOs for more generous managed care plans such as PPOs and POSs (AHA, 2016). Although health care growth has consistently outpaced economy-wide growth since the 1960s, it was during the managed care era that the two came closest to converging (Catlin & Cowan, 2015). But as the managed care heyday ended and costs diverged, policymakers again looked for ways to restrain spending.

Consumer-Directed Health Care, 2000s

In the early 2000s, employers experimented with high-deductible health plans as a way to impose financial accountability on consumers, encouraging them to shop for care. Enrollment in high-deductible health plans has been steadily increasing (AHA, 2016). But these plans have not been successful in reducing costs, because consumers are not well-equipped with information they need to shop—such as provider price and quality—and generally only the healthiest consumers have enrolled (Barry, Cullen, Galusha, Slade, & Busch, 2008; Brot-Goldberg, Chandra, Handel, & Kolstad, 2015; Greene, Hibbard, Dixon, & Tusler, 2006).

Payment for Quality- and Value-Based Care—2010s

Today, public and private payers have turned their focus to paying providers for *value*. The goal is to both limit costs and to incentivize high-quality care. Some see cost and quality as tradeoffs, while others believe that excellent care can be provided efficiently and within a budget. Value-based initiatives have ranged from bonuses to physicians for complying with certain quality standards to non-payment for preventable hospital readmissions in the Medicare program. We will discuss these initiatives in more detail later in this chapter.

PAYMENTS TO PROVIDERS

All insurers have different provider reimbursement policies. Medicare's reimbursement policy differs from state Medicaid policies, which differ from those of private plans. While FFS Medicare's provider payment policy is standard across the country, each state sets its own Medicaid policy. Florida, for example, pays physicians for Medicaid patients in a different way than Massachusetts. And each private plan has its own reimbursement policy as well, although because they look to Medicare for guidance, there are many similarities across private plans.

While a provider group may contract exclusively with one insurer, this arrangement is uncommon. More commonly, a provider has multiple contracts, and may be reimbursed in multiple ways. One hospital, for example, may receive FFS, per diem, and bundled payment from different plans. Table 8-1 shows the different types of payments made to different types of providers.

There are generally two separate reimbursements for care delivered in a hospital, ambulatory surgery center, or other health care facility (but not in a physician's office). The insurer pays a facility fee

TABLE 8-1 **Common Payment Mechanisms to Providers**

	Traditional Medicare	Private Payers, State Medicaid Programs, Medicare Part C
Hospital Inpatient	IPPS*	FFS, per diem, PPS-like system, bundled payment
Hospital Outpatient	OPPS	FFS, PPS-like system, bundled payment
Physician	RBRVS (FFS)	FFS, capitation, salary
Other Inpatient	Various (usually prospective)	FFS, per diem, PPS-like system, bundled payment
Other Outpatient	Various (usually prospective)	FFS, PPS-like system, bundled payment

* Bundled payments are used for certain episodes of care.

to the hospital or ambulatory surgery center and a professional fee to the physician who performed the services. For example, if you get spine surgery at a hospital, then your insurance company may pay a per diem to the hospital and a fee (based on the negotiated fee schedule) to the physician.

Payment to Hospitals

Private payers, state Medicaid programs, and Medicare Part C plans pay hospitals for inpatient and outpatient care in a variety of ways, primarily per diem, FFS, or a modified version of Medicare's PPS system, which is a severity-adjusted payment per admission. Some payers are also beginning to experiment with bundled payments for certain procedures.

Under the Medicare Inpatient PPS (IPPS), admissions are categorized by severity. The system groups together related diagnoses, called diagnosis-related groups (DRGs), and then ranks these groups based on expected resource use and clinical intensity. Payment is higher for more intensive DRGs, such as surgical procedures, and lower for less intensive DRGs, such as a fever. Medicare also adjusts inpatient hospital payment by area-level wages because, for example, the cost of living is higher in California than in Mississippi, and so payment must be higher in California to reflect this difference. Payment is also higher for hospitals that treat a disproportionate share of Medicaid and uninsured payments, for hospitals that train medical residents, and for unusually costly admissions.

Like payment for inpatient services, Medicare payments for hospital-based outpatient services were originally cost based, but rising spending led Medicare to implement prospective payment. The Outpatient Prospective Payment System (OPPS) groups outpatient service codes with similar clinical intensity and cost, with higher payments for more intensive groups, and lower payments for less intensive groups. These groups of service codes are called Ambulatory Payment Classifications (APCs), and are analogous to inpatient DRGs. Similar to IPPS payments, OPPS payments are adjusted for geographic factors and hospital characteristics such as rural sole community hospital (SCH) status, cancer center status, and unusually costly visits.

Payments to Physicians

To curb health care spending growth, Medicare took various measures to limit physician fee increases throughout the 1970s and 1980s, and as a result beneficiaries found it difficult to find participating physicians (Feldstein, 2015). To address both spending growth and access, in 1992 Medicare implemented the Resource-Based Relative Value Scale (RBRVS), a modified FFS system that pays higher fees for more intensive services and lower fees for less intensive services. (While the DRG system and the RBRVS system sound similar, the RBRVS system is more retrospective, because payments increase if physicians perform more services per visit, while the DRG system is more prospective, because payments do not increase if hospitals perform more services per admission.) The RBRVS fee rises with physician time required to perform the procedure or consultation, practice costs (including malpractice) associated with the physician specialty, and training costs associated with the specialty (Hsiao, Braun, Yntema, & Becker, 1988). RBRVS weights are updated every year under the guidance of the RVS Update Committee (RUC), which makes recommendations about these fees to the Centers for Medicare and Medicaid Services (CMS), which administers the Medicare and Medicaid programs.

As part of the 1997 Balanced Budget Act, Congress aimed to control Medicare physician spending by linking it to the sustainable growth rate (SGR), a formula based on economy-wide growth and the demand for Medicare services. Under this system, Medicare paid physicians a bonus if they collectively remained within the SGR, but imposed cuts (limits to fee increases) if spending surpassed the SGR. By 2002, spending had surpassed the target and physicians were threatened with cuts. But Congress did not follow through with this threat, and instead overrode the impending cuts with a piece of legislation known as the "doc fix." In fact, because spending over the years so frequently surpassed the SGR, Congress passed many subsequent doc fixes (Wynne, 2015). In 2015 the Medicare Access and CHIP Reauthorization Act (MACRA) replaced the SGR with modest rate increases tied to value.

As with other payment policies, the private market has adopted elements of Medicare payment policy for physicians. Many private insurers that pay FFS, such as PPO and POS plans, use the RBRVS to weight fees, though their fees are generally higher. But the private market has also diverged somewhat from Medicare with regard to physician payment. Around the same time as the RBRVS, HMO plans were on the rise and predominantly paid capitation or salary. FFS has always been the dominant payment model for physicians under traditional Medicare, but private plans under Part C use a variety of reimbursement methods.

While private insurers, even HMOs, still generally pay hospitals per diem or FFS, some physicians team up with hospitals to accept a global capitation, a budget for both physician and hospital services. This type of payment mechanism is rare because it leaves physicians at risk for care that is arguably out of their control, so capitated physicians more commonly accept partial capitation, in payment covers only some services, such as checkups, vaccinations, and screenings, but not specialty or hospital care.

Payment to Other Types of Providers

With the exception of physicians, FFS Medicare reimburses most providers via prospective payment systems. (The name *FFS Medicare* to refer to Medicare Parts A and B now really only refers to the RBRVS system for physicians under Part B, since Medicare has mostly abandoned FFS for other providers.) Ambulatory surgical centers (ASCs), which provide only outpatient care, receive payment through the ASC PPS. Like the OPPS, the basis of the ASC PPS is the APC code. Skilled nursing facilities (SNFs) are reimbursed through the SNF PPS, which are paid per diem, adjusted by Resource Utilization Groups (RUGs)—categories of patients' clinical attributes and functional abilities. Medicare also pays home health agencies through a prospective payment system in increments of 60-day episodes. It categorizes beneficiaries into Home Health Resource Groups (HHRGs) based on their clinical and functional severity and pays higher amounts for the 60-day episode for those in higher HHRGs. Medicare has also implemented prospective payment systems for inpatient psychiatric care, laboratory services, and inpatient rehabilitation services. While the details vary depending on the program, each system reimburses providers a prospectively determined amount that is then adjusted for geographic, clinical, and facility characteristics.

Private payers, state Medicaid programs, and Medicare Part C plans reimburse facilities in myriad ways. For outpatient care such as ASCs and laboratory services, insurers will often pay FFS or model a prospective reimbursement system after Medicare's. For inpatient care, such as SNFs, per diem is also an option. Every contract is different and depends on the conditions of the market.

RISK ADJUSTMENT

Providers that accept capitation rely on appropriate risk adjustment of these payments to remain financially solvent. Risk adjustment is higher payment for patients expected to cost more, and lower payment for patients expected to cost less. Let's illustrate this concept with an example.

Suppose that an HMO pays $20 per member per month to a primary care practice. This amount may not seem like much. But now suppose that the average practice has a panel of 1,500 patients—patients who have signed up with the practice as their primary care "gatekeeper." Then each month the operating budget is $20 × 1,500 = $30,000. Most of the 1,500 patients will not have to come in that month, so $30,000 should be sufficient to cover the cost of the 500 patients or so who do come in for routine care, and the 150 or so who will need additional tests or procedures.

But now consider Dr. Wegman, a geriatrician who has set up his practice in a poor area of town to serve its neediest elderly residents, many whom are chronically ill. While the practice similarly maintains a panel of about 1,500 patients, most need to come in each month, so the practice sees 1,000 patients, not 500. Further, a greater percentage need testing, putting further pressure on the $30,000 budget.

In contrast, Dr. Kendall, a doctor of adolescent medicine, has set up shop in a young, trendy neighborhood. She also has a panel of 1,500 patients, but usually only sees about 250 per month. Most do not need extensive testing. In general, her patients come in for acute injuries that require referrals to a specialist or because they need prescription medications, which are not capitated.

Clearly, it is not "fair" that both practices continue to get paid $20 per member per month. Dr. Wegman's practice sees higher-cost (riskier) patients, while Dr. Kendall's practice sees lower cost (less risky) patients. But risk adjustment has proven difficult in practice. Dr. Wegman's and Dr. Kendall's practices are two extremes meant to illustrate an idea, but in reality, it is difficult to predict differences in expenditures across providers.

There are various methods for adjusting risk. Under prospective risk adjustment, insurers compensate providers based on estimated expenses. In the example above, an HMO might estimate that Dr. Wegman's practice costs will be higher in the upcoming month compared to Dr. Kendall's, based on past spending and area demographics. At the start of the month, then, Dr. Wegman would receive a payment that is higher than $20 per member per month, and Dr. Kendall would receive a payment that is lower. Under concurrent risk adjustment, insurers compensate providers based on actual incurred expenses, rather than estimated expenses. Again using the example above, both practices might receive a $20 capitation at the beginning of the month, but at the end of the month, Dr. Wegman's practice would receive additional compensation.

In both prospective and retrospective risk adjustment, insurers must decide what factors make patients "risky." In particular, they must decide what factors should be considered within the physician's control (and thus not part of the risk-adjustment calculation) and what factors should be considered outside of the physician's control. Demographics such as age and sex are clearly out of the physician's control, and are thus almost always factored into any risk adjustment calculation because they also usually affect costs. Comorbidities (concurrent diseases) drive higher costs, and may have manifested before the patients joined the practice, but insurers would like to encourage physicians to manage these diseases. One way to encourage them to do so is by not factoring them into risk adjustment. This tactic may backfire, however, and can incentivize physicians to cream-skim by treating more highly profitable patients, avoiding less profitable patients, or both (Ellis, 1998; Friesner & Rosenman, 2009). For example, if insurers wanted to encourage physician groups to manage diabetes by not adjusting for severity of illness, then groups may seek out patients with well-managed diabetes, since these patients would surely cost less. Many more factors are outside of a physician's control than can be captured using claims data or data from electronic health records.

Figure 8-3 illustrates the difficulty that insurers have in adjusting risk. There are myriad components that influence health other than health care, such as a person's environment, genetics, and attitude and beliefs about health. Standardized data on these factors are not readily available, and thus insurers cannot fully adjust for them.

Payments to health plans are themselves risk adjusted so that plans attracting "good risks" fund plans that attract "bad risks." CMS prospectively risk adjusts payments to private Medicare plans (parts C and D) and concurrently risk adjusts payments to private health plans in the individual and small group markets, both inside and outside of the exchanges. Imagine a system in which a plan unexpectedly attracts costly enrollees one year, but no risk adjustment system is in place. The next year, the plan will have to fund the deficit by raising premiums, which will cause some healthy enrollees to leave. The plan will then be even worse off and have

to raise premiums even more, and so on, and so forth. This phenomenon is called a death spiral and is not theoretical. It has been documented many times (Cutler & Reber, 1998; Polyakova, 2015).

It is then up to each individual plan to adjust payments to providers. Capitations should be appropriately risk adjusted so that providers treating sick patients do not become insolvent. Performance bonuses to providers should be risk adjusted so that providers do not have an incentive to "game" the system by treating only patients for whom it is easy to meet quality measures.

VALUE-BASED PAYMENT AND ALTERNATIVE PAYMENT MODELS

In the 20th century, payers have developed new value-based payment models that incentivize both cost containment and improved quality. While FFS encourages volume and intensity, capitation encourages efficiency. Other payment models lie

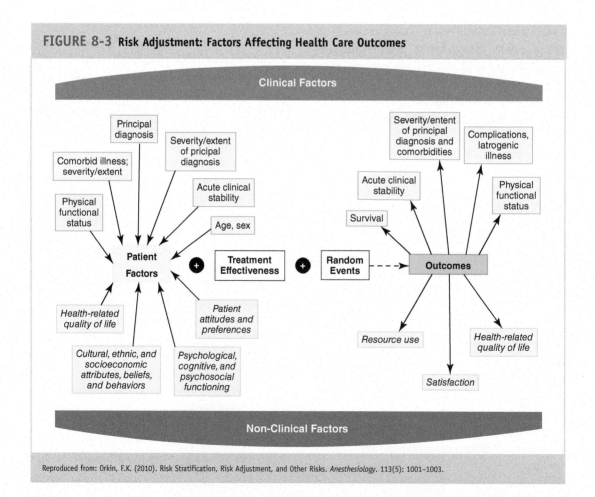

FIGURE 8-3 Risk Adjustment: Factors Affecting Health Care Outcomes

Reproduced from: Orkin, F.K. (2010). Risk Stratification, Risk Adjustment, and Other Risks. *Anesthesiology.* 113(5): 1001–1003.

between these extremes, but none explicitly incorporates quality. New value-based payment models were largely a response to a 2001 report released by the Institute of Medicine (IOM) called *Crossing the Quality Chasm*, which called on policymakers to make the U.S. health care system more safe, effective, patient-centered, timely, efficient, and equitable (IOM, 2001).

Early Value-Based Payment: Pay-for-Reporting and Pay-for-Performance

Value-based payment (VBP) is a payment strategy that rewards providers for quality and cost containment, rather than volume. Among the earliest incarnations of value-based payment were pay-for-reporting and pay-for-performance programs. Pay-for-reporting incentivizes providers, usually with a bonus or penalty, for reporting data on quality indicators. An early example was the Medicare Reporting Hospital Quality Data for Annual Payment Update (RHQDAPU) Program, which is now known as the Hospital Inpatient Quality Reporting Program (IQR). Pay-for-performance took this concept a step further, conditioning bonus and penalty payments on how providers performed on certain quality indicators. These indicators might include *process* measures such as staff immunization rates, *outcome* measures such as mortality rates, or *structural* measures such as the implementation of an electronic medical record (EMR). Later, these programs also incorporated measures of *patient experience*, such as waiting times for an appointment.

Evidence on the efficacy of these earlier programs is mixed. Pay-for-performance may have improved quality, even cost-effectively, but sometimes at the expense of other facets of quality that were not measured or paid for (Eijkenaar, Emmert, Scheppach, & Schöffski, 2013). In addition, most effects have been found to be small in magnitude (Li, Hurley, DeCicca, & Buckley, 2014; Rosenthal, Frank, Li, & Epstein, 2005). Furthermore, there is evidence that these programs tend to reward physicians who already performed well prior to implementation (Rosenthal et al., 2005), raising the concern that they may further reinforce disparities in quality by failing to invest where improvements are truly needed.

Today's Value-Based Payment: Bundled Payment, Accountable Care Organizations, Patient-Centered Medical Homes

Today's value-based payment programs aim to limit costs while simultaneously promoting quality. Bundled payments encourage providers to limit themselves to a budget for certain costly services that have historically varied widely in price, such as knee, hip, and spine surgeries. Usually the bundled payment is only for the facility fee, and physicians are paid separately, but if the providers agree, then the professional fee may be included as well. Bundling the two payments together aligns the financial incentives of hospitals and physicians, who might otherwise be paid in different ways. For example, a hospital paid on a per diem basis may aim to reduce costs and admit less severely ill patients, whereas a physician paid using FFS may aim to care for the neediest patients and err on the side of providing every laboratory test, image, and procedure necessary (Epstein et al., 1986).

Both public and private payers are experimenting with bundled payments, though this mechanism does not represent a large proportion of payments (Delbanco, 2014), since it is only appropriate for well-defined episodes of care, such as surgeries, and only necessary for care with large pricing variations. As with capitation, providers must be able to deliver care efficiently and recruit a sufficient volume of patients to remain profitable.

The movement toward value-based care has resulted in payment models that span provider categories. Primary care providers are increasingly financially accountable for patients who enter the hospital; hospitals are increasingly accountable for discharged patients. The ACA authorized Medicare to pay groups of providers, called accountable care organizations (ACOs), to manage the care of large populations of Medicare beneficiaries. ACOs are responsible for meeting quality standards including vaccinations and screenings, care coordination, patient ratings, and clinical indicators for their patients. Medicare will pay its usual fees to the ACO providers, but if at the end of the year the ACO has saved money compared to a predetermined benchmark, then it may share in the savings. ACOs may also elect to share in the risk for losses—in other words, if they do not save money, they will have to make payments to Medicare. The incentive to participate in this "double-sided risk" option is that ACOs that save money share in a greater proportion of the savings. As with many Medicare policies, the private market has followed suit and begun to pay its own ACOs to manage populations of privately insured individuals.

ACOs are responsible for managing patient care throughout the year, but *which* patients? Medicare could guess which ACO might be the best fit based on which providers beneficiaries have used in the past, and assign them to this ACO for the upcoming year—this method of assigning patients to an ACO is called prospective attribution. Alternatively, Medicare could wait a year and determine where patients actually used care, then assign patients to the ACO that they used most frequently for the prior year; this method is called retrospective attribution. Medicare chose prospective attribution, with some retrospective adjustment. No method of assignment perfectly captures how beneficiaries use care. Because beneficiaries are free to use any provider who participates in Medicare, no ACO has full control over the care of any of their patients. Yet an ACO is still responsible for the health and costs of attributed patients who obtain care from an outside provider.

Just as with payments to health plans and providers, payments to ACOs must be appropriately risk adjusted in order for these organizations to compete on a level playing field. Some ACOs are primary care providers, while others are multispecialty physician practices. Still others are large local networks of hospitals and physicians. The current evidence evaluating ACO performance paints a mixed picture. Some ACOs have been able to improve quality while generating cost savings. Other ACOs have generated losses and been forced to dissolve (Vogus & Singer, 2016). **Figure 8-4** shows the relationship among the different parties in the ACO.

Patient-centered medical homes (PCMH) are another type of value-based payment system. A PCMH is not only a physical location but also a model of primary care delivery in which the medical home is financially responsible for the health care needs of its patients (Agency

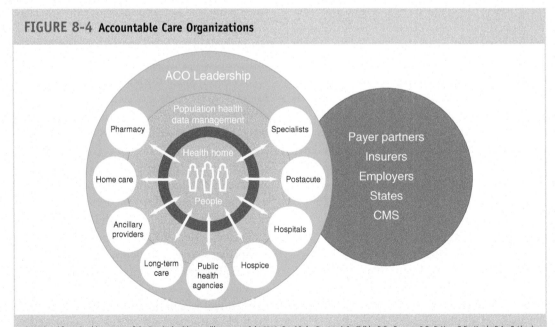

FIGURE 8-4 Accountable Care Organizations

for Healthcare Research and Quality [AHRQ], 2016). It differs from an ACO in that it is just one primary care practice, not a group of providers. As with other value-based payment systems, both public and private payers are encouraging the PCMH model by making incentive payments to practices that serve as a medical home,

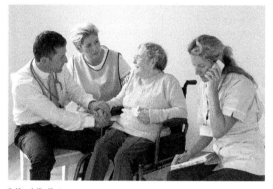
SolStock/E+/Getty

especially for patients with chronic conditions. The goal is to have these patients sign up for a medical home to improve the quality and lower the cost of their care.

In 2015 MACRA (the legislation that repealed the SGR formula), streamlined previously existing Medicare physician quality incentive programs into one program, the Quality Payment Program. Instead of linking Medicare physician payment to the SGR, MACRA links payment to value, but physicians have a choice about how Medicare can make this link. The Merit-based Incentive Payment System (MIPS) is similar to earlier pay-for-performance systems, and links pay to quality, cost, clinical practice improvement, and electronic health records. Alternatively, physicians may participate in an Alternative Payment Model (APM), such as bundled payment, an ACO, or a PCMH (CMS, 2016).

Summary

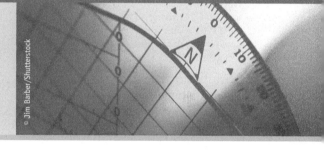
© Jim Barber/Shutterstock

Provider payment mechanisms profoundly affect what types of consumers can access what types of care. Hospitals flooded the market when reimbursed at cost for every service they provided, but slowed down when paid a flat rate per admission, and began closing and merging when forced to compete on price.

While health care cost growth has actually been declining over time, it is almost always higher than economic growth (Catlin & Cowan, 2015). Therefore, each year, health spending occupies a greater share of the economy; in 2014, it was almost 18 percent (CMS, 2015).

How much spending is "too much" is a topic for another book, but in order to reduce wasteful spending within that 18 percent, payers have developed value-based payments to providers to encourage efficiency in the delivery of medical care. They aim to reward providers for delivering high-value care and penalize them for delivering low-value care.

Appropriate risk adjustment and patient attribution are key to the functioning of these new payment systems. Providers cannot be held responsible for patients that mostly visit other providers. Practices that treat risky populations should be compensated to ensure patient access to care. Insurers with sick enrollees must receive higher payments to avoid a death spiral in the market for insurance. Payments must be carefully designed to consider their effects on cost, quality, and access to care.

References

Agency for Healthcare Research and Quality (AHRQ). (2016). *Defining the PCMH*. Retrieved from https://pcmh.ahrq.gov/page/defining-pcmh

American Hospital Association (AHA). (2016). *Trends affecting hospitals and health systems: Distribution of employer-sponsored health insurance enrollment by type of plan, 1988–2015*. Retrieved from http://www.aha.org/research/reports/tw/chartbook/ch1.shtml

Bamezai, A., Zwanzigier, J., Melnick, G. A., & Mann, J. M. (1999). Price competition and hospital cost growth in the United States (1989–1994). *Health Economics, 8*(3), 233–243.

Barry, C. L., Cullen, M. R., Galusha, D., Slade, M. D., & Busch, S. H. (2008). Who chooses a consumer-directed health plan? *Health Affairs, 27*(6), 1671–1679.

Blendon, R. J., Brodie, M., Benson, J. M., Altman, D. E., Levitt, L., Hoff, T., & Hugick, L. (1998). Understanding the managed care backlash. *Health Affairs, 17*(4), 80–94.

Brot-Goldberg, Z. C., Chandra, A., Handel, B. R., & Kolstad, J. T. (2015). *What does a deductible do? The impact of cost-sharing on health care prices, quantities, and spending dynamics*. NBER Working Paper No. 21632.

Catlin, A., & Cowan, C. (2015). *History of health spending in the United States, 1960–2013*. Retrieved from https://www.cms.gov/Research-Statistics-Data-and-Systems/Statistics-Trends-and-Reports/NationalHealthExpendData/Downloads/HistoricalNHEPaper.pdf

Centers for Medicare and Medicaid Services (CMS). (2015). *National health expenditure data*. Retrieved from https://www.cms.gov/Research-Statistics-Data-and-systems/Statistics-Trends-and-reports/NationalHealthExpendData/index.html

Centers for Medicare and Medicaid Services (CMS). (2016). *Quality payment program: System reform, Medicare payment reform, & MACRA*. Retrieved from https://www.cms.gov/Medicare/Quality-Initiatives-Patient-Assessment-Instruments/Value-Based-Programs/MACRA-MIPS-and-APMs/MACRA-MIPS-and-APMs.html

Conover, C. J., & Sloan, F. A. (1998). Does removing certificate-of-need regulations lead to a surge in health care spending? *Journal of Health Politics, Policy, and Law, 23*(3), 455–481.

Cutler, D. M., & Reber, S. J. (1998). Paying for health insurance: The trade-off between competition and adverse selection. *Quarterly Journal of Economics, 113*(2), 433–466.

Delbanco, S. (2014). *The payment reform landscape: Bundled payment*. Retrieved from http://healthaffairs.org/blog/2014/07/02/the-payment-reform-landscape-bundled-payment/

Eijkenaar, F., Emmert, M., Scheppach, M., & Schöffski, O. (2013). Effects of pay for performance in health care: A systematic review of systematic reviews. *Health Policy, 110*(2-3), 115–130.

Ellis, R. P. (1998). Creaming, skimping and dumping: Provider competition on the intensive and extensive margins. *Journal of Health Economics, 17*(5), 537–555.

Ellis, R. P., & McGuire, T. G. (1996). Hospital response to prospective payment: Moral hazard, selection, and practice-style effects. *Journal of Health Economics, 15*(3), 257–277.

Epstein, A. M., Begg, C. B., & McNeil, B. J. (1986). The use of ambulatory testing in prepaid and fee-for-service group practices. *New England Journal of Medicine, 314*(17), 1089–1094.

Feldstein, P. J. (2015). *Health policy issues: An economic perspective* (6th ed.). Chicago, IL: Health Administration Press.

Finkelstein, A. (2007). The aggregate effects of health insurance: Evidence from the introduction of Medicare. *The Quarterly Journal of Economics, 122*(1), 1–37.

Friesner, D. L., & Rosenman, R. (2009). Do hospitals practice cream skimming? *Health Services Management Research, 22*(1), 39–49.

Gold, M., Chu, K., Felt, S., Harrington, M., & Lake, T. (1993). Effects of selected cost-containment efforts: 1971–1993. *Health Care Financing Review, 14*(3), 183–225.

Grabowski, D. C., Ohsfeldt, R. L., & Morrisey, M. A. (2003). The effects of CON repeal on Medicaid nursing home and long-term care expenditures. *Inquiry, 40*(2), 146–157.

Greene, J., Hibbard, J. H., Dixon, A., & Tusler, M. (2006). Which consumers are ready for consumer-directed health plans? *Journal of Consumer Policy, 29*(3), 247–262.

Gruber, J., & Owings, M. (1996). Physician financial incentives and cesarean section delivery. *RAND Journal of Economics, 27*(1), 99–123.

Hospital Cost Containment Act, H.R. 6575/S. 1391, 95th Congress, 1st Session (1977).

Hospital Cost Containment Act, H.R. 2626/S. 570, 96th Congress, 1st Session (1979).

Hsiao, W. C., Braun, P., Yntema, D., & Becker, E. R. (1988). Estimating physicians' work for a resource-based relative-value scale. *The New England Journal of Medicine, 319*(13), 835–841.

Institute of Medicine (IOM). (2001). *Crossing the quality chasm: A new health system for the 21st century*. Washington, DC: National Academy Press

Li, J., Hurley, J., DeCicca, P., & Buckley, G. (2014). Physician response to pay-for-performance: Evidence from a natural experiment. *Health Economics, 23*(8), 962–978.

McGlynn, E. A., Asch, S. M., Adams, J., Keesey, J., Hicks, J., DeCristofaro, A., & Kerr, E. A. (2003). The quality of health care delivered to adults in the United States. *The New England Journal of Medicine, 348*(26), 2635–2645.

Miller, H. D. (2009). From volume to value: Better ways to pay for health care. *Health Affairs, 28*(5), 1418–1428.

Mitchell, M., & Koopman, C. (2014). *40 years of certificate-of-need laws across America.* Mercatus Center, George Washington University. Retrieved from http://mercatus.org/publication/40-years-certificate-need-laws-across-america

Polyakova, M. (2015). *Regulation of insurance with adverse selection and switching costs: Evidence from Medicare Part D.* NBER Working Paper No. 21541.

Rosenthal, M. B., Frank, R. G., Li, Z., & Epstein, A. M. (2005). Early experience with pay-for-performance: From concept to practice. *JAMA, 294*(14), 1788–1793.

Starr, P. (1982). *Social transformation of American medicine: The rise of a sovereign profession and the making of a vast industry.* Boulder, CO: Basic Books.

Vogus, T. J., & Singer, S. J. (2016). Unpacking accountable care using organization theory to understand the adoption, implementation, spread, and performance of accountable care organizations. *Medical Care Research and Review*, doi: 10.1177/1077558716640410

Wynne, B. (2015). *May the era of Medicare's doc fix (1997–2015) rest in peace. Now what?* Retrieved from http://healthaffairs.org/blog/2015/04/14/may-the-era-of-medicares-doc-fix-1997-2015-rest-in-peace-now-what/

CHAPTER 9

Claims and Reimbursement for Providers

Fernando A. Wilson, PhD and Jim P. Stimpson, PhD

LEARNING OBJECTIVES

- How do providers claim reimbursement for services from insurers?
- What are the differences between government and private insurers in claiming reimbursement?
- What options do providers have to resolve reimbursement disputes?

INTRODUCTION

When you step into your doctor's office, the first thing the receptionist will ask you for is your insurance information. This step is the first in a sometimes long and complex process in your provider receiving reimbursement for the visit. In this chapter, we will discuss how providers submit claims and receive reimbursement for medical services.

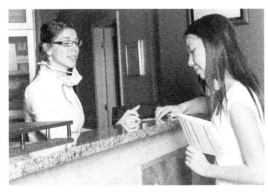

© Lopolo/Shutterstock

DIAGNOSIS AND PROCEDURE CODING SYSTEMS

Given the significant expense of many medical procedures, patients rarely pay for services directly in cash. This means that providers must wait for reimbursement for these services, sometimes long after they are provided. As a result, quickly submitting insurance claims, or requests for reimbursement, is a crucial task for providers, particularly for costly medical services. These claims must also be as accurate as possible; mistakes may delay reimbursement for services, result in underpayment, or worse, may subject the provider to financial penalties for fraud.

Imagine that you are experiencing a sharp pain in your chest as you're working in your garden one weekend. You quickly use your cell phone to call 911, and are soon on your way by ambulance to the local emergency department. This first point of contact with the health care system is the beginning of a chain of services that the health care provider must track and eventually report to your insurer in order to make a claim. Your diagnosis (or diagnoses) and each procedure performed on you must be assigned a number or code selected from one or more standardized lists.

Two of these lists are the International Classification of Diseases, 10th Revision (ICD-10) Clinical Modification (CM) codes and Procedure Coding System (PCS) codes. The ICD-10 coding system was first developed by the World Health Organization (WHO) more than 20 years ago, and the most recent version became effective in October 2015 (WHO, n.d.). The U.S. Department of Health and Human Services requires use of the ICD-10 coding system by all health care organizations covered under the Health Insurance Portability and Accountability Act (HIPAA) (National Center for Health Statistics [NCHS], 2015). We will discuss HIPAA later in this chapter. The ICD-10 includes a range of 68,000 possible diagnoses and 87,000 medical procedures, and ICD-10-CM and ICD-10-PCS codes contain up to seven digits using alphanumeric characters (see Figure 9-1).

For example, after arriving in the emergency room (ER), your physician concludes that you are suffering from *angina pectoris*, a symptom of coronary heart disease. The billing department for the ER must find the most appropriate ICD-10-CM code corresponding to this diagnosis. In your case, this code would start with "I20," denoting angina pectoris. Different forms of angina pectoris will require additional digits to your code; for example, "I20.0" denotes "unstable angina" while "I20.1" denotes "angina pectoris with documented spasm." You may also have other diagnoses as well. The physician may also find that you have hypertension; this will

require more codes, such as "I10," which denotes "essential or primary hypertension." If you tell your physician that you use tobacco and are not physically active, the codes "Z72.0" and "Z72.3" may be added to your record. A family history of heart disease that included sudden cardiac death will be recorded as "Z82.41," and so on. As you can see, a single patient may end up with a large number of codes that describe his or her medical condition, comorbidities, health behaviors, family or personal health history, exposure to environmental hazards, and many other factors that ultimately impact the patient's health and treatment.

In general, the first three digits in an ICD-10-CM code represent the broad category of the health issue, the fourth digit denotes the origin or etiology of the issue, a fifth digit denotes the affected body part, and the sixth digit denotes the severity of the health issue. There may also be a seventh digit to provide even more specificity to the illness or other health problem. Similarly, all procedures used in treating you in the ER must be matched to their corresponding codes in ICD-10-PCS. If your physician uses a chest x-ray to see what is going on with your heart, this will be coded as B for "imaging," 2 for "heart," 0 for "plain radiography," and 6 for "heart, right and left," or "B206." Each digit corresponds to a section, body system, type, body part, or other qualifiers and characteristics associated with a procedure. However, the ICD-10 coding system is not the only coding system used.

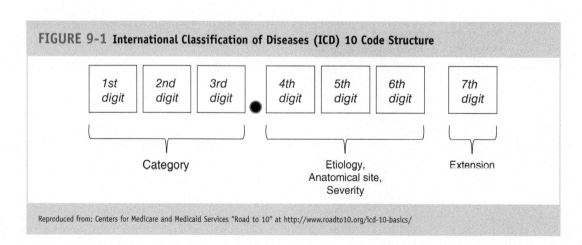

FIGURE 9-1 International Classification of Diseases (ICD) 10 Code Structure

| 1st digit | 2nd digit | 3rd digit | | 4th digit | 5th digit | 6th digit | 7th digit |

Category — Etiology, Anatomical site, Severity — Extension

Another important system that is maintained by the American Medical Association (AMA) uses Current Procedural Terminology (CPT) codes to identify procedures and services delivered by physicians, hospitals, and other providers to treat patients. Like the ICD-10, CPT codes help standardize the range of procedures that may be given to patients into about 7,800 five-digit items (see Table 9-1). Given an ICD-10-CM diagnosis code of, say, angina pectoris, there are specific procedures that are likely to be utilized by the physician to help make the diagnosis, monitor the illness, and, if possible, treat it. Each procedure will have a unique CPT code and a related, detailed description of each code. The use of an electrocardiogram (ECG), for example, may have a CPT code of either 0178T (if it had "64 leads or greater, with graphic presentation and analysis; with interpretation and report") or a code of 93005 (if it was a "routine ECG with at least 12 leads; tracing only, without interpretation and report").

Another coding system that is based on the CPT system is called the Healthcare Common Procedure Coding System (HCPCS). The HCPCS system uses two levels for its coding: Level I codes are the CPT codes described previously, and Level II codes cover other services and procedures not included in the CPT system, such as ambulance services and certain medical supplies, durable equipment, and devices such as prosthetics and orthotics (Centers for Medicare and Medicaid Services [CMS], 2013).

Physicians will also record CPT codes for "evaluation and management" (E/M) of a patient. These codes (99201, 99202, 99203, 99204, 99205) are differentiated by the severity of the patient visit (ranging from minor to high severity) and the amount of time in minutes spent face-to-face with the patient (ranging from 10 to 60 minutes). A short visit for a minor health issue will generally involve a "problem-focused" examination and "straightforward" decision making on the part of the treating physician. Longer visits are associated with comprehensive examinations and "high-complexity" decision making.

Unfortunately for the physician, there is a degree of subjectivity in determining severity and complexity of a visit, and thus appropriate documentation to support the selection of a particular E/M code for a visit is important. One study of 600 physicians found that one-third of physicians undercoded their established patients (King, Sharp, and Lipsky, 2001). Unlike "upcoding," in which claims are submitted with codes that result in higher-than-warranted reimbursements, undercoding or "downcoding" involves codes that underreport the complexity of a case. For example, a physician may record an E/M code denoting low complexity in medical decision making when the patient required moderate or high complexity. As a result, undercoding forgoes potentially higher reimbursements for services. Reasons for undercoding may involve errors in coding or a decision by the physician to avoid risks from accusations of upcoding, particularly when the choice of code involves subjectivity. Interestingly, in the same study, over 80 percent of the physicians tended to upcode using E/M codes when seeing new patients (King et al., 2001).

TABLE 9-1 Current Procedural Terminology (CPT) Code Categories

Category	Description
I	Five-digit code with descriptors for a procedure or service. Codes range from 00100 to 99499.
II	Optional alphanumeric codes with supplemental information to Category I codes. Codes range from 0001F to 7025F.
III	Interim codes for emerging technology, procedures, and services.

Data from: http://www.medicalbillingandcoding.org/intro-to-cpt/

Modifier codes may also be included as part of the CPT/HCPCS coding in order to note unusual circumstances or issues involving the service. These are two-digit alphanumeric codes. A prolonged E/M service beyond the highest level of E/M coding (code 99205) would have a modifier code of "21." For telehealth-related health care services, delivering a service "via interactive audio and video telecommunication systems" would require the modifier code "GT." Ambulance transport of a patient suffering from an acute health event or injury may have the modifiers "S" denoting "scene of accident or acute event" together with "H" denoting "hospital," or "SH." The modifiers will help determine the reimbursement for the service that a provider will receive. Returning to our telehealth example, if a provider provides a patient evaluation session using asynchronous technologies such as email associated with the modifier "GQ," the provider is unlikely to be reimbursed for this service by many insurers, including for Medicare patients.

In practice, given the depth, range, and complexity of these coding systems—and the need for accurate coding, as mentioned earlier—the billing departments for health care providers rely on electronic health information systems, and large providers such as hospitals may also employ coders to review and verify that appropriate diagnosis and procedure codes are being used for each patient. The next iteration of coding—ICD-11—is currently in development by the World Health Organization for release in 2018, for which ICD-10 is the "foundational building block" (WHO, n.d.; CMS, 2015c). Adoption of ICD-11 in the United States will likely take several years, if not decades; the transition to ICD-10 from ICD-9 occurred more than 20 years after ICD-10 was finalized by the WHO (WHO, n.d.).

FILING CLAIMS

Nearly all claims—94 percent according to one survey—are submitted electronically (America's Health Insurance Plans [AHIP], 2013). HIPAA and subsequent laws such as the Health Information Technology for Economic and Clinical Health Act (HITECH) and the Affordable Care Act (ACA) created national standards for the electronic transmission of health care transactions, data security, and privacy protections. All commercial and government health plans and health care providers that accept electronic health care transactions are required to follow these standards. Although commercial insurers generally follow Medicare's lead regarding coding of diagnoses and procedures, they may differ in the processes providers must use to submit claims for reimbursement. Because of these differences, electronic health care claims are typically sent to a clearinghouse first. The clearinghouse checks the claims for errors and formats the claims according to insurers' standards before they are securely forwarded to them. Furthermore, the clearinghouse identifies errors that may have otherwise delayed reimbursements.

The Medicare Program

There are a number of steps and requirements that providers must fulfill in order to be eligible to treat and submit claims for Medicare beneficiaries. The first step that a prospective Medicare provider must complete is applying for a National Provider Identifier, or NPI (CMS, 2015a). The NPI is a 10-digit number that uniquely identifies each health care provider and is used in administrative and financial transactions with Medicare. After receiving an NPI, the health care provider may apply for enrollment into the Medicare program either online via the Provider Enrollment, Chain, and Ownership System (PECOS) or using a paper form, CMS-855. To participate in Medicare, a provider must agree to accept Medicare fees for all services covered by Medicare for all beneficiaries. That is, the provider cannot accept Medicare fees for some patients but charge higher fees for others.

However, a provider may also be a "non-participating provider" in Medicare. Physicians are allowed to "opt out" of Medicare, but they must do so for all beneficiaries and all services. In this case, non-participating providers may choose whether to submit a Medicare claim, but will receive lower reimbursement compared to participating providers. Non-participating providers who do not submit a claim to Medicare may privately contract with beneficiaries for their services. Medicare beneficiaries may receive some reimbursement for using these providers, but coverage will not be as generous as for a participating provider.

To file a claim, providers use Form 837P for electronic submission of claims to a Medicare Administrative Contractor (MAC). A MAC is a private insurance company that is contracted to process Medicare Part A and B claims or durable medical equipment claims for a geographical area. Providers report a Medicare patient's identifying information (e.g., name, ID number, address, birth date), date of illness, injury or pregnancy, diagnoses (ICD-10), date and place of service, CPT/HCPCS codes with any modifiers, charges in dollars, provider ID number, and other information related to the patient and services rendered. After a claim is filed, the provider will receive a Remittance Advice (RA) listing adjustments made to the reimbursement. These adjustments may include denial of the claim; zero, partial, or reduced payment; penalties; or additional or supplemental payments. In these circumstances, the provider has the option of requesting a reopening of the claim if a minor clerical error was made, or filing a formal appeal with Medicare.

Electronic submission of claims is required under the Administrative Simplification Compliance Act (ASCA). Paper submission of claims is only allowed when providers qualify for an exception to the ASCA, for example, when the provider has fewer than 10 full-time employees or the computer system is disabled, preventing electronic submission of claims (CMS, 2014). In these instances, providers may use either the CMS-1500 form or, for hospital providers, the CMS-1450 (also known as UB-04) form.

Medicaid

Unlike Medicare, which is a national program with consistent eligibility criteria, Medicaid is a state-managed program whose eligibility and covered services vary substantially across states. Because Medicaid is state managed, providers should conform to both state and federal guidelines for beneficiary claims. Similar to our discussion of filing Medicare claims, providers will need ICD-10 and HCPCS Levels I and II codes. Recall that HCPCS Level I codes are also CPT codes. In addition, two-digit place–of-service codes must be provided, which identify where services were rendered, for example, office, inpatient or outpatient hospital, skilled nursing facility, and so on.

Furthermore, Medicaid is the "payer of last resort"; that is, claims must be filed with all other third-party payers before submitting a Medicaid claim (CMS, 2007). This is called the "third-party liability" rule (CMS, 2007). The process of enrolling as a Medicaid provider and filing claims for beneficiaries is determined by each state, and thus the specific information required from providers will vary. For example, physicians seeking to enroll in Medicaid may be asked to report their NPI, type of practice, contact information, medical license number, specialty and taxonomy code, board certification, demographic information, proof of liability insurance, hospital privileges, and other information.

Commercial Insurance

The requirements and process for submitting claims for commercial insurance plans such as UnitedHealthcare, BlueCross/BlueShield, Aetna, and others vary across these plans. In general, commercial insurers follow the same diagnosis and procedure code systems (e.g., CPT and HCPCS) as Medicare. There may be substantial differences in what services are covered and the reimbursements for these services across insurers. For example, UnitedHealthcare follows Medicare policy in reimbursing for services provided via telehealth. Claims using synchronous audio and video technologies must use a modifier code "GT" in addition to the CPT/HCPCS code for the service (UnitedHealthcare, 2015).

Workers' Compensation

Workers' compensation, or "workers' comp," is a state-managed program that provides medical and other benefits to employees who are injured while working. In return for these benefits, the injured employee forgoes his right to sue the employer for damages. Each state workers' comp program has its own process for providers to submit claims. Reimbursements are based on worker compensation fee schedules established by each state to reimburse health care providers. In general, to submit a claim, the provider reports the employee's and employer's contact info, date and time of injury, and diagnosis (with ICD code), in addition to other information.

COLLECTING REIMBURSEMENTS AND HANDLING DISPUTES

We previously discussed the claim process. After submitting a claim, the next steps from the perspective of the provider are collecting the money from the claim and handling disputes with the payer. The provider may dispute how a bill was paid by an insurance company, and a patient may appeal the decision of what portion of the medial bill an insurer is willing to pay.

Collecting Reimbursements

After receiving a claim from a health care provider, the insurer evaluates the claim and issues an explanation of benefits (EOB) form to the patient and provider, along with reimbursement to the provider. EOB forms vary in format and content across insurers, but typically include the following information: type of service provided, dates of service, charges submitted by the provider, provider discount from charges, the amount paid by the insurer to the provider, and remaining patient financial responsibility (see Figure 9-2). The latter includes amounts due to the patient's deductible, coinsurance or copayment, and charges not covered by insurance.

FIGURE 9-2 Example of Explanation of Benefits

Pay your bills and keep any paperwork. Some providers will not see you if you have unpaid medical bills. You may be able to go online to look up your own health information, such as screening and test results or prescribed medications. This can help you take charge of managing your health.

Reading your Explanation of Benefits (EOB)
After you visit your provider, you may receive an Explanations of Benefits (EOB) from your insurer. This is an overview of the total charges for your visit and how much you and your health plan will have to pay. An EOB is NOT A BILL and helps to make sure that only you and your family are using your coverage. You may get a bill separately from the provider.

APPEALS AND GRIEVANCES
If you have a complaint or are dissatisfied with a denial of coverage for claims under your health plan, you may be able to appeal or file a grievance. For questions about your rights, or assistance, you can contact your insurance plan or state Medicaid or CHIP program. If you think you were charged for tests or services your coverage is supposed to pay for, keep the bill and call the phone number on your insurance card or plan documentation right away. Insurance companies have call and support centers to help plann members.

Here's an example of an Expalanation of Benefits
Your insurance plan's or Medicaid or CHIP agency's **Customer Service Number** may be near the plan's logo or no the back of your EOB.

Explanation of Benefits (EOB)   Customer service: 1-800-123-4567

Insurance plan logo

Statement date: XXXXXX
Document number: XXXXXXXXXXXXXXXX
THIS IS NOT A BILL

Member name:
Address:
City, State, Zip:

Subscriber number: XXXXXXXX   ID: XXXXXXXX   Group: ABCDE   Group number: XXXXX

Patient name: Date received:				Provider: ⑤ Payee:				Claim number: XXXXXXXXX Date paid: XXXXXXXX		
	Claim Detail			What your provider can charge you		Your responsibility			Total Claim Cost	
Line No.	Date of Service	Service Description ①	Claim status	Provider Charges ②	Allowed Charges ③	Co-Pay	Deduct-ible	Co-Insurance	Paid by insurer ④	What You Owe ⑥	Remark Code ⑦
1	3/20/14–3/20/14	Medical care	Paid	$31.60	$2.15	$0.00	$0.00	$0.00	$2.15	$0.00	PDC
2	3/20/14–3/20/14	Medical care	Paid	$375.00	$118.12	$35.00	$0.00	$0.00	$83.12	$35.00	PDC
			Total	$406.60	$120.27	$35.00	$0.00	$0.00	$85.27	$35.00	

Remark Code: PDC—Billed amount is higher than the maximum payment insurance allows. The payment is for the allowed amount.

① **Service Description** is a description of the health care services you received, like a medical visit, lab tests, or screenings.

② **Provider Charges** is the amount your provider bills for your visit.

③ **Allowed Charges** is the amount your provider will be reimbursed; this may not be the same as the Provider Charges.

④ **Paid by Insurer** is the amount your insurance plan will pay to your provider.

⑤ **Payee** is the person who will receive any reimbursement for over-paying the claim.

⑥ **What You Owe** is the amount the patient or insurance plan member owes after your insurer has paid everything else. You may have already paid a portion of this amount, and payments made directly to your provider may not be subtracted from this amount.

⑦ **Remark Code** is a note from the insurance plan that explains more about the costs, charges, and paid amounts for your visit.

Contact your health plan if you have questions about your EOB.

CMS Product No.
11819 June 2014

Any outstanding balance that the patient does not pay becomes an accounts receivable for the provider. The larger the volume of patient services provided, the greater the balance of accounts receivable, which may total millions of dollars for large providers. A considerable amount of time may pass between the date of service, the processing of a claim, and the receipt of reimbursements for the service. For hospitals, the average number of days between a patient discharge and receipt of reimbursements from the patient and the insurers, if any, is 50 days (Ellison, 2014).

In order for a provider to pay employees and suppliers—and ultimately maintain its financial viability—effective patient accounts receivable management is crucial for health care providers. The movement toward electronic claims increased the speed that providers submit claims to third-party payers after treating patients, and decreased delays in processing claims. One survey of private insurance plans found that nearly 40 percent of paper-based claims, but only 8 percent of electronic claims, were received by the payer more than 60 days after the date of service. In addition, after they were received by the payer, just 79 percent of paper claims were processed (i.e., were paid, denied, or pending further information) within 14 days compared to 93 percent of electronic claims (AHIP, 2013).

A large majority of unpaid claims go uncollected. Each year, uncompensated care costs health care providers $84.9 billion, and accounts for 6 percent of hospital expenses in the United States (Coughlin, Holahan, Caswell, & McGrath, 2014; American Hospital Association [AHA], 2015b). Health care providers must determine whether to classify unpaid claims as charitable care or bad debt. Each provider will have their own criteria for this determination, and, for hospitals, written financial assistance policies are mandated under the ACA (Internal Revenue Service [IRS], 2016).

For Medicare beneficiaries who are unable to pay their coinsurance, the Medicare program reimburses hospital providers for a percentage of the bad debt. However, this percentage was reduced from 70 percent to 65 percent for non-critical access hospitals and from 100 percent to 65 percent for critical access hospitals under the Middle Class Tax Relief and Job Creation Act of 2012 (AHA, 2015a). Providers may engage the services of collections agencies for unpaid medical bills, but the recovery rate for these bills is low. The Association of Credit and Collection Professionals reports that only 15 cents out of each dollar is recovered for unpaid hospital bills (ACA International, n.d).

It is expected that total costs from uncompensated care may decline as more patients become eligible for Medicaid or sign up for private health insurance under the ACA. About 11 million more individuals were enrolled in Medicaid and CHIP beginning in 2014, primarily in states choosing to expand Medicaid eligibility under the ACA (Kaiser Commission on Medicaid and the Uninsured [KCMU], 2015).

Billing Disputes

Billing disputes arise and may delay reimbursements. Patients may dispute a medical bill for perceived or actual errors in billing. Providers may also dispute or appeal an insurer's decision regarding reimbursement of a claim. Each insurer will have their own procedures for filing an appeal, but in general, providers will need to file a written appeal stating reasons for the appeal and include supporting documents such as medical records and notes in addition to the patient's EOB. Aetna's process for appeals, for example, includes three stages: the initial request for reconsideration of the reimbursement or coding decision followed by two levels of appeals (Aetna, n.d.). Medicare has five levels to its appeals process for Part A or B claims, beginning with redetermination of the claim by the MAC, and possibly ending with judicial review by a U.S. District Court (CMS, 2015b). However, there is a minimum "amount in controversy" (AIC) that is required to proceed from Level 2 to 3 or from Level 4 to 5 in the Medicare appeals process. For Medicaid claims, each state program has its own process for providers to submit appeals. In general, the process of appealing claims decisions requires a significant investment of time on the part of the health care provider, and thus providers may be reluctant to file an appeal, particularly if the disputed amount is small.

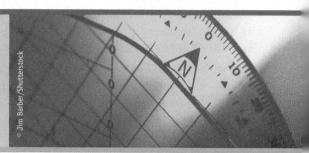

Summary

In this chapter, we reviewed the process of creating and submitting a claim for services rendered during a medical event. This included a review of the major diagnosis and procedure coding systems including International Classification of Diseases, 10th Revision (ICD-10), the American Medical Association's Current Procedural Terminology (CPT) system, and the Healthcare Common Procedure Coding System (HCPCS). Avoiding potential errors in the use of these systems is an important challenge for health care providers. We discussed the procedures for submitting claims to Medicare and other public and private insurers. Finally, we examined the collection of reimbursements from insurers and patients, including receipt of the Explanation of Benefits (EOB) form, receipt of funds, and billing disputes.

References

ACA International. (n.d.). *Healthcare collection statistics.* Retrieved from http://www.acainternational.org/products-healthcare-collection-statistics-5434.aspx

Aetna. (n.d.). *Disputes and appeals overview.* Retrieved from https://www.aetna.com/health-care-professionals/disputes-appeals/disputes-appeals-overview.html

American Hospital Association (AHA). (2015a, September 8). *Assistance to low-income Medicare beneficiaries (bad debt).* Retrieved from http://www.aha.org/content/13/fs-baddebt.pdf

American Hospital Association (AHA). (2015b, January). *Uncompensated hospital care cost fact sheet.* Retrieved from http://www.aha.org/content/15/uncompensated carefactsheet.pdf

America's Health Insurance Plans (AHIP). (2013, February). *An updated survey of health insurance claims receipt and processing times, 2011.* Washington, DC: Center for Policy and Research.

Centers for Medicare and Medicaid Services (CMS). (2007). *Third party liability in the Medicaid program.* Retrieved from https://www.cms.gov/regulations-and-guidance/legislation/deficitreductionact/downloads/tpl.pdf

Centers for Medicare and Medicaid Services (CMS). (2013, July 22). *HCPCS coding questions.* Retrieved from https://www.cms.gov/Medicare/Coding/MedHCPCSGenInfo/HCPCS_Coding_Questions.html

Centers for Medicare and Medicaid Services (CMS). (2014, October). *Medicare billing: 837P and form CMS-1500* (ICN 006976). Retrieved from https://www.cms.gov/Outreach-and-Education/Medicare-Learning-Network-MLN/MLNProducts/Downloads/837P-CMS-1500.pdf

Centers for Medicare and Medicaid Services (CMS). (2015a). *Medicare claim submission guidelines.* Retrieved from http://www.nacns.org/docs/CMS_ReimbursementClaim.pdf

Centers for Medicare and Medicaid Services (CMS). (2015b, February). *Medicare Parts A & B appeals process.* Retrieved from https://www.cms.gov/Outreach-and-Education/Medicare-Learning-Network-MLN/MLNProducts/downloads/MedicareAppealsprocess.pdf

Centers for Medicare and Medicaid Services (CMS). (2015c, February 25). *Transitioning to ICD-10.* Retrieved from https://www.cms.gov/Newsroom/MediaReleaseDatabase/Fact-sheets/2015-Fact-sheets-items/2015-02-25.html

Coughlin, T. A., Holahan, J., Caswell, K., & McGrath, M. (2014, May 30). *Uncompensated care for the uninsured in 2013: A detailed examination.* Retrieved from http://kff.org/uninsured/report/uncompensated-care-for-the-uninsured-in-2013-a-detailed-examination/

Ellison, A. (2014, October 1). *200 hospital benchmarks.* Retrieved from http://www.beckershospitalreview.com/lists/200-hospital-benchmarks.html

Internal Revenue Service (IRS). (n.d.). *New Requirements for 501(c)(3) hospitals under the Affordable Care Act.* Retrieved from https://www.irs.gov/charities-non-profits/charitable-organizations/new-requirements-for-501c3-hospitals-under-the-affordable-care-act

Kaiser Commission on Medicaid and the Uninsured (KCMU). (2015, March). *Recent trends in Medicaid and CHIP enrollment as of January 2015: Early findings from the CMS performance indicator project.* Retrieved http://files.kff.org/attachment/issue-brief-recent-trends-in-medicaid-and-chip-enrollment-as-of-january-2015-early-findings-from-the-cms-performance-indicator-project

King, M. S., Sharp, L., & Lipsky, M. S. (2001). Accuracy of CPT evaluation and management coding by family physicians. *Journal of the American Board of Family Medicine, 14*(3), 184–192.

National Center for Health Statistics (NCHS). (2015). *International Classification of Diseases, (ICD-10-CM/PCS) transition—Background*. Retrieved from http://www.cdc.gov/nchs/icd/icd10cm_pcs_background.htm

UnitedHealthcare. (2015). *Telemedicine policy*. Retrieved from https://www.unitedhealthcareonline.com/ccmcontent/ProviderII/UHC/en-US/Assets/ProviderStaticFiles/ProviderStaticFilesHtml/ReimbursementPolicies/Telemedicine_2016C.pdf

World Health Organization (WHO). (n.d.). *International Classification of Diseases*. Retrieved from http://www.who.int/classifications/icd/en/

CHAPTER 10

Benefits to People with Disabilities

Sara M. Ingram, MPA

Sara M. Ingram, MPA

LEARNING OBJECTIVES

- What are the differences between the social and medical definitions of disability?
- What are the eligibility criteria and benefits for SSDI and SSI?
- What are the eligibility criteria and benefits of workers' compensation programs?

INTRODUCTION

Just as health insurance does not insure against poor health, disability insurance does not insure against disability. In this chapter we outline several benefit programs that insure against financial hardship because of a person's inability to work due to a disabling condition. We also discuss the health insurance and medical coverage available to people who receive benefits through these programs.

People with disabilities who are uninsured may face substantial unmet health needs (Mahmoudi & Meade, 2015; Yee & Breslin, 2010). One way to fill this gap is through the Social Security Administration (SSA) programs, which may qualify this population for Medicare or Medicaid coverage with monthly subsidies. Another way is through state level workers' compensation or federal programs for specific conditions, all with differing health insurance coverage. Each of

these programs are explained in this chapter, but first we must define disability.

DEFINING DISABILITY

There are many ways to define **disability**, both theoretically and clinically. Of course, there are different degrees of disability, but how disability is framed can influence how a person with a disability is treated in society or by another person.

The medical model views disability as a problem with the individual that can be fixed, whereas the social model views disability as a problem of social and environmental barriers that are imposed on individuals. For example, suppose a classmate is in a terrible car crash. Thankfully,

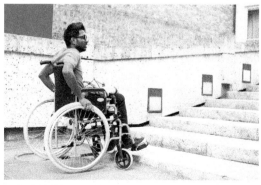

© Michaelpuche/Shutterstock

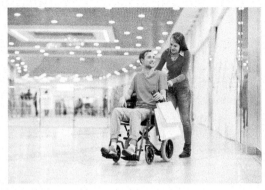

© Pressmaster/Shutterstock

everyone survived and now your classmate uses a wheelchair to get around. What if the only way to get to class is by a flight of stairs? The medical model perspective is that your classmate is the problem, but the social model perspective argues that the stairs are the problem. Take away the stairs and everyone can get to class.

So how do organizations and agencies define disability? The World Health Organization (WHO) follows a social model by defining disability as a complex phenomenon that is influenced by more than the individual's health (WHO, 2016). The Social Security Administration considers a person disabled if they cannot engage in substantial gainful activity due to a medically determinable physical or mental impairment that has lasted or is expected to last for at least one year, or is expected to result in death (Social Security Administration [SSA], n.d.b).

Another way to define disability is by how a person functions in activities of daily living

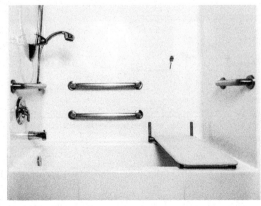

© Ben Carlson/Shutterstock

(ADL) or instrumental activities of daily living (iADL). ADLs include basic self-care such as bathing, dressing, and eating, and iADLs include behaviors such as shopping, socializing, and driving. The SSA may ask about ADLs and iADLs to supplement clinical diagnoses of disability in determining eligibility for benefits (SSA, n.d.a).

Another way to think about disability is that it is common. The SSA projects that more than one in four people who are 20 years old now will be disabled before they are 67 (Altman & Kingson, 2015). How many people do you know who wear glasses or contact lenses to see better? In the United States and all over the world, it is estimated that 60 percent of people either already do or should wear glasses to improve their eyesight (Bruggink, 2013). Rather than thinking about disability as atypical, it is really quite normal.

Even though disability is prevalent, there are significant health and other notable disparities between people with and without disabilities. For example, people with disabilities have a high incidence of secondary health conditions because of their disability (White, Gutierrez, & Seekins, 1996). Also, 32 percent of working-age people with disabilities are employed compared to 72 percent of non-disabled people (United States Department of Labor, n.d.b). The lower employment rate means that people with disabilities tend to be poor (Mahmoudi & Meade, 2015). These differences point to the importance of benefits available to people with disabilities.

People with disabilities constitute a disproportionate share of expenditures for Medicaid. They represent 43 percent of costs but just 15 percent of beneficiaries. Compare this number to non-disabled children, who represent 21 percent of costs, but 49 percent of beneficiaries (Morrisey, 2013). However, it is also important to note that not all people with disabilities have health insurance coverage through government programs. In fact, 41 percent of working-age people with disabilities have health insurance from private insurers (Smith & Medalia, 2015).

PROGRAMS ADMINISTERED BY THE SOCIAL SECURITY ADMINISTRATION

Most working-age people with disabilities have some type of health coverage. Nearly 90 percent of people with disabilities have health insurance and of those, more than half have government-provided health insurance coverage (Smith & Medalia, 2015). There are two types of disability programs available through the SSA: Social Security Disability Insurance and Supplemental Security Income.

Social Security Disability Insurance (SSDI) provides benefits to individuals with disabilities, and in some cases to family members of the benefit recipient, if that person worked a certain number of years paying Social Security Taxes. Two years after SSDI benefits are awarded, recipients are automatically enrolled in Medicare Parts A and B (Centers for Medicare and Medicaid Services [CMS], n.d.b). SSDI is also for adults who have had their disability since before the age of 22 and are eligible for benefits through their parents' income history; we discuss this more later in this chapter.

Social Security Income (SSI), on the other hand, is a means-tested program that supplies benefits based on financial need to individuals and their dependents. People on SSI are immediately enrolled in Medicaid. Although both SSDI and SSI originate from the SSA, they are separate programs for different categories of people with disabilities that are funded by distinct sources.

Some key distinctions between SSDI and SSI are highlighted in Table 10-1.

Applying for SSDI or SSI

To apply to receive SSDI or SSI benefits, one must first provide evidence that they have a medically determinable physical or mental impairment, and second they must meet the substantial gainful activity level. Claimants must apply directly with medical records and other proof of disability. The primary difference between SSDI and SSI is the previous work requirement for SSDI and the income level for SSI. When individuals apply for SSDI, they are also screened for SSI eligibility. Because the time to receive benefits is shorter for SSI, some people may be put in this program while they are waiting for SSDI benefits (The ALS Association, 2016). Additionally, a person may concurrently be in both programs (SSA, 2016a). It should be noted that the SSDI monthly benefit

TABLE 10-1 **Key Differences Between SSDI and SSI**

	SSDI	SSI
Must have paid Social Security tax to qualify?	Yes.	No.
Disability benefits for children?	Only adult children at least 18 years old and disabled before age 22.	Children of any age.
Waiting period before benefits begin?	For adults 5 months, for children no.	No.
Health insurance comes with disability benefits?	Yes, Medicare after 2 years.	Yes, Medicaid starts immediately in most states.
Can be "presumed disabled" before actual approval of benefits?	No.	Yes, up to 6 months before decision. Claimant does not have to return payments if deemed not disabled.
Minimum duration of disability?	12 months.	12 months (blind claimants are exempt from duration requirement).
Benefits to non-U.S. citizens?	Yes.	Generally no, but with some exceptions.

Data from: Morton, David (2010). Comparing SSDI and SSI. Nolo's guide to social security disability: Getting and keeping your benefits. *Nolo*. p. 11.

is generally higher and has fewer periodic reviews than SSI. Therefore, SSDI is generally considered a more desirable program compared to SSI and the application process is more rigorous. Not everyone who applies to either program is awarded with benefits.

The SSA suggests that a person who wants to apply for benefits use the online disability planner at https://www.ssa.gov/planners/disability/. The planner will provide applicants with the following information about the program (SSA, n.d.a):

- How you can qualify and apply for benefits
- What happens if your application is approved
- Who can receive benefits on your earnings record
- What you need to know about receiving disability benefits
- When Medicare coverage starts for Social Security disability beneficiaries

The SSA "Blue Book" is an extensive listing of impairments for adults (Part A) and children (Part B) that may be considered eligible disabilities, but the list does not cover every condition, nor do listed conditions guarantee benefits (SSA, n.d.c, n.d.d). The SSA encourages those who feel they qualify for benefits to apply either online, by phone, or in person at a local Social Security Office. According to the SSA, processing an application will take several months.

For applicants who are awarded with either benefit program, both SSDI and SSI have incentives for beneficiaries to return to work. Once the SSA pays the beneficiary a certain amount, the agency may reduce or even discontinue benefits, including reductions in Medicare and Medicaid coverage. Details on incentive-to-work programs for SSDI and SSI recipients are not covered in this chapter, but information can be found in the SSA document *Working While Disabled: How We Can Help.*

Applicants rejected from disability benefits may file an appeal. The Office of Adjudication and Review (ODAR) manages claim hearings.

In general, there are four levels of appeal (Social Security Administration, 2015a):

- Reconsideration
- Hearing by an administrative law judge
- Review by the Appeals Council
- Federal Court review

Social Security Disability Insurance

The SSDI program goes by other names. It is sometimes called "Disability Insurance" or "DI," "Social Security benefits," "Social Security Disability Benefits," "Social Security Disability Program," "Social Security Disability" or "SSD," "Disability Benefits," or in context simply "Disability." For the purpose of this chapter, we will refer to it by Social Security Disability Insurance and by its acronym, SSDI.

As previously explained, SSDI is for people with disabilities who have worked and paid into Social Security through income taxes. An applicant's work history will be reviewed along with their medically determinable physical or mental impairment that must have lasted a year or more or be expected to continue for at least that long or until death. Work history is commensurate with age. In general, to qualify for SSDI, applicants must have worked between a year and half (for those whose disability began before age 28) and 9.5 years (for those whose disability began before age 60). Because our concern here is health insurance, it is important to stress that those awarded SSDI must wait to become eligible for Medicare coverage until 2 years after the SSDI benefit is awarded.

If the SSA finds that a claimant is qualified, then it will pass on the application to the Disability Determination Services (DDS) office in the state where the applicant lives. This state-level agency takes over the disability eligibility determination for the SSA and gathers and manages all medical reports and related information. The local DDS office does this by contacting the applicant's doctors and other related professionals.

A person's doctor can make a case for eligibility, but even if the doctor believes that the applicant's disabling condition makes his or her patient eligible for SSDI, it is the DDS office who is responsible for making the determination. If the DDS office cannot make a decision about eligibility from the inquiry, then the state office can request that the claimant go for a special examination. The SSA pays for the cost of the exam and travel to the examination.

After the DDS office makes a decision, the SSA will send the applicant a letter either granting benefits or rejecting the application. If the application is accepted, the letter will state the effective date and the monthly amount awarded, which is based on average lifetime earnings. Because a person's condition can change over time, continuing disability review can occur after one, three, or seven years depending on the original reason for awarding benefits. In general, if the same condition persists, there will not be a break in benefits.

Some adults with disabilities who have had their impairment since before the age of 22 may be entitled to SSDI under the "Child's Benefit," sometimes called "Disabled Adult Child" or "DAC" benefit. It is available to adults who have not worked under SSDI eligibility criteria, but whose parents did. A beneficiaries' parent(s) must be receiving retirement benefits, on SSDI themselves, or be deceased. (SSA, 2016b).

As shown in **Figure 10-1**, SSDI claims fluctuate over time with changes to eligibility requirements, state funding for workers' compensation programs, and workforce participation (Milligan, 2012; Reno, Williams, & Sengupta, 2003/2004). A recipient of SSDI can age-out of the program and transition to Social Security benefits. In this case, the funding for that person switches from the Disability Insurance Trust Fund to the Old-Age and Survivors Insurance (OASI) Trust Fund (Altman & Kingson, 2015; SSA, 2005/2006).

FIGURE 10-1 Trends in SSDI Applications and Accepted Claims

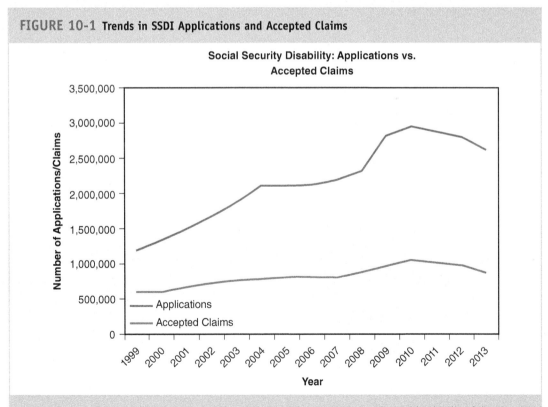

Supplemental Security Income

Eligibility for Supplemental Security Income, sometimes referred to as "SSI disability benefits," is determined based on an applicant's household income and assets and whether the applicant meets SSA's definition of disability. After reaching age 65, a person on SSI can remain in the program and receive Social Security benefits. Non-disabled people 65 and over who fall below the income and asset thresholds may also be eligible for SSI, but there are some differences in benefits compared to those awarded to disabled beneficiaries.

Some children who are disabled and from low-income households may also be eligible for SSI, though eligibility determination will be different for adults because the SSA usually makes disability determinations based on the ability to work. Like adults, children may qualify for SSI if they have had a disability, or are expected to have a disability, for a year or until death. The disability must severely limit the child's activities. Children in special education are not automatically eligible for SSI and children with disabilities who are not in special education are not necessarily ineligible (SSA, 2016b; Netter, 2016).

When a child is awarded with SSI benefits, the SSA will provide the parents or guardians with information on where the recipient can receive health care services. States refer to these services by different names, but are usually called Children's Special Health Services, Children's Medical Services, or Handicapped Children's Program. The SSA will continue to grant benefits to children with medical conditions that will not improve. The SSA performs periodic reviews for recipients until 18 years of age and for infants with low birth weights until their first birthday (SSA, 2016b).

In most states, children who receive SSI payments qualify for Medicaid; in many states, Medicaid enrollment comes automatically with SSI eligibility. In general, Medicaid eligibility is more generous for children than for adults, even those not receiving SSI benefits (SSA, 2016b).

Supplements to SSA Programs

There are some conditions that fall outside the criteria and rules for SSA programs. The SSA uses the Quick Disability Determination process to screen these cases that should be expedited.

Compassionate Allowances

For certain conditions, including many cancers, early-onset Alzheimer's disease, and stroke, the SSA expedites benefits under Compassionate Allowances.

Blind or Low Vision

People who are blind or have low vision are eligible for SSDI or SSI at a higher rate of benefits. The SSA defines a person as blind if vision cannot be corrected to better than 20/200 in at least one eye or if a person's visual field is 20 degrees or less in the better eye (SSA, 2016c). Work rules differ for blind individuals compared to other benefit recipients.

End-Stage Renal Disease

Individuals with end-stage renal disease, also called kidney failure, who are undergoing dialysis, are on a kidney transplant list, or who have received a transplant, are eligible for Medicare coverage starting either at the first month or three months after dialysis begins (CMS, n.d.a).

Terminal Illness

Often referred to as "TERI cases," the Social Security Administration describes a person with a terminal illness as a medical condition that is untreatable and expected to result in death (SSA, 2015b). The Disability Determination Services expedites terminal applicants. Several conditions are categorized as terminal illness, such as Lou Gehrig's Disease, also known as Amyotrophic Lateral Sclerosis (ALS), and liver cancer. If a person is diagnosed with ALS, Medicare is available as soon as SSDI benefits are awarded (The ALS Association, 2016).

Navigating SSDI and SSI Applications and Appeals

Applying for SSDI and SSI can be intimidating for many people. According to the SSA, an applicant may appoint a qualified representative for the application and appeals processes.

The representative cannot charge a fee without getting approval from the SSA (SSA, n.d.e) and attorneys work on contingency, so they only collect a fee when applicants are awarded SSDI (Dickey, 2016).

As we noted previously, there are several levels of appeal. Fewer than 50 percent of applicants for SSDI are awarded benefits at the first level; however, applicants can increase the chance of success with each level of appeal (SSA, n.d.f). Legal counsel can improve odds of success of being awarded benefits as applicants advance to higher stages of the appeal process. Thus, while the process may be daunting, it may be worth the time and effort to appeal.

There are several organizations that support SSDI applicants (see Table 10-2). The National Alliance on Mental Illness (NAMI) receives about 10,000 calls a year related to SSDI benefits (Venuti, 2013). The private non-attorney service company Allsup assists individuals and organizations with SSDI applications. The National Organization of Social Security Claimants' Representatives (NOSSCR) is an association for attorneys and advocates who represent people with disabilities and acts as a referral service for applicants during the adjudication process. Finally, local department of aging offices may also be contacted for support. It should be noted that the SSA will not assist a claimant with the appeals process.

WORKERS' COMPENSATION AND FEDERAL PROGRAMS FOR WORKERS

There are two types of benefits paid to employees who are injured on the job or have a disabling condition because of their work. Workers' compensation is a state-administered program with many variances in required coverage from state to state. There are also federally administered programs for certain types of workers. We outline each of these here.

Workers' Compensation

State workers' compensation programs and federally administered programs for certain types of workers, typically referred to as "workers' comp," are benefits paid to employees who are injured on the job or acquired a disabling condition because of their work. This benefit program started as part of the Industrial Revolution as work on railroads and in mines became increasingly dangerous. By 1915, 32 states required employers to have workers' compensation programs (Morrisey, 2013), and now all do except Oklahoma and Texas.

For all states with a workers' compensation program, required coverage depends on the type of worker and the employer. All participating states provide short-term disability, but only some provide long-term disability. Traumatic injuries are covered in all participating state programs, but eligibility for other conditions varies by state.

TABLE 10-2 Selected Organizations That Support SSDI Applicants

Administration for Community Living	http://www.acl.gov/
Allsup	https://www.allsup.com/
Disabled In Action: Links	http://www.disabledinaction.org/links.html
Kessler Foundation: Resources and Educational Materials	https://kesslerfoundation.org/consumersandfamilies/resourcesandeducationalmaterials
National Council on Disability	http://www.ncd.gov/
National Council on Independent Living	http://www.ncil.org/
The National Alliance on Mental Illness	http://www.nami.org/
The National Organization of Social Security Claimants' Representatives	https://www.nosscr.org/

For example, New York state requires coverage for both on- and off-the-job injuries for workers, but Texas does not mandate private employers to have workers' compensation coverage (New York State, n.d.a, n.d.b; Texas Department of Insurance, 2016).

Federal Programs Under the Office of Workers' Compensation

The Office of Workers' Compensation, under the United States Department of Labor, oversees several disability compensation programs for workers that have varying levels of health insurance coverage.

Energy Employees Occupational Illness Compensation

The Energy Employees Occupational Illness Compensation (EEOIC) program covers employees of the Department of Energy and related agencies who are diagnosed with health conditions from exposure to radiation, beryllium, or silica. There are several local resource centers throughout the country that assist with applications to one of four EEOIC District Offices. These regional EEOIC District Offices determine eligibility and process claims. Final Adjudication Branch offices, located within the four District Offices, independently review the decisions (U.S. Department of Labor, n.d.a).

A benefit recipient is entitled to reasonable cost medical coverage for accepted health conditions by medical providers who are enrolled in EEOIC. Illnesses due to the primary diagnosis are also covered. Once a person is enrolled in the program, a benefits card is issued that includes the diagnosis code for all applicable health conditions. Not all services are covered, and some medical expenses may be covered, but require approval. Most prescription drugs are covered. Only EEOIC should be billed for treatment of the accepted conditions (U.S Department of Labor, n.d.c).

Division of Federal Employees' Compensation

The Division of Federal Employees' Compensation (DFEC) provides medical and other benefits to all federal employees for occupational-related injury or illness. This includes postal workers and federal employees working in and out of the United States. Entitlements are made through determinations using the American Medical Association Guides to the Evaluation of Permanent Impairment. The DFEC makes decisions on claims, manages existing cases, pays medical bills, and assists employees to return to work. Claims are made to 1 of 12 district offices. According to DFEC, decisions are made within 45 days for traumatic injury claims. Decisions for occupational illnesses, depending on complexity, may take from 90 days to 10 months. Medical bills can be submitted by providers or by claimants, and will be processed within 1 month of receipt (U.S. Department of Labor, n.d.d, n.d.e).

Longshore and Harbor Workers' Compensation

The Longshore and Harbor Workers' Compensation (LHWC) provides workers compensation benefits under four laws: Longshore and Harbor Workers' Compensation Act (LHWCA); Defense Base Act (DBA); Non-Appropriated Fund Instrumentalities Act (NAFIA); and Outer Continental Shelf Lands Act (OCSLA). Applicants do not apply for benefits through LHWC, rather it serves to provide assistance to beneficiaries for employers it authorizes and regulates. Employees falling under the jurisdiction of LHWC that become disabled or injured should contact their employer, or its insurance company, who will cover medical costs.

Black Lung Benefits Act

Coal miners who become disabled due to coal workers' pneumoconiosis (CWP), or black lung disease are eligible for medical coverage related to this diagnosis through the Black Lung Benefits Act (BLBA). These benefits include prescription drugs, hospital services, and doctors' visits. Other benefits are available with a doctor's prescription, such as home oxygen and pulmonary rehabilitation.

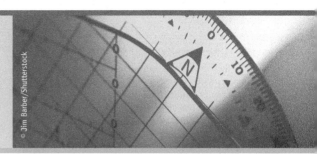

Summary

Disability insurance protects against financial insecurity because of a person's inability to work due to a disabling condition. Definitions of disability can determine a person's eligibility to receive benefits and health insurance coverage or medical care from some programs. We have explained what makes people with disabilities eligible for SSDI and SSI, the two programs administered by the SSA, and how to apply for benefits and appeal decisions. We gave an overview of state-level workers' compensation and you learned about the four federal programs for certain types of workers. While SSDI is an "earned" benefit, financed by payroll taxes, SSI is financed by general revenues. Worker's compensation, on the other hand, is paid directly by employers, though employees likely bear some cost by earning lower wages.

References

The ALS Association. (2016). *A professional's guide to assisting families with obtaining government benefits: What benefits are available to the disabled through Social Security?* Retrieved from http://www.alsa.org/als-care/resources/publications-videos/factsheets/professionals-guide-govt-benefits.html

Altman, N., & Kingson, E. (2015). *Social Security works!: Why Social Security isn't going broke and how expanding it will help us all.* New York, NY: The New Press.

Bruggink, J. W. (2013). *More than 6 in 10 people wear glasses or contact lenses.* Retrieved from https://www.cbs.nl/en-gb/news/2013/38/more-than-6-in-10-people-wear-glasses-or-contact-lenses

Centers for Medicare & Medicaid Services (CMS). (n.d.a). *How to sign up for Medicare if you have End-Stage Renal Disease (ESRD).* Retrieved from https://www.medicare.gov/people-like-me/esrd/getting-medicare-with-esrd.html#collapse-3166

Centers for Medicare & Medicaid Services (CMS). (n.d.b). *You may get Part A & Part B automatically if you have a disability.* Retrieved from https://www.medicare.gov/people-like-me/disability/get-a-and-b-automatically-disability.html

Dickey, E. (2016). *How much does a Social Security Disability lawyer cost?* Retrieved from http://www.nolo.com/legal-encyclopedia/how-much-does-social-security-disability-lawyer-cost.html

Mahmoudi, E., & Meade, M. A. (2015). Physical disabilities: Analysis of a representative national sample for a ten-year period. *Disability and Health Journal, 8,* 182–190.

Milligan, K. (2012). The long-run growth of disability insurance in the United States. In D. A. Wise (Ed.), *Social Security programs and retirement around the world: Historical trends in mortality and health, employment, and disability insurance participation and reforms* (pp. 359–389). Chicago, IL: University of Chicago Press. Retrieved from http://www.nber.org/chapters/c12391.pdf

Morrisey, M. (2013). *Health insurance* (2nd ed.). Chicago, IL: Health Administration Press.

Netter, L. (2016). *Disability benefits for children.* Retrieved from http://www.disabilitysecrets.com/page6-4.html

New York State Workers' Compensation Board. (n.d.a). *What are disability benefits?* Retrieved from http://www.wcb.ny.gov/content/main/offthejob/IntroToLaw_DB.jsp

New York State Workers' Compensation Board. (n.d.b). *Understanding workers' compensation insurance.* Retrieved from http://www.wcb.ny.gov/content/main/Employers/understandInsurance.jsp

Reno, C. V., Williams, T., & Sengupta, I. (2003/2004). Workers' compensation, Social Security Disability Insurance, and the offset: A fact sheet. *Social Security Bulletin, 65*(4). Retrieved from https://www.ssa.gov/policy/docs/ssb/v65n4/v65n4p3.html

Smith, J. C., & Medalia, C. (2015). *Health insurance coverage in the United States: 2014 current population reports.* U.S. Department of Commerce, Economics and Statistics Administration, U.S. Census Bureau. Retrieved from http://www.census.gov/content/dam/Census/library/publications/2015/demo/p60-253.pdf

Social Security Administration (SSA). (2005/2006). A primer: Social Security Act programs to assist the disabled. *Social Security Bulletin, 66*(3). Retrieved from https://www.ssa.gov/policy/docs/ssb/v66n3/v66n3p53.html

Social Security Administration (SSA). (2015a). *The appeals process.* SSA Publication No. 05-10041. Retrieved from https://www.ssa.gov/pubs/EN-05-10041.pdf

Social Security Administration (SSA). (2015b). *Program Operations Manual System (POMS): DI 23020.045 terminal illness (TERI) cases.* Retrieved from https://secure.ssa.gov/poms.nsf/lnx/0423020045

Social Security Administration (SSA). (2016a). *2016 Red Book: Example of concurrent benefits with employment supports*. Retrieved from https://www.ssa.gov/redbook/eng/supportsexample.htm

Social Security Administration (SSA). (2016b). *Benefits for children with disabilities*. SSA Publication No. 05-10026. Retrieved from https://www.ssa.gov/pubs/EN-05-10026.pdf

Social Security Administration (SSA). (2016c). *If you're blind or have low vision—How we can help*. SSA Publication No. 05-10052. Retrieved from https://www.ssa.gov/pubs/EN-05-10052.pdf

Social Security Administration (SSA). (n.d.a). *Disability planner: Social Security protection if you become disabled*. Retrieved from https://www.ssa.gov/planners/disability/

Social Security Administration (SSA). (n.d.b). *Disability planner: What we mean by disability*. Retrieved from https://www.ssa.gov/planners/disability/dqualify4.html

Social Security Administration (SSA). (n.d.c). *Medical/professional relations, disability evaluation under Social Security, listing of impairments—Adult listings (Part A)*. Retrieved from https://www.ssa.gov/disability/professionals/bluebook/AdultListings.htm

Social Security Administration (SSA). (n.d.d). *Medical/professional relations, disability evaluation under Social Security, listing of impairments—Childhood listings (Part B)*. Retrieved from https://www.ssa.gov/disability/professionals/bluebook/ChildhoodListings.htm

Social Security Administration (SSA). (n.d.e). *Representing Social Security claimants*. Retrieved from https://www.ssa.gov/representation/index.htm

Social Security Administration (SSA). (n.d.f). *Selected data from Social Security's disability program*. Retrieved from https://www.ssa.gov/oact/STATS/dibStat.html#f2

Texas Department of Insurance. (2016, July). *Workers' compensation insurance*. Retrieved from http://www.tdi.texas.gov/pubs/consumer/cb030.html

U.S. Department of Labor. (n.d.a). *Division of Energy employees occupational illness compensation (DEEOIC)*. Retrieved from https://www.dol.gov/owcp/energy/regs/compliance/roles.htm

U.S. Department of Labor. (n.d.b). *Economic picture of the disability community project: Key points on disability and occupational projections tables*. Retrieved from https://www.dol.gov/odep/pdf/20141022-KeyPoints.pdf

U.S. Department of Labor. (n.d.c). *How will my EEOICP medical benefits be paid?* Division of Energy Employees Occupational Illness Compensation. Retrieved from https://www.dol.gov/owcp/energy/regs/compliance/brochure/medicalqaform.pdf

U.S. Department of Labor. (n.d.d). *Information for injured workers and their representatives*. Division of Federal Employees' Compensation (DFEC). Retrieved from https://www.dol.gov/owcp/dfec/regs/compliance/infoinjuredwrkers.htm

U.S. Department of Labor. (n.d.c). *Medical provider*. Division of Federal Employees' Compensation (DFEC). Retrieved from https://www.dol.gov/owcp/dfec/medicalprovider.htm

Venuti, T. (2013). *Understanding Social Security Disability Insurance*. National Alliance on Mental Illness. Retrieved from https://www.nami.org/About-NAMI/NAMI-News/Understanding-Social-Security-Disability-Insurance

White, G. W, Gutierrez, R. T., & Seekins, T. (1996). Preventing and managing secondary conditions: A proposed role for independent living centers. *The Journal of Rehabilitation*, *62*(3), 14.

World Health Organization (WHO). (2016). *Health topics: Disabilities*. Retrieved from http://www.who.int/topics/disabilities/en/

Yee, S., & Breslin, M. L. (2010). Achieving accessible health care for people with disabilities: Why the ADA is only part of the solution. *Disability and Health Journal*, *3*, 253–261.

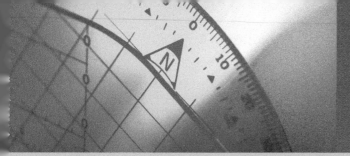

CHAPTER 11

Long-Term Care

Sarah R. Swanson BS Ed and Jim P. Stimpson, PhD

LEARNING OBJECTIVES

- What is long-term care, and how does it get financed?
- Who needs long-term services and supports?
- What challenges does the United States face in the coming decades in providing long-term care?

INTRODUCTION

Individuals with disabilities and seniors sometimes need assistance to complete daily activities. Their needs may include long-term services and supports. This chapter will provide a basic overview of long-term care, including how it gets financed, who it supports, where it is provided, and who provides it, as well as the expenses that comprise long-term care. This chapter will also discuss federal and state financing reforms to extend long-term care coverage to more individuals.

WHAT IS LONG-TERM CARE?

Long-term care is assistance with everyday medical and social tasks for individuals with chronic conditions. Most long-term care is not medical care but instead provides assistance with basic personal tasks of everyday life. Long-term services and supports can be provided through nursing facility care, adult daycare programs, home health aide services, personal care services, transportation, and employment supports, as well as assistance provided by a family caregiver. Care may be informal (unpaid) or formal (paid) care (Reaves & Musumeci, 2015).

FINANCING OF LONG-TERM CARE

Because the United States does not have a national program that provides long-term care, family caregivers make up the backbone of the long-term care system. However, the single largest financing source for long-term care is Medicaid. Medicare and private insurers generally provide much more limited coverage than Medicaid for long-term care services. In 2013 the United States spent $338.8 billion on long-term care. Medicaid paid for 43 percent of this care, the largest share by far. Next, Medicare paid 22 percent, as this program has some limited coverage, which we will discuss. Out-of-pocket funds accounted for 17 percent of spending, while private insurance accounted for just 6 percent. Other sources of publically funded care constituted 7 percent of spending and included programs such as the Veterans Administration and the Children's Health Insurance Program. Other private sources, including philanthropic programs and other types of insurance, constituted 6 percent of spending (Colello & Talaga, 2015). See **Figure 11-1** for a breakdown of long-term care spending. See **Table 11-1** for a list of the estimated monthly costs associated with long-term care.

FIGURE 11-1 Long-Term Care Spending

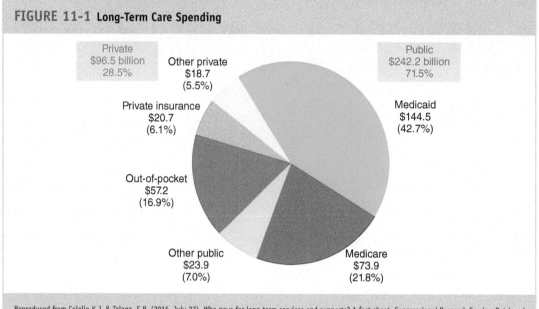

Medicaid

Medicaid is the largest payer of long-term care. Medicaid provides coverage to low-income individuals, especially low-income seniors and individuals with disabilities. Although coverage varies by state, Medicaid, unlike private coverage or Medicare, generally covers institutional long-term care and community-based services, though not all providers accept Medicaid as a form of payment. Medicaid also provides extra help for millions of low-income Medicare beneficiaries, known as "dual eligibles," assisting them with Medicare premiums and cost-sharing and covering additional services, especially long-term care, that Medicare excludes or limits (The Henry J. Kaiser Family Foundation [KFF], 2013).

While nursing home or institutional care has always been a required benefit for Medicaid (Colello, 2013), individuals with disabilities and advocates have pushed back against this institutional bias and demanded coverage for home- and community-based services (HCBS) (National Council on Independent Living, n.d.). The National Council on Independent Living advocates that individuals should be allowed to remain in their homes, that long-term care services should allow for choice, and that HCBS are less expensive than institutional care. Subsequent reforms have been successful in allowing states to cover HCBS. The 1990 passage of the

TABLE 11-1 Estimated Monthly Cost of Long-Term Care

United States (National Median)	
Monthly Cost	2016
Home Health Care	
Homemaker Services	$3,813
Homemaker Health Aide	$3,861
Adult Day Health Care	
Adult Day Health Care	$1,473
Assisted Living Facility	
Private, One Bedroom	$3,628
Nursing Home Care	
Semi-Private Room	$6,844
Private Room	$7,698

Data from: Genworth. Compare Long Term Care Costs Across the United States. Genworth Cost of Care Survey. Retrieved from https://www.genworth.com/about-us/industry -expertise/cost-of-care.html

Americans with Disabilities Act (ADA) and the 1999 Supreme Court ruling in Olmstead v. L.C. helped reinforce the rights of individuals with disabilities to obtain care in their desired setting.

Lois Curtis and Elaine Wilson were two women with mental illness and intellectual and developmental disabilities who voluntary entered a state psychiatric hospital in Georgia for treatment. Upon completion of their treatment, they were told that there were no services available in a less restrictive setting and the women were held at the hospital. They filed suit seeking alternative placement. After a five-year court battle, the case was heard by the United States Supreme Court. In 1999, the court ruled that the unjustified institutional isolation of people with disabilities is a form of unlawful discrimination and violates the ADA. The Olmstead ruling established precedent for the delivery of state-based services—specifically that there must be choice, and that individuals with disabilities must be served in the least restrictive environment, which supports the movement toward HCBS (Department of Justice, 2016).

State Variation in Medicaid

States can offer a variety of medical and non-medical services under various Medicaid waiver programs, such as 1915(c) waivers, 1115 Demonstration waivers, and through the Medicaid state plan. Under Medicaid, the state will pay a portion of these costs, which will be matched by the federal government. While there are required Medicaid services, states have flexibility in the design and eligibility. Waiver services can include case management (i.e., supports and service coordination), home-maker services, home health aide, personal care, adult day health services, habilitation (both day and residential), employment supports, and respite care. States may also propose other types of services that may assist in diverting or transitioning individuals from institutional settings into their homes and community (Centers for Medicare and Medicaid Services [CMS], n.d.a).

Medicaid is a means-tested program, but states may adopt special rules to provide services for individuals who require long-term care. For example, states may offer a Medicaid buy-in for working people with disabilities so that they can work without losing their benefits, such as Supplemental Security Income (SSI) and Medicaid (CMS, n.d.b). States may extend financial eligibility for people who need long-term care up to 300 percent of the SSI level through the special income rule. Additionally, the Affordable Care Act (ACA) provides states with an option to provide HCBS to people with functional limitations but who do not yet require an institutional level of care (Reaves & Musumeci, 2015). The ACA also provides increased financial incentives for states to shift more long-term care services out of institutional settings and into the community (KFF, 2013).

Medicare

Medicare provides only limited coverage for long-term care. For example, it pays for care in a nursing home or skilled nursing facility for only up to 100 days after a hospitalization. It covers home health services only for beneficiaries who are homebound, but does not cover personal care services (CMS, n.d.c). Hospice care is covered for individuals who have a terminal illness (CMS, 2016).

For additional information about the Medicare Program, individuals can contact the State Health Insurance Assistance Program (SHIP) in their state. SHIPs provide free counseling about Medicare plans and coverage benefits. Additionally, the SHIP National Technical Assistance Center serves as a central source of information for and about the national State Health Insurance Assistance Program. The center serves as a resource to each of the state programs and also to the general public.

Private Health Insurance

While actual coverage amounts vary by plan, most private health insurance plans will pay for institutional care after a hospitalization or injury,

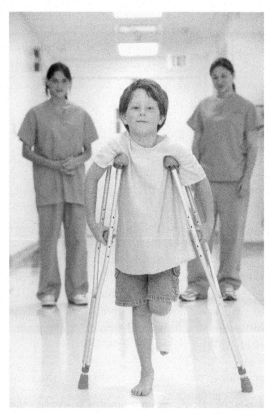

© Blend Images/Shutterstock

but, like Medicare, will not pay for long-term care (United States Department of Health and Human Services [HHS], n.d.a). An important provision of the ACA included rehabilitation and habilitation as essential health benefit categories. While rehabilitation was a widely recognized health service, habilitation was often not covered because it was considered an educational service. Habilitation is defined as a service or device that helps an individual learn or maintain skills. This new coverage category is especially important for children who are not hitting developmental milestones such as walking or talking and may benefit from therapies to help them improve or maintain skills.

Private Long-Term Care Insurance

Long-term care insurance policies are specifically designed to reimburse policyholders for long-term care services that are not covered by health insurance. Premiums are determined by the policy holder's age, health status, and benefits.

The applicant will sometimes be required to undergo a medical exam.

Most individuals buy long-term care policies from an insurance agent, a financial planner, or broker (HHS, n.d.d). However, long-term care policies may also be purchased through an employer or union. Typically, when employers offer this benefit, they do not pay a portion of the premium but have negotiated a favorable group rate (HHS, n.d.d).

Private long-term care insurance initially began as nursing facility insurance and has been available for about 30 years; however, the market for this insurance product is relatively small. Fewer than nine million Americans have private long-term care insurance coverage, and the average annual premium for an individual policy is $2,283 (Reaves & Musumeci, 2015). Concerns about long-term care insurance prices and lack of understanding of long-term care expenses and financing have likely limited wider adoption of these insurance policies.

Other Financing for Long-Term Care

Other mechanisms are available to finance long-term care. Reverse mortgages, for example, allow seniors to receive cash against the value of their home without selling it. Individuals are required to pay back the loan when they move or sell their home, so a drop in the value of their home may make it difficult to pay back the loan. Further, if the loan is in a spouse's name and the spouse dies, then the balance of the loan is due and may force the living heir out of their home (Huffman, 2015; Rosenblatt, 2012). While reverse mortgages can help finance long-term care, individuals must understand the risks and benefits.

Some life insurance plans offer an accelerated, pre-tax death benefit that individuals may use prior to death. Additionally, some plans allow beneficiaries to buy out benefits for cash, or, if beneficiaries are terminally ill, to sell their plans to a third party (HHS, n.d.c). Exercising these options may impact Medicaid eligibility and have adverse tax implications. Some insurance companies are combining long-term care policies with life insurance through special riders so that beneficiaries do not have to give up their death benefits to finance long-term care.

Finally, annuities are contracts in which individuals give an insurance company money that is later distributed back to the person over time. Annuity contracts traditionally provide a guaranteed distribution of income over time until death or a specified date, whichever comes first (HHS, n.d.b). This income distribution can be used to help finance long-term care costs.

WHO NEEDS LONG-TERM SERVICES AND SUPPORTS?

More than 12 million Americans with functional impairments relied on some form of long-term services and supports (LTSS) provided either in their home and community or in an institution (U.S. Senate Report to Congress, 2013). People who rely on LTSS are almost equally split between adults who are age 65 and older (56 percent) and adults under 65 (44 percent). However, people with disabilities who need LTSS most often reside in HCBS compared to the elderly. Children under the age of 18 often live with their families and are a small percentage of the total population requiring LTSS, but can have substantial needs that will last a lifetime.

Seniors

The United States Congressional Budget Office (CBO) estimates that the percentage of the total U.S. population over 65 years of age will continue to grow (Hagen, 2013). The federal government estimates that about half of Americans turning 65 today will develop a disability serious enough to require LTSS. While most will likely only need assistance for less than two years and will spend relatively little on their care, about one in six older adults will spend at least $100,000 out-of-pocket for future LTSS (Favreault & Dey, 2015). One insurer estimated that the average cost was $91,250 per year for a nursing facility, $45,720 per year for home health care, and $17,940 for adult day health care (Reaves & Musumeci, 2015). Strategies to finance long-term care and to give seniors a choice in their care setting will be priorities as the population ages.

Children with Severe Disabilities

Special considerations are often needed to ensure coverage of children with disabilities whose family income disqualifies them from public program eligibility. For example, states may elect to extend Medicaid coverage to children with significant disabilities regardless of family income, or allow Medicaid to help cover expenses that the family's private health insurance does not (Dembner, 2012).

Family Caregivers

Family caregivers provide the largest source of long-term care support in the United States today (Reaves & Musumeci, 2015). This informal (unpaid) care has a significant impact on our economy. It is estimated that the value of family caregivers is $470 billion per year—as big as the world's largest company, and bigger than Medicaid (Reinhard, Feinberg, Choula, & Houser, 2015). (See **Figure 11-2.**) More than 65 million people provide approximately 20 hours per week of care for a chronically ill, disabled, or aged family member or friend. Many of these family caregivers provide care for both an aging parent and their children. Among working caregivers providing care to a family member or friend, 69 percent report the need to rearrange their work schedule, decrease their hours, or take unpaid leave in order to meet their caregiving responsibilities (Feinberg, Reinhard, Houser, & Choula, 2011).

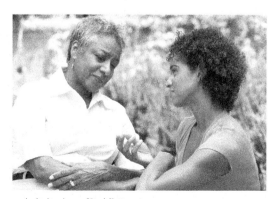

monkeybusinessimages/iStock/Getty

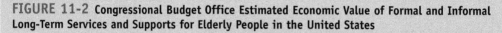

FIGURE 11-2 Congressional Budget Office Estimated Economic Value of Formal and Informal Long-Term Services and Supports for Elderly People in the United States

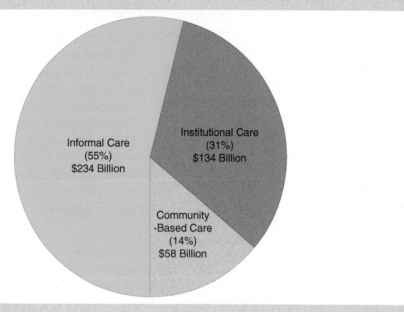

Our aging population further highlights the growing demand of caregivers available to support those in need of long-term services and supports. While in 2010 there were seven caregivers for every person over the age of 80 in need of LTSS, by 2030 this number is expected to decrease to five, and by 2050, to just three (Redfoot, Feinberg, & Houser, 2013).

Caregiving can be emotionally and physically stressful. Caregivers may have numerous responsibilities, including jobs and children. There are various ways to relieve the burden of caregiver stress. For example, caregiver "respite" is short-term relief provided by a substitute paid or unpaid caregiver. The Family Medical Leave Act (FMLA) is a federal law that protects family caregivers from losing their employment. FMLA allows eligible employees to take up to 12 weeks of unpaid time off each year to provide care for a child, spouse, or parent. The law applies to all public agencies and employers with more than 50 employees (United States Department of Labor, n.d.).

LONG-TERM CARE REFORM

Federal and state reforms have focused on financing long-term care insurance as the population ages. The Community Living Assistance Services and Supports (CLASS) Act, a provision of the ACA, was intended to be a voluntary national long-term care insurance program. Congress repealed the CLASS Act, however, after the Department of Health and Human Services determined that the program was not financially viable as written (American Association for Long-Term Care Insurance, 2013).

Some states are experimenting with new mechanisms to provide LTSS to dual-eligible beneficiaries. For example, states that provide Medicaid through managed care organizations may integrate LTSS with Medicaid (Smith et al., 2015; Musumeci, 2014). There is limited evidence on the impact of managed care on LTSS (KFF, 2011) therefore strong evaluation metrics are needed to ensure accessibility and quality (Dembner, 2012).

Because family caregivers are the backbone of our long-term care system, identifying ways to support them is needed. One of the recommendations of the Commission on Long-term Care's Report to Congress included expanding the role of Aging and Disability Resource Centers (ADRCs), and its enhanced counseling program to insure that individuals in need of LTSS and their families understand the programs and eligibility available to them (U.S. Senate Report to Congress, 2013).

Further, employers must have more awareness of the needs of their workers who are family caregivers, as well as strategies that they can implement to better support them. Respecting A Caregivers Time (ReACT) is an employer-focused coalition of more than 30 companies and non-profit organizations dedicated to addressing the challenges faced by employee caregivers and reducing the impact on the companies that employ them. Two simple strategies that ReACT recommends are offering flex-time or evaluating employees for their work rather than the time that they are present (Wagner, Lindemer, Yokum, & DeFreest, 2012).

Given that so few Americans understand LTSS and have not adequately prepared for their own long-term care needs, educational outreach and strategies to help Americans save for long-term care or purchase long-term care policies could help. For example, the majority of Americans 50 years and older believe that making the premiums for private long-term care policies tax deductible or allowing individuals to purchase policies pre-tax would encourage more individuals to purchase a policy (LifePlans, Inc., 2014).

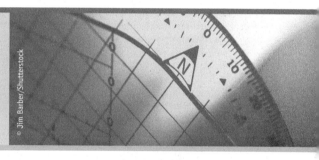

© Jim Barber/Shutterstock

Summary

Long-term care is costly, and most health insurance plans have limited coverage. Eligibility for Medicaid, the largest payer of long-term care, depends largely on income and assets and varies by state. Many people have not enacted a savings plan for LTSS, and rely on family caregiving. With the increasing aging population and their long-term care needs, future efforts should focus on encouraging individuals to save for long-term care, and to purchase a long-term care policy. States should work to identify strategies to help individuals in need of LTSS remain in their homes and community rather than institutional settings.

References

American Association for Long-Term Care Insurance. (2013, January 3). *CLASS Act information.* Retrieved from http://www.aaltci.org/long-term-care-insurance/learning-center/CLASS-Act.php

Centers for Medicare & Medicaid Services (CMS). (n.d.a). *1915c home and community-based waivers.* Retrieved from https://www.medicaid.gov/medicaid-chip-program-information/by-topics/waivers/home-and-community-based-1915-c-waivers.html

Centers for Medicare & Medicaid Services (CMS). (n.d.b). *Medicaid employment initiatives.* Retrieved from https://www.medicaid.gov/Medicaid-cHIP-program-information/by-topics/delivery-systems/grant-programs/employment-initiatives.html

Centers for Medicare & Medicaid Services (CMS). (n.d.c). *Your Medicare coverage: Home health services.* Retrieved from https://www.medicare.gov/coverage/home-health-services.html

Centers for Medicare & Medicaid Services (CMS). (2016, February). *Medicare hospice benefits.* Retrieved from https://www.medicare.gov/Pubs/pdf/02154.pdf

Colello, K. J. (2013, December 5). Medicaid coverage of long-term services and supports. Retrieved from https://www.fas.org/sgp/crs/misc/R43328.pdf

Colello, K. J., & Talaga, S. R. (2015, July 27). *Who pays for long-term services and supports? A fact sheet.* Retrieved from https://www.fas.org/sgp/crs/misc/R43483.pdf

Dembner, A. (2012, November). *Putting consumers first: Promising practices for Medicaid managed long-term services and supports*. Retrieved from http://www.communitycatalyst.org/doc-store/publications/putting_consumers_first_LTSSmanagedcare.pdf

Favreault, M., & Dey, J. (2015, February). *Long-term services and supports for older Americans: Risks and financing research brief*. Retrieved from https://aspe.hhs.gov/basic-report/long-term-services-and-supports-older-americans-risks-and-financing-research-brief

Feinberg, L., Reinhard, S. C., Houser, A., & Choula, R. (2011). *Valuing the invaluable: 2011 Update-the growing contributions and costs of family caregiving*. Washington, DC: AARP Public Policy Institute.

Hagen, S. (2013, June). *Rising demand for long-term services and supports for elderly people*. Congressional Budget Office. Retrieved from https://www.cbo.gov/sites/default/files/113th-congress-2013-2014/reports/44363-LTC.pdf

Huffman, M. (2015, January). *A reverse mortgage should always be in both spouses' names*. Retrieved from https://www.consumeraffairs.com/news/a-reverse-mortgage-should-always-be-in-both-spouses-names-010915.html

LifePlans, Inc. (2014, November). *The benefits of long-term care insurance and what they mean for long-term care financing*. America's Health Insurance Plans. Retrieved from https://www.ahip.org/wp-content/uploads/2014/11/LifePlans_The_Benefits_LTC_Insurance_Report_2014.pdf

Musumeci, M. B. (2014, November). Key themes in capitated Medicaid managed long-term services and supports waivers. Retrieved from http://kff.org/medicaid/issue-brief/key-themes-in-capitated-medicaid-managed-long-term-services-and-supports-waivers/

National Council on Independent Living. (n.d.). About independent living. Retrieved from http://www.ncil.org/about/aboutil/

Reaves, E. L., & Musumeci, M. B. (2015, December). *Medicaid and long-term services and supports: A primer*. Retrieved from http://kff.org/medicaid/report/medicaid-and-long-term-services-and-supports-a-primer

Redfoot, D., Feinberg, L., & Houser, A. (2013, August). *The aging of the baby boom and the growing care gap: A look at future declines in the availability of family caregivers*. American Association of Retired Persons Public Policy Institute. Retrieved from http://www.aarp.org/home-family/caregiving/info-08-2013/the-aging-of-the-baby-boom-and-the-growing-care-gap-AARP-ppi-ltc.html

Reinhard, S. C., Feinberg, L. F., Choula, R., & Houser, A. (2015). *Valuing the invaluable: 2015 update*. American Association of Retired Persons. Retrieved from http://www.aarp.org/content/dam/aarp/ppi/2015/valuing-the-invaluable-2015-update-new.pdf

Rosenblatt, C. (2012, July). The hidden truths about reverse mortgages. *Forbes*. Retrieved from http://www.forbes.com/sites/carolynrosenblatt/2012/07/23/hidden-truths-about-reverse-mortgages/2/#51ebeb2417b2

Smith, V. K., Gifford, K., Ellis, E., Health Management Associates, Rudowitz, R., Snyder, L., & Hinton, E. (2015, October). *Medicaid reforms to expand coverage, control costs and improve care: Results from a 50-state Medicaid budget survey for state fiscal years 2015 and 2016*. Retrieved from http://kff.org/medicaid/report/medicaid-reforms-to-expand-coverage-control-costs-and-improve-care-results-from-a-50-state-medicaid-budget-survey-for-state-fiscal-years-2015-and-2016/

The Henry J. Kaiser Family Foundation (KFF). (2013, March). *Medicaid: A primer*. Retrieved from https://kaiserfamilyfoundation.files.wordpress.com/2010/06/7334-05.pdf

The Henry J. Kaiser Family Foundation. (2011, October). *Medicaid and the uninsured*. Retrieved from https://www.aucd.org/docs/annual_mtg_2012/KFF_MLTSS_Key_Issues.pdf

United States Department of Health and Human Services (HHS). (n.d.a). *Coverage limits charts*. Retrieved from http://longtermcare.gov/costs-how-to-pay/what-is-covered-by-health-disability-insurance/coverage-limits-chart/

United States Department of Health and Human Services (HHS). (n.d.b). *Glossary*. Retrieved from http://longtermcare.gov/the-basics/glossary/#Annuity

United States Department of Health and Human Services (HHS). (n.d.c). *Using life insurance to pay for long-term care*. Retrieved from http://longtermcare.gov/costs-how-to-pay/using-life-insurance-to-pay-for-long-term-care/

United States Department of Health and Human Services (HHS). (n.d.d). *Where to look for long-term care insurance*. Retrieved from http://longtermcare.gov/costs-how-to-pay/what-is-long-term-care-insurance/where-to-look-for-long-term-care-insurance/

United States Department of Justice. (2016, July 28). *Olmstead: Community integration for everyone*. United States Department of Justice. Retrieved from https://www.ada.gov/olmstead/index.htm

United States Department of Labor. (n.d.). *FLMA (Family & Medical Leave Act)*. Retrieved from https://www.dol.gov/general/topic/benefits-leave/fmla

United States Senate Report to Congress. (2013, September). *Commission on long-term care report to congress*. Retrieved from http://ltccommission.org/ltccommission/wp-content/uploads/2013/12/Commission-on-Long-Term-Care-Final-Report-9-26-13.pdf

Wagner, D. L., Lindemer, A., Yokum, K.N., DeFreest, M. (2012, March). *Best practices in workplace eldercare*. National Alliance for Caregiving. Retrieved from http://www.caregiving.org/pdf/research/BestPracticesEldercareFINAL.pdf

CHAPTER 12

Retiree Benefits

Kate E. Trout, MPH

LEARNING OBJECTIVES

- What are different types of retiree benefits offered by employers and the government?
- What retiree benefit obligations are unfunded, and why is it a problem?
- What are characteristics of firms that offer retiree benefits?

INTRODUCTION

By 2050, 22 percent of the U.S. population is projected to be 65 years or older, up from 15 percent in 2015 (He, Goodkind, & Kowal, 2016). Commensurate with this increase in the elderly population, health care and long-term care costs are expected to rise (de Meijer, Wouterse, Polder, & Koopmanschap, 2013; Olivares-Tirado, Tamiya, Kashiwagi, & Kashiwagi, 2011; Rechel, Doyle, Grundy, & McKee, 2009). Older populations have higher rates of chronic diseases and comorbidities that may strain both public and household resources (He et al., 2016; National Institute on Aging and U.S. Department of State, 2007; Tsai, 2010). This chapter will discuss retiree health benefits, as well as other types of benefits that can provide financial support for individuals who have stopped working.

TYPES OF RETIREE BENEFITS

Retiree Health Benefits

The major source of health insurance for retirees, 65 years of age and older, is Medicare. Retirees may also temporarily stay on their employer's health insurance plan for 18 months through the Consolidated Omnibus Budget Reconciliation Act (COBRA). But some employers offer benefits to retirees, which can be advantageous to workers who retiree before age 65, or who would like insurance that covers benefits that Medicare generally does not, such as prescription drugs. **Retiree health benefits** are more common in the public sector; in the private sector, only 18 percent of individuals were employed in firms that offered retiree benefits (Fronstin & Adams, 2012).

There are also differences in the level of coverage among employers. Among large firms (firms with 200 or more employees) offering retiree health benefits, 2 percent covered only the cost prescription drugs. Many drop benefits for retirees once they become eligible for Medicare. And retiree health plans may not be as generous as employee health plans. Understanding retiree benefits is important for employees planning their retirement.

There are several sources of retiree health coverage for both Medicare-eligible and non-Medicare-eligible retirees (**Figures 12-1** and **12-2**). Medicare-eligible retirees, those 65 years or older, are automatically enrolled in Medicare Part A, and may choose Part B. They may supplement Medicare benefits with Medigap. If their employer offers retiree benefits, then they will have this option as well. Younger retirees may continue coverage temporarily through COBRA but will then have to find coverage elsewhere, such as through the health insurance exchange or directly from a health insurance company—that is, in the individual market for health insurance. And if they are offered retiree benefits, then this will be an option as well. Both types of beneficiaries may also be able to enroll in a spouse's insurance.

While retiree health coverage may draw talented and motivated employees, the proportion of firms offering these benefits has substantially decreased over time in the United States. Only 23 percent of large firms (firms with 200 or more employees) offered retiree health benefits in 2015 compared to 66 percent in 1988 (Claxton et al., 2015). As health care costs rise and the elderly live longer, employers may find it increasingly difficult to fund retiree health benefits.

Coordination of Benefits

Early retirees are those who retiree before age 65. Employers may offer them retiree health benefits (**Figure 12-3**). Medicare-eligible retirees are those who retire at age 65 or later. Employers are less likely to offer these retirees health benefits, but if they do, Medicare and the private health plan must decide on coordination of benefits, or rules about who pays first in what situation. Coordination of benefits rules must be implemented whenever an individual has more than one type of insurance; for example, for dual eligibles (Medicare usually pays first for dual eligibles, and Medicaid second). For Medicare-eligible retirees, Medicare usually pays first, and the private plan second. For example, the private plan might cover some leftover out-of-pocket expenses, or a benefit that was not covered by Medicare, such as an outpatient prescription drug.

Social Security

Individuals who have worked for 10 years and paid federal Social Security taxes are eligible to collect Social Security income in proportion to their lifetime earnings. While retirees may claim discounted benefits as early as age 62, full benefits are not available until age 67. Social Security is the primary income for the majority of the elderly population,

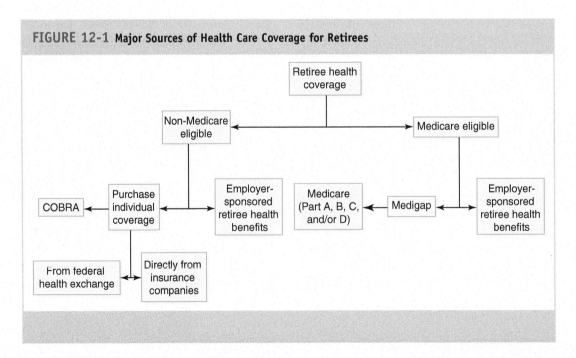

FIGURE 12-1 Major Sources of Health Care Coverage for Retirees

FIGURE 12-2 Income Distribution for Elderly Population Showing Social Security Is the Primary Source of Income for Elderly with Below-Average Incomes

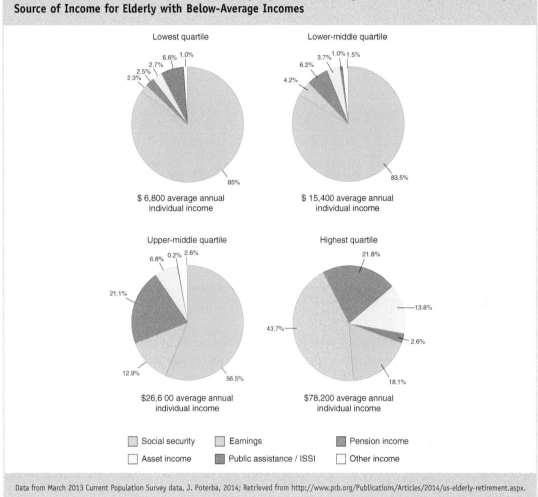

Lowest quartile

6.6% 1.0%
2.7%
2.5%
2.3%
85%

$ 6,800 average annual individual income

Lower-middle quartile

3.7% 1.0% 1.5%
6.2%
4.2%
83.5%

$ 15,400 average annual individual income

Upper-middle quartile

6.8% 0.2% 2.6%
21.1%
12.9%
56.5%

$26,6 00 average annual individual income

Highest quartile

21.8%
13.8%
43.7%
2.6%
18.1%

$78,200 average annual individual income

☐ Social security   ☐ Earnings   ▨ Pension income
☐ Asset income   ▨ Public assistance / ISSI   ☐ Other income

Data from March 2013 Current Population Survey data, J. Poterba, 2014; Retrieved from http://www.prb.org/Publications/Articles/2014/us-elderly-retirement.aspx.

and is therefore an important income source to cover out-of-pocket medical costs. In 2010, the maximum Social Security benefit was $2,346 per month (Social Security Administration [SSA], 2010), while average monthly household spending on health care (including premiums) was $395 (Cubanski, Swoope, Damico, & Neuman, 2014), almost one-fifth of the *maximum* Social Security benefit. Health care costs may therefore represent a substantial portion of income for seniors.

Pensions from Employers

Some employers offer private pension plans to their employees. When you are hired, you may be asked to choose a plan, or you may be defaulted into a plan. In general, there are two types of pension plans. **Defined benefit plans** are plans that guarantee the employee a predefined amount (or benefit) upon retirement. The retirement benefit depends on the employee's salary or wage, years of service to the firm, and sometimes also Social Security eligibility. The employee must contribute to the pension fund and remain employed for a certain number of years before the full benefits can be received under the plan. The benefits in private-sector defined benefit plans are insured under the Pension Benefit Guaranty Corporation (PBGC) and offer some protection in case the employer cannot cover the cost of benefits (PBGC, 2000).

Alternatively, defined contribution plans are plans in which employees and employers contribute regularly to investment accounts, and benefits

FIGURE 12-3 **Large Firms Offering Retiree Health benefits, 1988–2015**

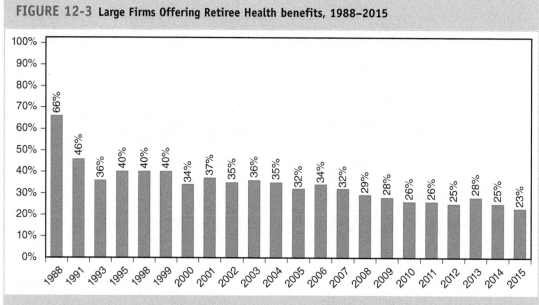

Reproduced using data from Kaiser/HRET Survey of Employer-Sponsored Health Benefits, 1999–2015; KPMG Survey of Employer-Sponsored Health Benefits, 1991, 1993, 1995, 1998; The Health Insurance Association of America (HIAA), 1988; Claxton et al., 2015.

depend on the performance of the account. As with defined contribution plans, the employer contribution usually depends on salary or wages (e.g., 3.5 percent of annual salary) and years of service to the firm. The government sets caps on employer and employee contributions to different types of defined contribution plans each year. Some examples of defined contribution plans include 401(k) plans, offered by for-profit firms, and 403(b) plans, offered at nonprofit firms and governmental organizations.

There are several benefits to a defined contribution plan. While defined contribution plans are portable from employer to employer if employees lose their jobs or leave the workforce, defined benefit plans stay with the employer. If an employee leaves a firm, then a defined contribution account can be rolled over to an IRA or transitioned to a new employer's retirement system. Further, in contrast to defined contribution plans, employees must work a certain number of years before defined benefit plans vest (before employees may claim benefits). If an employee leaves the firm before the defined benefit plan vests, then the employee also surrenders the benefits.

Yet defined contribution plans also have risks. Primarily, while defined benefit plans offer a known monthly income upon retirement, defined

contribution plans depend on the performance of the investment account, which can be higher or lower than a defined benefit plan. Employer contributions to profit-sharing plans and stock ownership plans may be modified based on the success of the company.

Much of the difference in value between defined benefit and defined contribution plans comes from variability across firms in the employer matching rate, the age of retirement, and the value of the defined benefit plan (Poterba, Rauh, Venti, & Wise, 2007). Insuring the value of a defined benefit plan is costly, so an employer with concerns about funding defined benefits in the future may not offer very generous benefits. New employees should not simply enroll into the default pension plan when they are hired but actively choose a plan and contribution level. Continuing employees who have not already done so should actively make this choice as well.

Designing pension plans that result in financial security for retirees is crucial to offset the high cost of health care and long-term care at the end of life. Ultimately, if pension plans are not enough, retirees may resort to using their Social Security income to cover these expenses or forgo needed care.

UNFUNDED RETIREE BENEFIT OBLIGATIONS

There is a substantial funding gap between what is set aside to pay for retiree benefits and the cost of these benefits, a problem known as unfunded retiree benefit obligations. These benefits may include the cost of retiree health care, as well as defined benefit pensions. Unfunded obligations in the private sector are about $425 billion for defined benefit pensions, and between $1 trillion and $3 trillion in state and local governments (Hanif et al., 2016). The largest unfunded liability in the United States is the Social Security pension system, which is estimated to be about $10 trillion (Hanif et al., 2016). As the baby boomers age, policymakers will have to find ways to fund the obligations to which retirees are entitled.

There are also unfunded health care obligations. The gap between states' assets and their retiree health insurance benefits for public sector workers is estimated to be more than $627 billion (The Pew Center on the States, 2012). In the public sector, city and state workers such as fire fighters, police officers, public educators, road and maintenance workers, bus drivers, and public hospital employees depend on the public sector retirement system. When these shortfalls exist, funding comes from tax resources that would otherwise be used for public services including education, parks, transit infrastructure, and libraries.

In the long run, employers may feel pressure to reduce or cut retiree benefits by reducing matching rates, raising the retirement age, or limiting defined benefits. The public sector may raise taxes or borrow money. Other public services may experience budget reductions in order to cover the unfunded liabilities. Unfunded obligations can create uncertainty for the public sector, for private employers, and for employees planning for retirement.

CHARACTERISTICS OF FIRMS THAT OFFER RETIREE BENEFITS

Retiree health benefits vary substantially by firm. Overall, large firms are more likely to offer retiree benefits compared to small firms because of differences in resources and budgets (Table 12-1).

TABLE 12-1 Characteristics of Large Firms Offering Retiree Health Benefits, 2015

All Large Firms (200 or More Workers)	
Firm size	
200–999 workers	20%*
1,000–4,999 workers	34%*
5,000 or more workers	42%*
Region	
Northeast	23%
Midwest	20%
South	23%
West	27%
Industry	
Agriculture/Mining/Construction	15%
Manufacturing	14%*
Transportation/Communications/Utilities	62%*
Wholesale	23%
Retail	12%
Finance	49%*
Service	20%
State/Local government	73%*
Health care	18%
All large firms (200 or more workers)	**23%**

*Estimate is statistically different from estimate for all other large firms not in the indicated size, region, or industry category ($p < 0.05$)

Reproduced using data from Kaiser/HRET Survey of Employer-Sponsored Health Benefits, 2015.

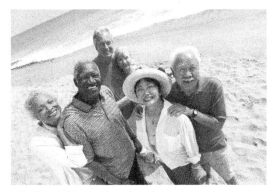

© bikeriderlondon/Shutterstock

In 2015, 72 percent of firms with fewer than 1,000 employees offered retiree health benefits to Medicare-age retirees, while 80 percent of firms with 5,000 or more employees offered such benefits. Even among large firms, however, the percentage of firms that offer retiree health benefits has decreased substantially over time (Claxton et al., 2015).

The public sector is much more likely than the private sector to offer retiree health benefits. In 2010, 63 percent of state governments offered retiree benefits to Medicare-eligible retirees, while just 6 percent of private sector firms offered such benefits. In comparison, 32 percent of firms with 1,000 or more employees offered retiree health benefits to Medicare-eligible retirees (Fronstin & Adams, 2012).

The characteristics of the workers in a firm are also associated with whether the firm offers retirement benefits (Table 12-2). A firm with older workers is more likely to offer retirement benefits, likely because firms that offer retirement benefits draw older workers, and also because older workers demand retirement benefits. Firms with union workers, who have the negotiating power of the union behind them, are also more likely to offer retirement benefits. Lastly, firms with higher-wage workers are also more likely to offer retirement benefits.

Such benefits may be necessary to recruit high-wage workers, who are willing to pay for them (Claxton et al., 2015).

IMPACT OF AGING ON THE LABOR FORCE

Due to the pressures faced by retirees, employees in the United States have increasingly delayed retirement. The United States is among the countries with the highest proportion of older workers participating in the labor force. As life expectancy grows, as people live longer, they must work longer as well. Other factors contributing to the aging labor force include uncertainty about the sufficiency and viability of public pension systems, increased reliance on defined contribution pension, later eligibility ages to receive retirement benefits, and changing social norms about exiting the labor force (Friedberg & Webb, 2005; Hasselhorn & Apt, 2015; Hurd & Rohwedder, 2011; Skugor, Muffels, & Wilthagen, 2012; van Dalen, Henkens, Henderikse, & Schippers, 2010). Especially since the Great Recession of 2007 to 2009, workers have delayed retirement or rejoined the workforce after retirement (Burtless & Bosworth, 2013). Greater personal savings, combined with policies to reform unfunded pensions, will be necessary to ensure financial stability for retirees (Poterba, 2014).

TABLE 12-2 Differences in Workers' Characteristics in Offering Retiree Health Benefits Among Large Firms in the United States

Characteristics	Differences in Characteristics	
	More likely to offer retiree health benefits	Less likely to offer retiree health benefits
Age of workers	Larger proportion of older workers in a firm (35% or more of workers are age 50 or older)	Smaller proportion of older workers in a firm (Less than 35% of workers are age 50 or older)
Unions	Some union workers in a firm	No union workers in a firm
Wage level	Larger proportion of higher wage level in a firm (35% or more earning $58,000 a year or more)	Lower proportion of higher wage level in a firm (Less than 35% earning $58,000 a year or more)
Medicare eligibility	"Early retiree" (under the age of 65 years)	Medicare eligible (65 years of age and older)

Reproduced using information from Kaiser/HRET Survey of Employer-Sponsored Health Benefits, 2015; Claxton et al., 2015.

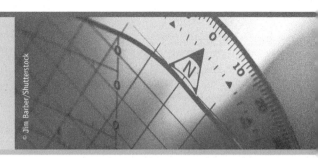

Summary

There are several types of benefits for retirees, including employer-sponsored retiree health insurance plans, Medicare coverage, defined benefit and defined contribution pension plans, and Social Security. There are various benefits and risks to defined benefit and defined contribution plans, but there is also substantial variation in the design of these plans across firms. While the public sector is much more likely to offer retiree benefits than the private sector, it also has much larger unfunded obligations, for which it will eventually need to raise revenue or cut benefits. As the population ages, so will the workforce, and individuals and policymakers will need to adjust to this change.

References

Burtless, G., & Bosworth, B. (2013, December 16). *Impact of the great recession on retirement trends in industrialized countries*. Washington, DC: The Brookings Institution. Retrieved from https://www.brookings.edu/research/impact-of-the-great-recession-on-retirement-trends-in-industrialized-countries/

Claxton, G., Rae, M., Long, M., Panchal, N., Damico, A., Kenward, K., & Whitmore, H. (2015). *Employer health benefits: 2015 Annual Survey*. Chicago, IL: Health Research & Educational Trust.

Cubanski, J., Swoope, C., Damico, A., & Neuman, T. (2014). *How much is enough? Out-of-pocket spending among Medicare beneficiaries: A chartbook*. Retrieved from http://files.kff.org/attachment/how-much-is-enough-out-of-pocket-spending-among-medicare-beneficiaries-a-chartbook-report

De Meijer, C., Wouterse, B., Polder, J., & Koopmanschap, M. (2013). The effect of population aging on health expenditure growth: A critical review. *European Journal on Ageing*, *10*(4), 353–361.

Friedberg, L., & Webb, A. (2005). Retirement and the evolution of pension structure. *The Journal of Human Resources*, *40*(2), 281–308.

Fronstin, P., & Adams, N. (2012). Employment-based retiree health benefits: Trends in access and coverage, 1997–2010. *ERBI Issue Brief, 377*. Retrieved from https://www.ebri.org/pdf/briefspdf/ebri_ib_10-2012_no377_rethlth.pdf

Hanif, F., Millard, C., Bass, E. J., Curmi, E., Deans, S., Lam, D., … Pittaway, N. (2016, March). The coming pensions crisis: Recommendations for keeping the global pensions system afloat. In K. Boyle (Ed.), *Citi GPS: Global Perspectives & Solutions*. Retrieved from: https://ir.citi.com/A44lKhe6CVSitfkypsON6kDXypHYjJ%2BENxq8FLMoTBde6kse9Kt9KQ%3D%3D

Hasselhorn, H. M., & Apt, W. (Eds.). (2015). *Understanding employment participation of older workers: Creating a knowledge base for future labour market challenges*. Berlin, Germany: Federal Ministry of Labour and Social Affairs and Federal Institute for Occupational Safety and Health.

He, W., Goodkind, D., & Kowal, P. (2016, March). *An aging world: 2015*. International population reports. U.S. Census Bureau, P95/16-1. Washington, DC: U.S. Government Publishing Office.

Hurd, M., & Rohwedder, S. (2011). Trends in labor force participation: How much is due to changes in pensions? *Journal of Population Ageing*, *4*(1–2), 81–96.

National Institute on Aging (NIA) and U.S. Department of State. (2007). *Why population aging matters: A global perspective*. National Institute on Aging of National Institutes on Health Publication 07-6134. Washington, DC: National Institute on Aging of National Institutes on Health.

Olivares-Tirado, P., Tamiya, N., Kashiwagi, M., & Kashiwagi, K. (2011). Predictors of the highest long-term care expenditures in Japan. *BioMedCentral Health Services Research*, *11*, 103.

Pension Benefit Guaranty Corporation (PBGC). (2000, January). *A predictable, secure pension plan for life: Defined benefit pensions*. Washington, DC: PBGC, Publication 1007.

The Pew Center on the States. (2012). *The widening gap update*. The Pew Charitable Trust: Washington, DC. Retrieved from: http://www.pewtrusts.org/~/media/legacy/uploadedfiles/pcs_assets/2012/pewpensionsupdatepdf.pdf

Poterba, J. M. (2014). Retirement security in an aging population. *American Economic Review: Papers & Proceedings*, *104*(5), 1–33.

Poterba, J., Rauh, J., Venti, S., & Wise, D. (2007). Defined contribution plans, defined benefit plans, and the accumulation of retirement wealth. *Journal of Public Economics*, *91*(10), 2062–2086. Retrieved from http://www.ncbi.nlm.nih.gov/pmc/articles/PMC2972552/

Rechel, B., Doyle, Y., Grundy, E., & McKee, M. (2009). *How can health systems respond to population ageing?* European Observatory on Health Systems and Policies, Policy Brief 10. Retrieved from http://www.euro.who.int/__data/assets/pdf_file/0004/64966/E92560.pdf

Skugor, D., Muffels, R., & Wilthagen, T. (2012). *Labour law, social norms and the early retirement decision.* Network for Studies on Pensions, Aging and Retirement Discussion Paper, 11, 2012-046. Retrieved from https://www.netspar.nl/en/publication/labour-law-social-norms-and-the-early-retirement-decision-an-empirical-study/

Social Security Administration. (2010). Fast facts and figures about social security: 2010. Retrieved from https://www.ssa.gov/policy/docs/chartbooks/fast_facts/2010/fast_facts10.html

Tsai, T. (2010). *More caregivers needed worldwide for the "oldest old."* Washington, DC: Population Reference Bureau.

van Dalen, H. P., Henkens, K., Henderikse, W., & Schippers, J. (2010). Do European employers support later retirement? *International Journal of Manpower, 31*(3), 360–373.

CHAPTER 13

A Global Comparison of U.S. Health Insurance

Gordon C. Shen, PhD, SM and Julia K. Duch, BA

LEARNING OBJECTIVES

- What are the defining characteristics of a national health system?
- How is universal health coverage practiced around the globe?
- How do the health systems of Germany, the United Kingdom, and Canada compare to the United States?
- How do health systems of low- and middle-income countries operate?
- What are the challenges of comparing national health systems?

INTRODUCTION

The United States spends more on health care than other countries, yet the American population ranks much lower than other developed countries in several health indicators such as life expectancy at birth and infant mortality (Organisation for Economic Co-operation and Development [OECD], 2016). Health is the result of many individual and environmental factors. Socioeconomic conditions, neighborhood factors, and the natural environment play large roles in shaping health. Genetics, lifestyle, and the medical care system also contribute to health. To what extent lower rankings in life expectancy and infant mortality are attributable to the health care system, or to social and environmental factors, requires further study.

The United States is a leader in biomedical research, develops cutting-edge medical technology, and has many highly specialized practitioners and academic teaching hospitals. But these innovations are costly, while basic health care can be difficult to access for some Americans. Therefore, an enduring problem for American policymakers is how to design a health insurance system that achieves the "triple aim" of quality and access at an affordable cost (Berwick, Nolan, & Whittington, 2008).

In this chapter, we define a national health system and we introduce universal health coverage as a concept that unifies all countries. We compare the essential features of the U.S. health system to those of other high-income countries, including Canada, the United Kingdom, and Germany. We will also briefly characterize how the governments of low- and middle-income countries provide health care. We will also discuss how it can be difficult to compare national health systems performance because of differences in data availability and collection methods across countries.

DEFINING HEALTH SYSTEMS

Health systems are made up of structural components that interact with one another to achieve health-related goals, including health status improvement, financial risk protection, and consumer satisfaction with care delivery (Hsiao, 2003). Although the World Health Organization [WHO, 2000] considers maximizing population health both the main goal of health systems and a human right, other actors operating within national health systems argue that health systems should also focus on affordability and patient satisfaction (Giedion, Alfonso, & Diaz, 2013; Moreno-Serra & Smith, 2012). Ideally, a good definition of a health system would allow us to compare health systems across countries, but we will describe later in the chapter how it can be challenging to compare health systems in countries with different economic, political, and social contexts.

Universal Health Coverage

The WHO encourages countries to achieve universal health coverage, which is defined as a health system that provides everyone with access to quality promotive, preventative, curative, and rehabilitative health services, while also protecting people from financial hardship related to paying for these services (U.N. Development Programme, 2015; WHO, 2015).

Universal health coverage (UHC) is more than just health insurance. It can be broken down into three objectives:

1. Equity in access to health services for all those who need services
2. Quality of health services that is adequate to improve health
3. Financial protection, ensuring that the cost of care does not put people at risk of financial hardship

Before the ACA, the United States stood out from many other high-income countries like Japan, the United Kingdom, and Sweden, all of which had enacted UHC-like legislation as early as the 1950s (Stuckler, Feigl, Basu, & McKee, 2010). Despite long-standing legislation in some countries, no country has been able to obtain true UHC in practice. While the concept of UHC and its intrinsic value are clear, the road

map to achieving the three objectives of UHC is not.

HEALTH SYSTEMS IN HIGH-INCOME COUNTRIES

We now describe the health care systems of Germany, the United Kingdom, and Canada, with a focus on the financing, delivery system, and benefit design.

Germany

The German social health insurance system is the oldest health system in the world. In 1883, Otto von Bismarck created a system of health insurance with a vision of building a strong nation, earning support from the working class, and defeating the opposing, socialist party from gaining majority power. The Bismarck Model emphasizes solidarity, and its goal was to reduce impoverishment due to disease, disability, or unemployment (Reichs Gesetzblatt, 1883).

The modern German health insurance system comprises private health insurance plans and public regional plans called "sickness funds" with a standard benefit package. About 85 percent of the German population is covered by one of the 132 sickness funds, while 11 percent is covered by private health insurance and 4 percent is covered by sector-specific governmental schemes (e.g., military) (Busse & Blümel, 2014). German residents are automatically enrolled in public sickness funds, which are financed by payroll taxes and supplemented by federal subsidies. The welfare system covers the cost for anyone who is unable to pay their premium. For most, public coverage is mandatory, but high earners, students, and some public workers may elect private coverage instead.

Sickness funds receive a risk-adjusted capitation for each enrollee, but generally pay physicians on a fee-for-service basis and hospitals on a case-based system, similar to diagnosis-related groups in the U.S. system. Both public and private health care providers offer inpatient and outpatient services, medications, rehabilitation therapy, and dental benefits. Out-of-pocket payments for services are nominal.

United Kingdom

The British National Health Service (NHS) has its roots in the National Insurance Act of 1911, which provided health insurance for workers. After World War II, as part of the larger state reconstruction, Sir William Beveridge extended this system to all residents in a publicly financed, publicly delivered system now known as the Beveridge Model. The National Health Services Act of 1946 dictated that the NHS would have two main functions: to provide universal insurance coverage and to provide comprehensive health care to residents of the United Kingdom.

The NHS is primarily financed through general tax revenues, including revenue from payroll taxes. In 2014, approximately 83.1 percent of NHS funding comes from general government sources, while the remaining 17 percent comes from private sources (WHO, 2014). The central government establishes benefits and disburses funds to regional health authorities, which in turn manage services in their respective areas. Patients must register with a general practitioner, who is the first point of contact in the health system. About 10 percent of residents forgo public insurance and instead purchase private insurance (Mossialos, Wenzl, Osborn, & Anderson, 2015). The benefits of purchasing private insurance are reduced wait times, access to more sophisticated (and more expensive) technology, and the ability to purchase access to extra services.

Most hospitals in the United Kingdom are public and owned by the NHS. Except for general practitioners, physicians who see NHS patients may also see patients privately. As in the United States, physicians are paid in a variety of ways— some fee-for-service, some capitation—and hospitals are paid per case. Unlike in the United States, however, there is a global budget for health care to control spending from year to year.

Canada

The Canadian Medicare program (not to be confused with the U.S. Medicare program), is, like the NHS, a tax-financed national health insurance system. Unlike the NHS, however, providers deliver care in mostly private settings. The Canadian Medical Care Act of 1968 had three key provisions:

1. Universal insurance coverage with a set of necessary medical services provided free of charge
2. A central regulatory authority overseeing hospitals
3. Governmental negotiation power for physician reimbursement rates

Canadian provinces and territories jointly fund and administer the Medicare program. They have autonomy to set reimbursement policy for providers, establish benefits, and set budgets. This governance arrangement gives provincial and territorial governments the authority to use resources that best suit the needs of people in their jurisdiction. Canadians also have the option of purchasing private insurance for services and amenities not offered in provincial health plans (Canadian Institute for Health Information [CIHI], 2014).

General tax revenues at both the provincial and federal levels fund the Canadian health insurance system. Some provinces pay hospitals case-based payments, while others pay a global budget. Physicians are mostly paid fee-for-service, though some are paid capitation (CIHI, 2014). Delivery system ownership varies by region, but, like in the United States, there is a mix of public and private hospitals, and mostly private physician practices.

Summary of High-Income Countries' Health Systems

We have compared the health care systems of three high-income countries based on several factors such as the role of private insurance, the ownership mix of the delivery system, and the role of government in health care spending. The U.K. health system is both publicly financed and mostly publicly delivered. The Canadian system is publicly financed but delivered in a mix of public and private settings. Germany has a mix of public and private insurance through the workplace, with support for those who do not work, and care is delivered in a mix of settings. Private insurance plays a much larger role in the United States, which distinguishes it from these other health care systems.

HEALTH SYSTEMS IN LOW- AND MIDDLE-INCOME COUNTRIES

Low- and middle-income countries face common challenges in achieving UHC. One challenge is the availability of resources. High-income countries, such as the United States, often have resources such as trained health workers and technology but struggle with creating equal access to these resources. On the other hand, low- and middle-income countries often have limited resources but strive to provide several vital health services nationwide, regardless of individuals' ability to pay.

Another challenge is the heavy reliance on out-of-pocket payments for health services, rather than insurance reimbursement, which has the potential to create inequities in access to services because out-of-pocket payments disproportionately burden low-income households. On average, out-of-pocket payments range from 30 percent to 56 percent of expenditures for low- and middle-income countries (WHO, 2014). In contrast, high-income countries finance their health systems with less than 15 percent out-of-pocket payments on average (WHO, 2014). As countries develop systems in support of UHC, the financial risk can be spread across the population and thereby reduce the risk of impoverishment from getting sick or injured.

Financing Health Systems in Low- and Middle-Income Countries

Achieving UHC is a dynamic process that depends on a country's political, economic, demographic, and health trends. Policymakers must make difficult choices in designing benefit packages, reimbursement decisions, and budgets. For governments to achieve UHC, they must consider ways in which they can increase resources and deliver care. Some governments do not have the resources or infrastructure to create a national health insurance program, and instead choose to subsidize health services with general revenues

and international aid (Escobar, Griffin, & Shaw, 2011). A tax-based system of insurance poses particular challenges for low- and middle-income countries because the infrastructure to collect taxes may be limited (Reeves et al., 2015). An alternative is voluntary health insurance, but this system generally yields low participation, inherently leaving gaps in coverage and excluding large segments of the population (Mills, 2014).

Development assistance for health has not increased in the past decade due to the shifting political and economic priorities of donors (Dieleman et al., 2016; Fan, Grépin, Shen, & Chen, 2014). As low- and middle-income countries grow their economies, they must increasingly rely on raising domestic funds. For many countries, health insurance, with its pool of prepaid premiums, is the next step to ensuring a stable revenue stream to pay for health services for a population.

There are two possible ways that governments can insure their residents. In a social health insurance scheme, workers and their employers make regular tax contributions that are managed by the government, which then reimburses providers and establishes benefits. Contributions are usually based on income to ensure that low-wage workers are not unduly burdened. Those who do not work, such as children, the elderly, the disabled, and spouses, are covered through general revenues or dependent coverage. China has experience with social health insurance (see **Box 13-1**).

Community-based health insurance, or mutual health insurance, on the other hand, is an insurance scheme in which members of a community (rather than an entire nation) voluntarily contribute premiums. These premiums are not usually based on income. Some community-based systems have expanded to better spread risk by combining funds from multiple communities or by integrating funds from community-based health insurance schemes into the funds from a national social health insurance scheme. Countries like Ghana, Rwanda, and Ethiopia have piloted and instituted community-based health insurance schemes to varying degrees of coverage and success. Ethiopia has experience with community-based health insurance (see **Box 13-2**).

BOX 13-1 China's Social Health Insurance Schemes

China launched its health care reform plan in 2009 with the intent of developing a "harmonious society" where "everyone enjoys equal access to basic health care and medical services," according to then Minister of Health Chen Zhu (Cheng, 2008). This reform is massive and transformational: massive because it covers the entire Chinese population of 1.34 billion people (and counting, or about 20 percent of the global population), and transformational in that they started with coverage expansion before moving onto broad-based changes in the health care and public health systems. The Chinese leadership committed an additional RMB 850 billion, or about US$125 billion, in the first three years of the reform to advance five interdependent areas: (1) expand coverage to insure more than 90 percent of the population; (2) establish a national essential medicines system; (3) improve the primary care delivery system; (4) make public health services available to all; and (5) pilot public hospital reforms. We will elaborate on the first area as it directly relates to health insurance.

China has taken significant strides toward UHC. Under Communist rule, China had a comprehensive system that emphasized primary care and public health. Market reforms that were introduced in 1978 destroyed that system and replaced it with a market-oriented health care system, resulting in a national insurance coverage rate of 23 percent in 2003 (Barber & Yao, 2010; Blumenthal & Hsiao, 2005). By 2011 over 95 percent of China's population had access to private health insurance or one of the three flagship social health insurance schemes: New Rural Cooperative Medical Scheme for rural residents, Urban Employees Basic Medical Insurance for urban employees, and Urban Residents Basic Medical Insurance for unemployed urban residents. Like the United States, the Chinese health insurance system is made up of distinct health insurance schemes and public and private health care providers.

China's extension of health coverage to its sizable population, and within a short period of time no less, can be considered a beacon of success. However, ongoing work is being done to expand the scope (i.e., comprehensiveness of benefit package) and depth (i.e., the degree of financial risk protection) of its health insurance system (Liang & Langenbrunner, 2013). The China National Health and Family Planning Commission reported increasing the average subsidy across the three public insurance plans to RMB320 (about USD $48.71) per individual per year, although the benefit package and quality of health services vary by province (Liu, Hsiao, & Eggleston, 1999; Wang, 2014). Furthermore, the Commission is overseeing pilots of catastrophic medical insurance schemes that would increase the reimbursement rate so that the majority of health expenses incurred for serious illnesses would be covered (Yip et al., 2012).

China's health insurance system emphasizes egalitarianism, or providing access to health care on equal terms for all citizens. The progress China has made over a short period time in health reform arguably complements its economic development plan. But China's UHC agenda remains incomplete: the National Health and Family Planning Commission is working through terms related to the second and third objectives of UHC (Global Hospital Management Survey—China [GHMS], 2014).

Note: References noted in the exhibits and in-text can be found in the end-of-chapter reference list.

Many low- and middle-income countries operate more than one insurance scheme to work toward UHC, borrowing features from established health care systems in other countries. For example, Ghana's National Health Insurance Scheme, established in 2003, is a mix of U.K.-like social health insurance, funded by payroll taxes as in Germany, supplemented by district-level health insurance schemes, as in Canada. In contrast, Rwanda's health care financing relies solely on community-based health insurance schemes, in which they have had success in covering most of the population.

We can begin to evaluate the global progress toward UHC by looking at the three dimensions of coverage: (1) Who is covered? (2) Which services are covered? and (3) What proportion of costs are covered? (See **Figure 13-1**.) There is substantial variability in enrollment in health insurance by country and region. In sub-Saharan Africa, Rwanda has enrolled over 90 percent of the population in their health insurance scheme, compared to just 54 percent in Ghana (Lagomarsino, Garabrant, Adyas, Muga, & Otoo, 2012). In South Asia, the Philippines have enrolled 76 percent of

BOX 13-2 Ethiopia's Community-Based Health Insurance Scheme

Ethiopia, like other low- and middle-income countries, has a large population who are informally employed. As a part of the government's health care financing reforms, the Ethiopian government began to explore a state-run health insurance scheme. In 2011, the Ethiopian government began to pilot a community-based health insurance scheme in 13 districts in 4 different regions in Ethiopia (Mebratie, Sparrow, Yilma, Alemu, & Bedi, 2015). The communities were given the option to join and help manage the scheme.

In the Ethiopian community-based health insurance scheme, households can volunteer to join and pay a monthly premium to access services. The monthly premium was set according to feasibility studies and amounted to around 2 to 3 percent of a household's monthly income. The government subsidizes the cost of the premium for the poorest 10 percent of the population, so that all members of a community have the ability to join the scheme.

Once enrolled in the scheme, each patient is given a photo identification book that identifies them as a member of the scheme and allows them to receive inpatient and outpatient care in public facilities. If a patient visits a public facility that is contracted in the scheme, there is no out-of-pocket payment at the time of the service utilization. Whereas if a patient visits a public facility outside of the scheme, they must pay upfront for the services but can file for reimbursement. To contain costs, scheme members must be referred by a primary care facility first before going to a hospital. If a member chooses to go to a hospital without a primary care referral, they are responsible for 50 percent of the cost of the services received (Mebratie et al., 2015). Finally, to ensure that money stays within the public sector, the plans do not allow patients to visit private facilities unless a particular service or drug is not available at the public facility.

The community-based health insurance reached 45.5 percent enrollment a year after starting the scheme, which is a high enrollment rate compared to other sub-Saharan African countries that have rolled out community-based health insurance. Because of its success within the first few years of its launch, the Ethiopian government planned to expand the pilot to 161 districts around Ethiopia.

The community-based health insurance intends to cover the informal employment sector, such as day laborers and farmers. The Ethiopian government has been separately planning a social health insurance scheme, in which the formally employed would be automatically enrolled in the scheme. The government hopes to integrate both schemes in the future to create a larger risk pool and more effective subsidization.

the targeted population, compared to just 42 percent in Vietnam (Lagomarsino et al., 2012). And in Latin America, Chile has managed to cover over 90 percent of the population, while Peru has covered only about 60 percent (Atun et al., 2015).

People in low- and middle-income countries often lack coverage for basic health care services. For example, 41 percent of people in sub-Saharan Africa, 58 percent in South Asia, and 64 percent of Europe and Central Asia have access to family planning services, compared to 80 percent in high-income countries (WHO, 2015). The median proportion of births attended by a skilled health worker is 62 percent across 75 countries that account for most maternal and child deaths globally (WHO, 2012).

The WHO advises that out-of-pocket spending constitute just 15 to 20 percent of total national health spending, and even countries that have implemented reforms, such as Ghana,

Vietnam, and the Philippines, have out-of-pocket costs that well exceed this threshold (WHO, 2005). Vietnam's out-of-pocket spending exceeds 50 percent (Bitran, 2012). A lack of financial protection for health care costs puts people at risk for poverty.

Summary of Low- and Middle-Income Countries' Health Systems

Low- and middle-income countries struggle to achieve UHC because of low levels of resources and inadequate infrastructure to efficiently distribute these resources. International financial aid for health care has not increased, leading countries to search for other means of raising revenue for health care and develop health insurance systems that are appropriate for their populations. Two possibilities are a social health insurance system, which is mandatory, and community-based systems, which are voluntary. Some low- and middle-income countries have had success with combinations of these

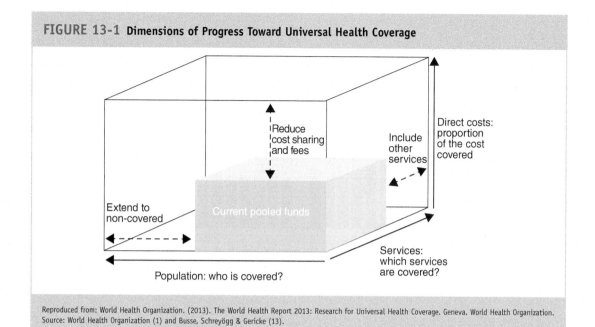

FIGURE 13-1 Dimensions of Progress Toward Universal Health Coverage

health insurance schemes. There is substantial variability across countries and regions in three dimensions of coverage: how much of the population is covered, which services are covered, and what proportion of costs are covered.

COMPARING HEALTH SYSTEM PERFORMANCE

Health care Spending

The United States spends more per person (per capita) and more as a share of the economy than other countries, as shown in **Figure 13-2** (Morgan & Canaud, 2015). All developed countries have increased medical spending over time, but as health care technology advanced in the 1970s, medical spending in the United States began to deviate from that of other countries (OECD, 2016). Innovations in health care have substantially improved the length and quality of life for many Americans suggesting that higher expenditures have yielded some value (Cutler, 2004). However, while other countries relied mostly on a single payer for health services that set prices for health care within a global budget, the United States had multiple payers with negotiated prices and no cap on services or costs.

The extent to which greater health spending improves population health outcomes is important in determining how to allocate health care resources. Spending is a combination of price, volume, and intensity of health care services. In addition to direct delivery of health care, any system requires administration. Compared to other countries, the United States has much higher prices (Anderson, Reinhardt, Hussey, & Petrosyan, 2003). Higher prices can attract a talented workforce, and may reflect more sophisticated technologies that are not as commonly used in countries that cap spending. On the other hand, they may reflect waste or misallocated funds. One study found that compared to Canada, the difference in spending on hospitals and physicians was primarily due to administration (39 percent), followed by higher physician incomes (31 percent), and finally, the greater intensity of medical services provided in the United States (14 percent) (Pozen & Cutler, 2010).

Public Opinion

American health care providers and patients are more dissatisfied with their health care system than their counterparts in other countries. In a recent international survey comparing the public's

FIGURE 13-2 Health Spending as a Percentage of Gross Domestic Product

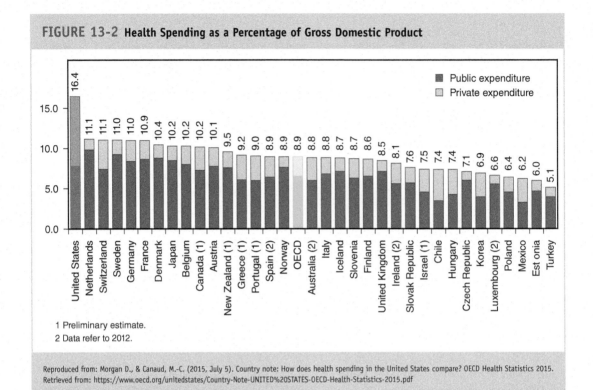

1 Preliminary estimate.
2 Data refer to 2012.

Reproduced from: Morgan D., & Canaud, M.-C. (2015, July 5). Country note: How does health spending in the United States compare? OECD Health Statistics 2015. Retrieved from: https://www.oecd.org/unitedstates/Country-Note-UNITED%20STATES-OECD-Health-Statistics-2015.pdf

views of the health care system in 10 countries, 75 percent of Americans reported that fundamental changes or a complete overhaul of the system were needed. France had the second highest dissatisfaction rate, with 60 percent reporting that major changes were needed, while less than 40 percent reported dissatisfaction in the United Kingdom (Mossialos et al., 2015).

In another survey comparing primary care physicians' views on the health care system, most primary care physicians were satisfied with practicing medicine (66 percent), and the rate of dissatisfaction was on par with countries such as Germany (36 percent) and the United Kingdom (33 percent). Norwegian primary care physicians reported the lowest rates of dissatisfaction (8 percent), even though a quarter found their jobs "very or extremely stressful," on par with Australia, Canada, the Netherlands, New Zealand, and Switzerland. Yet Norwegian physicians also reported the lowest rates of burdens with administrative or insurance issues (9 percent). The highest rate was in the Netherlands, where 60 percent of physicians reported that administrative burdens or insurance were a major problem; the United States was the next highest, at 54 percent (Osborn et al., 2015).

Survey results also indicate that U.S. adults are more likely than adults in many other high-income countries to not see a doctor because of cost, not fill a prescription or skip doses because of cost, and have problems paying medical bills, especially uninsured adults. Although most countries outperform the United States in affordability, the United States tends to rank better in disease management and access to specialty care. Compared to other countries, the United States has fewer gaps in hospital discharge planning and in chronic care management for older adults, in part because private insurance plans have developed innovative disease management programs for older populations. The United States also has lower wait times for specialty care on average (Schoen, Osborn, How, Doty, & Peugh, 2009).

Challenges of Comparing Health Systems

Even with data on national health spending and public satisfaction, the economic, political, and social complexity of countries makes it difficult to compare health systems (Shen, 2014). Only certain measures of health system performance are made available from various organizations. For example, while we have patient-reported information comparing medical error rates across countries, we cannot validate these errors, nor do we know the nature of these errors (Schoen et al., 2007). Further, data may be collected in different ways from different countries. The OECD collects data on health care spending, but countries may have different conventions for accounting for such spending, and especially for dividing such spending into categories such as public versus private, or out-of-pocket versus insurance.

International comparisons of public opinion are difficult for two reasons. First, people's expectations for their health care system may be different in each country. For example, if those in Canada hold their system to a higher standard than those in Norway, then Canadians might rank their health system lower, even if it performed equally to Norway's. Second, public satisfaction can be influenced by factors outside of the health care setting, such as the political climate and news media reporting at the time of the survey (Papanicolas, Cylus, & Smith, 2013). The ACA expanded health insurance to the U.S. population, which will likely affect future evaluations of the health care system. Other countries also continue to introduce insurance and delivery system reforms that will impact surveys of public opinion on the access to and quality of health care services.

Another important consideration in comparing health systems by health care spending is that medical care alone has limited impact on life expectancy and quality of life (Bunker, Frazier, & Mosteller, 1994; Cohen, Preston, & Crimmins, 2011; Cutler, Rosen, & Vijan, 2006; McKinlay & McKinlay, 1977). The totality of population health has to do more with the interaction of personal genetic composition, social networks, health behavior, medical care, and environmental exposures (Galea, Tracy, Hoggatt, DiMaggio, & Karpati, 2011; Institute of Medicine [IOM], 2000). Public health achievements such as tobacco control, seat belt laws, food fortification with micronutrients, and pollution controls for water and air have significantly reduced the global burden of disease, especially when compared to the impact of innovations in medical technology (Bradley & Taylor, 2013; Murray & Lopez, 1996).

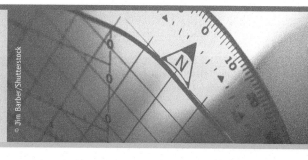

Summary

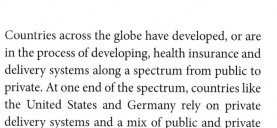

Countries across the globe have developed, or are in the process of developing, health insurance and delivery systems along a spectrum from public to private. At one end of the spectrum, countries like the United States and Germany rely on private delivery systems and a mix of public and private payers. At the other end, countries like the United Kingdom provide services that are mostly publicly financed and delivered in public settings.

At either end of the spectrum, countries face different types of challenges. The United States struggles to ensure equal access to and quality of services for people in different types of insurance plans, and to enroll the uninsured. Single payer countries such as the United Kingdom face challenges such as long waiting times for specialty care and elective surgery, as well as underfunded health care infrastructure.

Low- and middle-income countries face particular challenges, as they frequently lack resources to support a social health insurance system. Some countries have combined social health insurance systems with voluntary community-based insurance schemes with some success; others have used community-based insurance alone. Domestic financing for health services will be essential for low- and middle-income countries to ensure a reliable delivery of basic health care services and to protect households from high levels of out-of-pocket spending.

References

Anderson, G. F., Reinhardt, U. E., Hussey, P. S., & Petrosyan, V. (2003, May). It's the prices, stupid: Why the United States is so different from other countries. *Health Affairs, 22*(3), 89–105.

Atun, R., De Andrade, L. O., Almeida, G., Cotlear, D., Dmytraczenko, T., Frenz, P.,... De Paula, J. B. (2015, April 3). Health-system reform and universal health coverage in Latin America. *The Lancet, 385*(9974), 1230–1247.

Barber, S. L., & Yao, L. (2010). *Health insurance systems in China: A briefing note.* World Health Report Background Paper 37. Retrieved from http://www.who.int/healthsystems /topics/financing/healthreport/37ChinaB_YFINAL.pdf

Berwick, D. M., Nolan, T. W., & Whittington, J. (2008, May 1). The triple aim: Care, health, and cost. *Health Affairs, 27*(3), 759–769.

Bitran, R. (2012, August). *Universal health coverage reforms: Patterns of income, spending and coverage in four developing countries.* Washington, DC: Results for Development Institute.

Blumenthal, D., & Hsiao, W. (2005, September 15). Privatization and its discontents—The evolving Chinese health care system. *New England Journal of Medicine, 353*(11), 1165–1170.

Bradley, E., & Taylor, L. (2013). *The American health care paradox: Why spending more is getting us less.* New York, NY: Public Affairs.

Bunker, J. P., Frazier, H. S., & Mosteller, F. (1994, January 1). Improving health: Measuring effects of medical care. *The Milbank Quarterly, 72*(2), 225–258.

Busse, R., & Blümel, M. (2014). Germany: Health system review. *Health Systems in Transition, 16*(2), 1–296.

Canadian Institute for Health Information (CIHI). (2014). *National health expenditure trends, 1974 to 2014.* Retrieved from https://www.cihi.ca/en/nhex_2014_report_en.pdf

Cheng, T. M. (2008, July 1). China's latest health reforms: A conversation with Chinese Health Minister Chen Zhu. *Health Affairs, 27*(4), 1103–1110.

Cohen, B., Preston, S. H., & Crimmins, E. M. (Eds.). (2011, June 27). *Explaining divergent levels of longevity in high-income countries.* Washington, DC: National Academies Press.

Cutler, D. M. (2004). *Your money or your life: Strong medicine for America's health care system.* Oxford: Oxford University Press.

Cutler, D. M., Rosen A. B., & Vijan, S. (2006, August 31). The value of medical spending in the United States, 1960–2000. *New England Journal of Medicine, 355*(9), 920–927.

Dieleman, J. L., Schneider, M. T., Haakenstad, A., Singh, L., Sadat, N., Birger, M.,... Murray, C. J. (2016, June). Development assistance for health: Past trends, associations, and the future of international financial flows for health. *The Lancet, 387*(10037), 2536–2544.

Escobar, M. L., Griffin, C. C., & Shaw R. P. (Eds.). (2011). *The impact of health insurance in low-and middle-income countries.* Washington, DC: Brookings Institution Press.

Fan, V. Y., Grépin, K. A., Shen, G. C., & Chen, L. (2014, June). Tracking the flow of health aid from BRICS countries. *Bulletin of the World Health Organization, 92*(6), 457–458.

Galea, S., Tracy, M., Hoggatt, K. J., DiMaggio, C., & Karpati, A. (2011, August). Estimated deaths attributable to social factors in the United States. *American Journal of Public Health, 101*(8), 1456–1465.

Giedion, U., Alfonso, E. A., & Díaz, Y. (2013). *The impact of universal coverage schemes in the developing world: A review of the existing evidence.* Retrieved from http://siteresources .worldbank.org/HEALTHNUTRITIONAND POPULATION/Images/IMPACTofUHCSchemesin DevelopingCountries-AReviewofExistingEvidence.pdf

Global Hospital Management Survey—China (GHMS). (2014). *Global hospital management survey-China: Management in health care report.* Retrieved from http://www .hbs.edu/faculty/conferences/2014-world-management -survey/Documents/GlobalHospital_Management _Survey_Horak.pdf

Hsiao, W. C. (2003). *What is a health system? Why should we care?* Harvard School of Public Health Working Paper. Retrieved from http://isites.harvard.edu/fs/docs/icb.topic 1418653.files/Hsiao%202003_What%20is%20a%20 Health%20System.pdf

Institute of Medicine (IOM). (2000). *Promoting health: Intervention strategies from social and behavioral research.* Washington, DC: National Academy Press.

Lagomarsino, G., Garabrant, A., Adyas, A., Muga, R., & Otoo, N. (2012, September 14). Moving towards universal health coverage: Health insurance reforms in nine developing countries in Africa and Asia. *The Lancet, 380*(9845), 933–943.

Liang, L., & Langenbrunner, J. (2013). *The long march to universal coverage: Lessons from China.* Washington, DC: World Bank.

Liu, Y., Hsiao, W. C., & Eggleston, K. (1999, November 30). Equity in health and health care: The Chinese experience. *Social Science & Medicine, 49*(10), 1349–1356.

McKinlay, J. B., & McKinlay, S. M. (1977, July 1). The questionable contribution of medical measures to the decline of mortality in the United States in the twentieth century. *The Milbank Memorial Fund Quarterly Health and Society, 55*(3), 405–428.

Mebratie, A. D., Sparrow, R., Yilma, Z., Alemu, G., & Bedi, A. S. (2015, October 31). Enrollment in Ethiopia's community-based health insurance scheme. *World Development, 74*, 58–76.

Mills, A. (2014). Health care systems in low-and middle-income countries. *New England Journal of Medicine, 370*(6), 552–557.

Moreno-Serra, R., & Smith, P. C. (2012, September). Does progress towards universal health coverage improve population health? *The Lancet, 380*(9845), 917–923.

Morgan, D., & Canaud, M.-C. (2015, July 5). *Country note: How does health spending in the United States compare?* OECD Health Statistics 2015. Retrieved from https://www.oecd.org/unitedstates/Country-Note-UNITED%20STATES-OECD-Health-Statistics-2015.pdf

Mossialos, E., Wenzl, M., Osborn, R., & Anderson, C. (Eds.). (2015, January). *International profiles of health care systems*. Washington, DC: The Commonwealth Fund.

Murray, C. J., & Lopez, A. D. (1996, May). *Global burden of disease*. Cambridge, MA: Harvard University Press.

Organisation for Economic Co-operation and Development (OECD). (2016). OECD health statistics 2016. Retrieved from http://www.oecd.org/els/health-systems/health-data.htm

Osborn, R., Moulds, D., Schneider, E. C., Doty, M. M., Squires, D., & Sarnak, D. O. (2015, December 1). Primary care physicians in ten countries report challenges caring for patients with complex health needs. *Health Affairs, 34*(12), 2104–2112.

Papanicolas, I., Cylus, J., & Smith, P. C. (2013, April 1). An analysis of survey data from eleven countries finds that "satisfaction" with health system performance means many things. *Health Affairs, 32*(4), 734–742.

Pozen, A., & Cutler, D. M. (2010). Medical spending differences in the United States and Canada: The role of prices, procedures, and administrative expenses. *Inquiry, 47*(2), 124–134.

Reeves, A., Gourtsoyannis, Y., Basu, S., McCoy, D., McKee, M., & Stuckler, D. (2015, July 24). Financing universal health coverage—Effects of alternative tax structures on public health systems: Cross-national modeling in 89 low-income and middle-income countries. *The Lancet, 386*(9990), 274–280.

Reichs Gesetzblatt. *Gesetz betreffend die Krakenvessicherung der Arberter*. Germany, 1883.

Schoen, C., Osborn, R., Doty, M. M., Bishop, M., Peugh, J., & Murukutla, N. (2007, November 1). Toward higher-performance health systems: Adults' health care experiences in seven countries, 2007. *Health Affairs, 26*(6), w717–734.

Schoen, C., Osborn, R., How, S. K., Doty, M. M., & Peugh, J. (2009, January 1). In chronic condition: Experiences of patients with complex health care needs, in eight countries, 2008. *Health Affairs, 28*(1), w1–6.

Shen, G. C. (2014). Cross-national diffusion of mental health policy. *International Journal of Health Policy and Management, 3*, 269–282.

Stuckler, D., Feigl, A. B., Basu, S., & McKee, M. (2010, November 16). The political economy of universal health coverage. In *Background paper for the global symposium on health systems research*. Geneva, Switzerland: World Health Organization.

U.N. Development Programme (UNDP). (2015). *Sustainable development goals: 17 goals to transform our world*. Retrieved from http://www.un.org/sustainabledevelopment/

Wang, H. H. (2014, August 30). China's new health department: Progress and priorities. *The Lancet, 384*(9945), 733–734.

World Health Organization (WHO). (2000). *The world health report 2000: Health systems: Improving performance*. Geneva, Switzerland: World Health Organization.

World Health Organization (WHO). (2005). *Designing health financing systems to reduce catastrophic health expenditure*. Geneva, Switzerland: World Health Organization.

World Health Organization (WHO). (2012). *Countdown to 2015: Accountability for maternal, newborn and child survival*. Geneva, Switzerland: World Health Organization.

World Health Organization (WHO). (2013). *The world health report 2013: Research for universal health coverage*. Geneva, Switzerland: World Health Organization.

World Health Organization (WHO). (2014). WHO global health expenditure database. Retrieved from http://apps.who.int/nha/database/Comparison_Report/Index/en

World Health Organization (WHO). (2015). *Tracking universal health coverage: First global monitoring report*. Geneva, Switzerland: World Health Organization.

Yip, W. C., Hsiao, W. C., Chen, W., Hu, S., Ma, J., & Maynard, A. (2012, March 9). Early appraisal of China's huge and complex health-care reforms. *The Lancet, 379*(9818), 833–842.

APPENDIX A

A Guide to Dental and Vision Insurance

Only some health insurance plans include dental and vision benefits. Usually, consumers must purchase stand-alone dental and vision plans if they wish to have these services covered by insurance.

DENTAL

Dental Coverage by Private Payers

Most private health insurance plans do not cover dentistry services. More commonly, consumers in the private market obtain dental coverage through stand-alone dental plans. There are two markets for these plans: the individual market and the group (employer-based) market.

Consumers may purchase stand-alone plans in the individual market both inside and outside of the state health insurance exchanges, but the Affordable Care Act (ACA) extended fewer consumer protections to these plans. For example, insurers may rescind dental coverage for reasons other than fraud, while rescissions for health insurance are illegal. In theory, state health insurance exchanges offer both integrated plans (health insurance plus dental insurance) and stand-alone plans, but integrated plans may not be available in all states. Consumers must have purchased health insurance in order to purchase a stand-alone dental plan in the exchange. As with outside of the exchanges, there are fewer consumer protections inside of the exchanges. For example, premium

and cost-sharing subsidies are not available for stand-alone plans. Yet the exchanges offer consumers a place to compare multiple dental insurance options at once.

The majority of employers offer stand-alone dental insurance. While an overwhelming majority (88 percent) of large employers (over 200 workers) offer stand-alone dental benefits, just over half (52 percent) of small firms (under 200 workers) offer stand-alone dental benefits (The Henry J. Kaiser Family Foundation [KFF], 2014) (see Table A-1).

Dental Coverage by Public Payers

Medicare does not cover dental procedures. Rather, Medicare beneficiaries must rely on private retiree benefits or stand-alone plans purchased in the individual market or through the exchanges. Some Medigap plans include dental insurance, as do some Medicare Advantage (Part C) plans.

While the CHIP program must cover dental benefits for low-income children, Medicaid need not cover dental benefits for low-income adults, so coverage varies across states. More information on state-by-state dental coverage under Medicaid can be found on the Medicaid website (Centers for Medicare and Medicaid Services [CMS], n.d.).

TABLE A-1 **Percentage of Firms Offering Health Benefits That Offer or Contribute to a Separate Benefits Plan Providing Dental or Vision Benefits, by Firm Size or Region, 2014**

	Separate Dental Benefits	Separate Vision Benefits
FIRM SIZE		
200–99 Workers	88%*	60%*
1,000–4,999 Workers	91*	76*
5,000 or More Workers	91*	75*
All Small Firms (3–199 Workers)	52%*	34%*
All Large Firms (200 or More Workers)	88%*	63%*
REGION		
Northeast	46%	30%
Midwest	60	41
South	59	39
West	45	39
ALL FIRMS	53%	35%

* Estimate is statistically different from estimate for all other firms not in the indicated size or region category (p < 0.05)
Reproduced from Kaiser/HRET Survey of Employer-Sponsored Health Benefits, 2014 (Exhibit 2.9 Page 47)

Types of Dental Plans

There are typically two types of private stand-alone dental plans—HMOs and PPOs. As with health insurance, dental HMOs have more restrictive provider networks and a primary dentist "gatekeeper." Further, dental HMOs usually do not pay for out-of-network benefits. Dental PPOs, on the other hand, have wider provider networks, do not require a primary dentist "gatekeeper," and generally offer out-of-network benefits at higher rates. Less common is indemnity dental insurance, which, like indemnity health insurance, has no restrictions on providers, but requires subscribers to pay out-of-pocket for services and then submit a claim for reimbursement for a portion of the fee. When these plans pay providers directly, they are called fee-for-service plans.

VISION

Vision Coverage by Private Payers

Vision insurance is coverage for vision correction, including eye exams, eyeglasses, and contact lenses.

As with dental insurance, most health insurance plans do not integrate vision correction. Instead, consumers may purchase stand-alone plans or combined dental–vision plans on the individual market outside of the exchanges (state exchanges do not offer vision benefits unless they are integrated into health insurance plans). Like dental benefits, however, stand-alone vision plans in the individual market are not subject to the consumer protections established by the ACA. Employers do not offer stand-alone vision benefits as commonly as dental. The offer rate is 63 percent for large firms, and 34 percent for small firms (KFF, 2014).

Vision Coverage by Public Payers

Traditional (fee-for-service) Medicare does not cover vision correction services except for those related to medical problems such as cataracts. However, it does cover vision services related to glaucoma and macular degeneration. Like with dental services, Medicare beneficiaries who wish to obtain vision correction insurance must do so through retiree benefits, Medigap, or through the individual market. Some Medicare Advantage plans may include vision benefits.

Similarly to dental services, CHIP must cover vision services for low-income children. The Medicaid program does not require vision correction services for low-income adults, however, so coverage varies from state to state.

Types of Vision Plans

Vision plans vary widely in benefits, but most cover an annual eye exam and eyewear (frames and lenses or contact lenses), limited to a certain dollar amount. Some also offer discounts on laser corrective surgery and hearing aids (which are corrective devices not usually covered by health insurance). While some vision plans are HMO-like, restricting coverage to network providers and requiring referrals for non-network providers, others are PPO-like, allowing referral-free visits to any provider.

References

Centers for Medicare and Medicaid Service (CMS). (n.d.). *Dental care*. Medicaid.gov. Retrieved from https://www.medicaid.gov/medicaid/benefits/dental/index.html

The Henry J. Kaiser Family Foundation (KFF). (2014). *2014 employer health benefits survey*. Retrieved from http://files.kff.org/attachment/2014-employer-health-benefits-survey-full-report

Marketplace Assister Toolkit
Standard Operating Procedures Manual for Assisters in the Individual Federally-facilitated Marketplaces

The following is an excerpt of the SOP manual. To view the full manual, go to the following link: https://marketplace.cms.gov/technical-assistance -resources/assister-sop-manual.pdf

PURPOSE OF THE MANUAL

The Standard Operating Procedures Manual for Assisters in the Individual Federally-facilitated Marketplaces is an instructional guide intended for assisters. In this Manual, the term "assisters" refers to certified application counselors (CACs), Navigators, and non-Navigator assistance personnel who help consumers in the Federally-facilitated Marketplaces. This Manual contains standard operating procedures (SOPs) for assister activities within a Federally-facilitated Marketplace for the individual market (also referred to in this document as an "Individual Federally-facilitated Marketplace," "Individual FFM," or "Individual Marketplace"). The SOPs reflect requirements, policies, and best practices under the Patient Protection and Affordable Care Act and the Health Care and Education Reconciliation Act of 2010 (referred to collectively as the Affordable Care Act), CMS regulations, and CMS guidance.

INDIVIDUAL MARKETPLACE SOPs

The SOPs contained in this section provide guidance to help you assist individuals who select and purchase health coverage through a Federally-facilitated

Marketplace for the individual market or who have questions about exemptions from the individual shared responsibility payment or requirement to maintain minimum essential coverage.

Each SOP adheres to the following general structure:

A. Introduction: Outlines general task(s) and describes the SOP topic.
B. Procedures: Provides step-by-step instructions, tables, and graphics to guide assisters as they help consumers complete Marketplace activities.
C. Next Steps: Identifies next steps or associated SOPs that assisters can reference to further assist consumers with Marketplace activities.

Assess Consumers' Knowledge & Needs
A. Introduction

This section will assist you in understanding the type of support consumers require so that you can assist them.

B. Procedures
1. Assess Consumers' Knowledge

As a best practice, have a conversation with consumers to gauge their knowledge of health coverage, the Affordable Care Act, and the

Marketplace. The Knowledge Checks and Sample Questions listed in **Exhibit B-1** provide ideas to help you start a conversation to assess consumers' understanding.

EXHIBIT B-1 Knowledge Assessment Guide

Knowledge Category	Knowledge Checks	Sample Questions
Health Coverage	Determine if consumers: • Understand the basics of health coverage. • Know that for individual market health insurance, consumers and insurance companies pay for health care. • Understand key terms, such as premiums, deductibles, coinsurance, and copayments. • Know that insurance companies contract with different networks of doctors, and that their health care provider may not be included in some insurance networks.	• What questions do you have about health coverage? • How have you managed your health care costs in the past? • Do you understand how premiums, deductibles, coinsurance, and copayments function? • Do you have a doctor you see regularly? How would you feel if you had to see a new or different doctor?
Affordable Care Act	Determine if consumers: • Are aware of the preventive services available to them without cost sharing when they have non-grandfathered coverage. • Understand that there are limits on the amount they will pay in cost sharing for essential health benefits each year (excluding grandfathered coverage). • Are aware that they can no longer be denied coverage or charged more for having a pre- existing medical condition. • Understand the individual shared responsibility payment. • Know the exemptions available from the individual shared responsibility payment and the requirement to maintain minimum essential coverage and how to apply for an exemption if they think they might be eligible.	• What questions do you have about how the Affordable Care Act can lower the cost of your coverage? • What questions do you have about the requirement to maintain minimum essential coverage? Do you understand the consequences for consumers who do not meet this requirement? • Are you aware that some consumers may be exempt from the requirement to maintain minimum essential coverage?
Marketplace	Determine if consumers: • Understand the eligibility requirements for health coverage, tax credits, and cost savings available through a Marketplace. • Are aware of the key dates for the Marketplace annual Open Enrollment period, during which any consumer can apply for health coverage. • Are aware of the different health coverage options. • Are aware of the available programs to lower the costs of health coverage. • Understand the essential health benefits covered by all QHPs offered through a Marketplace (as well as most individual and small group coverage outside the Marketplace).	• What questions do you have about applying for and enrolling in health coverage through a Marketplace? • Are you aware of the start and end dates for the Marketplace annual Open Enrollment period? • How can I help you apply for health coverage through a Marketplace? • What questions do you have about the health coverage available through a Marketplace? • What are your concerns about paying for coverage? • Are you aware of the types of services covered by health coverage available through a Marketplace?

Reproduced from the Center for Medicare and Medicaid Services Marketplace Assister Toolkit

2. Assess Consumers' Needs

Step 1. As a best practice, have conversations with consumers to learn about their health coverage status, any questions they might have about the enrollment process, and problems they might have with completing their Marketplace applications. During this discussion, you should attempt to find out:

a. Whether consumers have existing health coverage and, if so, whether that coverage continues to meet their needs (e.g., if it is ending, benefits are changing, costs are changing);

b. Who is in need of health coverage (e.g., consumers and/or family members);

c. Whether consumers have started the Marketplace eligibility application process, and if they have, what stage in the application process they have reached (e.g., submitted the application, received an eligibility determination, ready to select a QHP);

d. How consumers intend to pay for the coverage (e.g., with advance payments of the premium tax credit, with personal income); and

e. What additional information, if any, consumers need to know about the Affordable Care Act, health coverage, or the Marketplaces (e.g., how to apply for an exemption to the individual shared responsibility payment or requirement to maintain minimum essential coverage, how to make changes to their account profile).

C. Next Steps

1. If consumers require additional information about health coverage, the Affordable Care Act, or the Marketplace, a good place to start is to refer to the resources on Marketplace.cms.gov.

2. If consumers are ready to begin eligibility and enrollment activities or have questions about exemptions from the individual shared responsibility payment or requirement to maintain minimum essential coverage, proceed to the appropriate SOP(s) in this Manual.

3. For more help answering consumers' specific questions, see the Frequently Asked Questions (FAQs) related to SOP-2 Assess Consumers' Knowledge & Needs [online].

Lower Costs of Coverage

A. Introduction

When consumers who apply for help lowering the costs of coverage receive their eligibility results, the Marketplace will inform them of their eligibility for options to lower their health plan costs through advance payments of the premium tax credit and/or cost-sharing reductions. If eligible, consumers can choose whether to apply advance payments of the premium tax credit to the cost of their health plans. When comparing plans, consumers select the amount of advance payments of the premium tax credit for which they are eligible that they want paid on their behalf to their chosen insurance provider. The amount of advance payments of the premium tax credit for which a consumer is eligible is based on the consumer's projected household income for the coming year and other factors. Consumers can also select health plans that apply cost-sharing reductions if they are eligible.

While assisting consumers with selecting the amount of advance payments of the premium tax credit or viewing a plan's cost-sharing reductions, remind consumers that they must accurately represent their household income information. Consumers generally are required to report all forms of household income, although Supplemental Security Income (SSI) and certain other items are not included in household income. Don't include child support payments, SSI, gifts, veteran's disability payments, worker's compensation, or proceeds from loans, such as student loans This SOP provides guidance on how to assist consumers with understanding advance payments of the premium tax credit and cost-sharing reductions.

B. Procedures

1. Select Advance Payments of the Premium Tax Credit

If consumers are eligible for advance payments of the premium tax credit, they have the option of using all, some, or none of the amount for which they are eligible to reduce their monthly premium cost. Before helping them make changes to their Marketplace accounts, make sure that consumers understand advance payments of premium tax credit. APTC is reconciled on tax returns, so using too much or too little of their credit can result in balances owed or refunds at tax time. **Exhibit B-2** provides information to help answer questions about advance payments of the premium tax credit available through the Marketplace.

2. Select the Amount of the Advance Payments of the Premium Tax Credit

If consumers are eligible for advance payments of the premium tax credit, the Marketplace will notify them of the maximum dollar amount available to them. Consumers can choose to apply the entire amount to their monthly health plan premiums or a lesser amount of their choice, including zero. Be sure to point out the differences between their eligibility for a certain amount of premium tax credit; and receiving advanced

---

EXHIBIT B-2 Common Premium Tax Credit Questions and Answers

Question	Answer
What is the premium tax credit?	• A tax credit that helps low- and moderate-income individuals afford health insurance.
What are advance payments of the premium tax credit?	• Individuals who meet certain criteria at the time of enrollment in a QHP may choose to have advance payments of the premium tax credit paid to their insurance provider to lower the cost of their monthly premiums. Consumers may choose to have some, none, or all of the advance payments of the premium tax credit for which they are eligible paid on their behalf.
How do advance payments of the premium tax credit affect individuals' tax returns?	• When consumers file their tax returns for the year, the actual amount of the premium tax credit they were eligible for is calculated. Consumers whose advance payments of the premium tax credit exceed their actual premium tax credit eligibility may be required to pay back all or a portion of the difference. Consumers whose advance payments of the premium tax credit is less than the amount they were eligible for will owe less in taxes or get a refund for the difference.
Who is eligible for advance payments of the premium tax credit?	To be eligible for a premium tax credit: • Consumers or family members, such as their spouse or dependent, must be enrolled in a QHP through the Marketplace for one or more months in which they were not eligible for other minimum essential coverage (MEC) such as Medicaid, CHIP, TRICARE, or affordable employer-sponsored coverage that meets the minimum value standard; • Consumers must file a joint tax return if married, unless the consumer is a victim of domestic abuse or spousal abandonment, and will not be claimed as a dependent on another taxpayer's tax return;[†] • In general, consumers must have household income between 100% and 400% of the federal poverty level (FPL) (see Appendix C: Federal Poverty Guidelines [online]);* and • Note that a premium tax credit is only allowed for months in which consumers pay their share of the premium by the due date of the consumers' tax return.

[†]Consumers who are married but living apart from their spouse and are unable to file a joint income tax return because of a case of spousal abandonment or domestic abuse can obtain advance payments of the premium tax credit and cost-sharing reduction as long as they are otherwise eligible. For more information, see the guidance available at: https://www.CMS.gov/CCIIO/Resources /Regulations-and- Guidance/Downloads/victims-domestic-violence-guidance-3-31-2014.pdf.

*Adult Consumers generally must have a household income between approximately 138% and 400% of the FPL (approximately $16,590 to $47,520 for an individual and $33,934 to $97,200 for a family of four; higher in Alaska and Hawaii) if they live in a state that has expanded Medicaid. Consumers living in a Medicaid expansion state whose household income is less than 100% FPL and who are not eligible for Medicaid due to immigration status may also be eligible for financial assistance through the Marketplace. See the Assister Guide to the Immigration Section of the Online Marketplace Application for more information on helping non-citizens through the Marketplace application process.

Reproduced from the Center for Medicare and Medicaid Services Marketplace Assister Toolkit

payments of the premium tax credit; and their premium tax credit.

Advance payments of the premium tax credit are based on estimates of the premium tax credit consumers may be allowed to claim when filing their tax return. Eligibility for the premium tax credit and the amount of the credit they are allowed is not determined until the consumer files a tax return.

Also point out that when filing their tax return for the year, consumers must reconcile or compare their advance payments of the premium tax credit with the premium tax credit they are allowed. Consumers whose advance payments of the premium tax credit exceed their actual premium tax credit will owe all or a portion of the difference to the IRS when filing their taxes. Consumers whose actual premium tax credit is more than their advance payments of the premium tax credit may get a credit on their taxes or get a refund for the difference. You can help consumers select the amount of advance payments of the premium tax credit to apply to their monthly premiums during plan selection after the initial application or when reporting a life change to the Marketplace.

For example, if a consumer will have an uncertain variable income, you may want to discuss the idea of claiming only part of the tax credit for which they are eligible as an advance payment. This may reduce the amount of money the consumer may owe at tax filing time in the event the consumer's actual income is higher than anticipated. However, it's important to remind consumers that you cannot provide tax advice within your capacity as an assister.

To help consumers select the amount of advance payments of the premium tax credit they would like to have paid on their behalf, complete the following steps:

Step 1. Help consumers review the amount of advance payments of the premium tax credit for which they are eligible. The amount of advance payments of the premium tax credit for which consumers are eligible can be found in the Eligibility Results table on their eligibility notice, as shown in **Exhibit B-3**. Explain that the amount shown on the table represents the amount of the advance payments of the premium tax credit for the entire family, not just the individual, on that particular row of the chart. For example, if a married couple is eligible for $300 of advance payments of the premium tax credit, the eligibility results table will show $300 after the husband's name and $300 after the wife's name. Even though the amount of $300 appears twice, the couple is not eligible for $600.

Explain to consumers that they have the option to use less than the total amount of the advance payments of the premium tax credit for which they are found eligible. The amount they use will lower the cost they will pay for QHP monthly premiums.

EXHIBIT B-3   What Are the Results of My Application?

Family Member(s)	Results	Next Steps
Andre Hill	• Eligible to purchase health coverage through the Marketplace, but more information is needed • Eligible for advance payments of the premium tax credit ($300 each month, which is $3,600 for the year), but more information is needed	• Send the Marketplace more information
Bridget Hill	• Eligible to purchase health coverage through the Marketplace, but more information is needed • Eligible for advance payments of the premium tax credit ($300 each month, which is $3,600 for the year), but more information is needed	• Send the Marketplace more information

Reproduced from the Center for Medicare and Medicaid Services Marketplace Assister Toolkit

Things You Should Know

Remind consumers that they must file taxes in the upcoming year if advance payments of the premium tax credit are paid on their behalf. Also inform consumers that they will be ineligible for advance payments of the premium tax credit in future years if advance payments of the premium tax credit are paid on their behalf but they do not file a federal tax return for the year.

Step 2. Describe the potential effects of adjusting advance payments of the premium tax credit amount, including:

a. Premium amount paid by consumers; and
b. Tax consequences (see Section on Potential Tax Consequences [online]).

Step 3. Explain when the advance payments of the premium tax credit take effect.

During Open Enrollment:

a. If consumers adjust advance payments of the premium tax credit between the 1st and 15th of the month, the change in premium takes effect on the first of the next month (e.g., if the change is made on December 8, the change in premium takes effect on January 1).
b. If consumers adjust advance payments of the premium tax credit between the 16th and the last day of the month, the change in premium takes effect on the first of the month following the next month (e.g., if the change is made on December 17, the change in premium takes effect on February 1).

Outside of Open Enrollment

a. If consumers adjust the amount of advance payments of the premium tax credit (APTC), the change generally takes effect the day the adjustment is made, unless the family simultaneously receives a Special Enrollment Period (SEP) determination, in which case the APTC change follows the SEP effective date.

Step 4. Help consumers select the amount of advance payments of the premium tax credit they would like to apply towards their monthly premium payments. Consumers' maximum amount of the advance payments of the premium tax credit cannot be more than the cost of their monthly premiums.

IMPORTANT: If the consumer is shopping for a plan, monthly premium costs will reflect the amount of APTC the consumer selected. Some consumers may wish to change the amount of advance payments of the premium tax credit they are using for an existing plan. These consumers should log in to their Marketplace accounts; select the plan they are currently enrolled in from the Plan Compare menu; and proceed to the Review and Confirm Plan Selection page to make the change.

Potential Tax Consequences   Before Navigators, non-Navigator assistance personnel, and certified application counselors provide assistance to consumers, they must provide consumers with a disclaimer stating that they are not acting as tax advisors or attorneys, and they cannot provide tax or legal advice within their capacities as Navigators, non-Navigator assistance personnel, and certified application counselors. However, these assister entities are expected to help consumers understand general information about the impact of Marketplace policies on consumer taxes.

Explain to consumers that the amount of the advance payments of the premium tax credit paid on their behalf will affect the amount they owe or the amount of their refund when they file their federal income tax return. Consumers for whom advance payments of the premium tax credit payments are made must file a tax return, even if they are not otherwise required to file taxes. On their tax return, the advanced payments of the premium tax credit they received will be compared to the actual premium tax credit they are allowed to claim on that return.

A consumer's maximum advance payments of the premium tax credit (APTC) depend on the consumer's projected household income and family size. However, the consumer must use his or her actual household income and family size in calculating the premium tax credit when filing his or her tax return to calculate the premium tax credit. If a consumer's actual household income differs from the projected household income amount, this may affect the amount the consumer will pay or receive as a credit or refund when filing the consumer's federal income tax return.

Consumer repayments of the excess advanced payments of the premium tax credit is limited to amounts based on their income and household size, as shown in **Exhibit B-4**.

If consumers' actual household incomes are less than they projected when they submitted their Marketplace application, or if consumers chose to have less than all of the advance payments of the premium tax credit for which they were eligible paid to the insurance provider, it is likely that the consumers' premium tax credit will be more than their advance payments of the premium tax credit. In that case, consumers will get a credit or a refund for the difference when they file a tax return for the year.

If a consumer's income is below 100% FPL, he or she may still be able to claim the premium tax credits at tax time if the individual had been enrolled in a Marketplace plan with APTC and had expected a household income between 100 and 400% FPL when the consumer initially enrolled in the plan. However, for the next plan year, the individual may be eligible for Medicaid and generally will not be eligible for APTC if household income for the next plan year is expected to remain below 100% FPL. Consumers should be encouraged to go back to the Marketplace to update their income information. If a consumer does appear to qualify for Medicaid, his or her application information will be sent directly to the consumer's State Medicaid office. The consumer will receive a notice of Medicaid eligibility later.

Note that as an Assister, you may educate consumers on the Marketplace-related components of the premium tax credit reconciliation process, and help them understand the availability of IRS resources on this process. However, you must inform consumers that you are not acting as a tax adviser or attorney when providing assistance as an assister and cannot provide tax or legal advice within your capacity as an assister.

Exhibit B-5 provides a reference on when consumers should contact the Marketplace Call Center or the IRS if they have questions about how their coverage status and/or Marketplace financial assistance will affect the tax filing process. Use this resource in your work with consumers to help them route their questions accordingly.

3. Select Plans with Cost-Sharing Reductions

In addition to premium tax credits, consumers may be eligible for financial assistance through the Marketplace in the form of cost-sharing

EXHIBIT B-4 Consumer APTC Repayment Limits

Household Income Percentage of Federal Poverty Line	Limitation Amount for Single, Married Filing Separately, and HOH Taxpayers	Limitation Amount for All Other Filing Statuses
Less than 200%	$300	$600
At least 200%, but less than 300%	$750	$1,500
At least 300%, but less than 400%	$1,250	$2,500
400% or more	No limit	No limit

Reproduced from the Center for Medicare and Medicaid Services Marketplace Assister Toolkit

EXHIBIT B-5 Where Consumers Can Direct Questions About the Tax Consequences of APTC and Marketplace Coverage

Marketplace Call Center Will Handle Questions Regarding:	Internal Revenue Service Will Handle Questions Regarding:

• Form 1095-A (Advance Premium Tax Credit)
 • Form 8962 (Premium Tax Credit) and how it works with Form 1095-A
 • Advance Premium Tax Credit versus Premium Tax Credit
 • Eligibility for Advance Premium Tax Credit
 • Exemptions (including who qualifies for exemptions, what to do if your exemption is pending, and how to get an Exemption Certificate Numbers (ECNs))
 • Handling problems with Form 1095-A (including missing or incorrect information and duplicate copies)
 • How the Tax Credit may Impact Consumers' Tax Refunds
 • Fees for Not Having Coverage (what it is, how much it will cost, and what it will be in future years)
 • Tax Assistance (including free file, which forms to fill out, where to get assistance with tax filing, and what the tax deadline is)
	• Help Filing Taxes
	 • Help Paying Taxes Owed to the IRS
	 • Questions Related to Tax Filing, such as:
	   ○ How long can I delay filing?
	   ○ What happens if I don't file?
	   ○ I filed my taxes prior to getting Form 1095-A. How do I amend my tax return?
	 • Questions on how to complete Form 8962 Premium Tax Credit
	 • Questions on how to complete Form 8965 Exemptions
	 • Questions about other tax forms

reductions ("income-based cost-sharing reductions" or CSRs). If consumers have household income between 100% and 250% FPL or are members of a federally recognized Indian tribe, they may be eligible for plans with cost-sharing reductions. Plans with income-based cost-sharing reductions reduce the amount that consumers have to pay out of pocket for health care (e.g., deductibles, copayments, and coinsurance), provided that the consumer chooses a Silver level QHP. Members of federally recognized tribes may take advantage of cost-sharing reductions at any health plan metal level. Eligible members of federally recognized Indian Tribes may receive their special cost sharing benefit in any Bronze, Silver, Gold or Platinum plan. The Marketplace will determine if consumers are eligible for cost-sharing reductions based on projected household income and family size; or membership in a federally recognized tribe. Exhibit B-6 provides information to help answer questions about cost-sharing reductions.

Consumers will find out if they are eligible for cost-sharing reductions by reviewing their onscreen eligibility results. It is important for those eligible for the most generous cost-sharing reductions provided, at the 94%/06 and 87%/05 level, to understand that if they use medical services, they may potentially save thousands of dollars but only by selecting a Silver plan.

If consumers are eligible for cost-sharing reductions, discuss the following topics.

Topic 1: Explain to consumers that they must choose a Silver category plan to take advantage of the cost-sharing reduction. If they qualify for a cost sharing reduction and do not choose a Silver level plan, they may owe more when they need health care. There is one exception to this rule: members of a federally recognized tribe may take advantage of cost-sharing reductions at any health plan metal level. Consumers who are eligible for cost-sharing reductions will see eligible plans indicated with an "Extra Savings" box in the corner. Topic 2: Explain that cost-sharing reductions may decrease the following costs:

• Deductibles;
• Coinsurance; and/or
• Copayments.

EXHIBIT B-6 Common Cost-Sharing Reductions Questions and Answers

Question	Answer
What is a cost-sharing reduction?	A discount that lowers the amount a consumer has to pay for deductibles, coinsurance, and copayments.
Who is eligible for cost-sharing reductions?	To be eligible for and utilize cost-sharing reductions, a consumer must: • Have a projected household income between 100% and 250% of the FPL[†]; or an American Indian with household income under 300% of the FPL. • Enroll in a Silver category QHP* through the Marketplace; and • Be eligible for the premium tax credit.

[†]Members of federally recognized tribes who have a household income below 300% of the FPL are exempt from cost-sharing and do not have to pay out-of-pocket costs for health coverage.

*Members of federally recognized tribes may take advantage of cost-sharing reductions at any health plan metal level.

Reproduced from the Center for Medicare and Medicaid Services Marketplace Assister Toolkit

Topic 3: Explain that cost-sharing reductions will not decrease the following costs:

- Monthly premiums;
- Balances billed by non-network providers; nor
- Amounts spent on non-covered services.

Topic 4: Explain that consumers need to be aware of their responsibility to notify the Marketplace within 30 days of any changes in their household income level or other application information that may affect their eligibility for cost-sharing reductions.

C. Next Steps

1. If consumers would like to compare plans or make plan selections, proceed to SOP - Compare, Save, & Select Health Plans.
2. If consumers need to report changes that affect their eligibility results, proceed to SOP—Report Life Changes.
3. If consumers believe that they are eligible for more advance payments of the premium tax credit or cost-sharing reductions, proceed to SOP - Request an Eligibility Appeal.
4. For more help answering consumers' specific questions, see Appendix A for Frequently Asked Questions (FAQs) related to SOP - Lower Costs of Coverage [online].

Pay Health Plan Premium

A. Introduction

This SOP provides guidance on how to assist consumers with making premium payments once they have selected a QHP. After the consumer has selected a QHP, the Marketplace will redirect the consumer to the QHP website—when applicable—or will instruct the consumer to contact the QHP issuer directly to make premium payments. Online premium payment is optional and not every health insurance company will accept online payments. Consumers should contact their health insurance company with any specific questions about acceptable methods or deadlines for premium payment. Please ensure that consumers understand that the individual Marketplace does not accept payments on behalf of insurance companies. All financial transactions that consumers need to make related to their Marketplace QHP coverage are handled directly by their insurance company, not the Marketplace.

QHP issuers in the FFMs are required to accept paper checks, cashier's checks, money orders, electronic fund transfers (EFTs), and all general-purpose prepaid debit cards as methods of payment. The insurance company must present all payment method options equally for a consumer to select the preferred payment method.

Insurance companies may accept payment of the initial premium by a method that is exclusive to the initial premium. For example, online payment ("payment redirect") may allow payment of the initial month's premium by credit card, even though the issuer does not accept credit cards as a method of payment for regular, monthly premiums.

Application of premium payment methods must not improperly discriminate against any consumer or group of consumers. Insurance companies may not offer a discount on premiums to individuals who elect a specific type of premium payment method (e.g., EFT). Additionally, issuers may not apply additional fees to a consumer based on payment method. For example, an issuer may not pass on administrative fees for processing a premium payment via credit card.

Before assisting consumers when they are making a payment, it's important to understand that consumers' financial payment information (e.g., bank account, debit cards, credit cards) must be kept private and secure, just like all consumer PII that you may encounter while helping a consumer. **Exhibit B-7** specifies appropriate and inappropriate activities related to assisting consumers with information about premium payments:

B. Procedures

1. Make a Premium Payment

If a consumer understands the requirement to make a premium payment and the available payment options, you can proceed with the following steps to help the consumer submit a premium payment:

Step 1. Assist consumers with navigating to their Enroll To-Do List on HealthCare.gov to view their selected QHP.

Step 2. Help consumers select how they would like to make payments:

a. Pay online/electronically, if available as an option.
b. Mail payments to the appropriate insurance company.

Step 3. If consumers wish to make electronic payments, they may click the "Pay for Health Plan" button (if available) to be redirected to their QHP issuer's website.

Step 4. Once consumers have navigated to their QHP issuer's website, you can complete the following steps to assist consumers:

a. Explain to consumers that their enrollment in a QHP is not complete until the insurance company receives the first premium payment.
b. Explain that consumers can follow the prompts on the insurance company's website to complete electronic payments, if available. Consumers should be sure to follow their insurance company's payment policies.
c. Encourage consumers to contact their insurance company's call center with questions about billing.
d. Remind consumers that to protect their PII, they should log out of the insurance company's website after making their premium payments.

EXHIBIT B-7 Premium Payment Assistance Do's and Don'ts

Do	Don't
• Assure consumers that the assister will protect any financial information consumers share with the assister, and that an Individual FFM does not collect their financial information, because they will make their payments directly to the issuer of the QHP they selected. • Keep any financial information that consumers give you private and secure. • Turn computers to face consumers to keep information private. • Ask consumers to enter their own financial information.	• Use consumers' financial information for personal gain. • Enter consumers' payment methods (e.g., credit card information) on their behalf unless the consumer requests assistance and is physically present in person.

Reproduced from the Center for Medicare and Medicaid Services Marketplace Assister Toolkit

Things You Should Know

- Insurance companies must accept methods of payment that include options for consumers that do not have bank accounts or credit cards.

Step 5. If consumers wish to pay their premiums by mail, you can complete the following steps:

a. Explain to consumers that enrollment in their QHP is not complete until the insurance company receives the first premium payment.

b. Direct consumers to the insurance company's call center if they need additional billing information. Consumers should note that it may take a day or two before their QHP selection shows up in the insurance company's system.

c. Encourage consumers to contact their insurance company's call center with questions about billing.

C. Next Steps

1. If consumers do not have their payment information with them (e.g., credit card or bank account routing info), they should access their insurance company's website or contact the insurance company's call center to make a payment at a later time.

2. If consumers have further questions or issues about premium payments, they should contact their insurance company's call center.

3. For more help answering consumers' specific questions, see Appendix A for Frequently Asked Questions (FAQs) related to SOP - Pay Health Plan Premium [online].

Request an Eligibility Appeal

A. Introduction

Assisters are not required to help consumers through the entire eligibility appeals process, and must not act as tax advisers or attorneys when providing assistance as Navigators, non-Navigator assistance personnel, or certified application counselors. This SOP provides guidance on how to assist consumers with understanding the process of filing Marketplace eligibility appeals. The Marketplace allows consumers to request an appeal of the following:

- Eligibility or redetermination of eligibility to: purchase a Marketplace QHP (including a catastrophic plan); a child only plan; or eligibility for an employer to participate in a SHOP employer plan.
- An eligibility determination for a special enrollment period.
- Eligibility or redetermination of eligibility for advance payments of the premium tax credit or cost-sharing reductions, including the amount of advance payments of the premium tax credit and cost-sharing reductions for which the consumer was determined or re-determined eligible. Note that consumers who have outstanding data matching issues (DMIs) will need to resolve those issues or wait for them to expire before they will be able to file an appeal regarding the eligibility determination for which there is a DMI. Consumers cannot appeal eligibility determinations that still have open DMIs.
- Eligibility for an exemption from the individual shared responsibility payment that is granted by the Marketplace.
- Eligibility for Medicaid or CHIP.
- Eligibility for Basic Health Programs.
- A Marketplace individual or SHOP application that had not been acted on with reasonable promptness such that the consumer did not receive timely notice of an eligibility determination.
- The appeal decision of a state-based appeals entity or the refusal of a state-based appeals

entity to vacate dismissal of an appeal request (that is, to reinstate the appeal).

Consumers may file appeals from Medicaid and CHIP determinations with FFM only under limited circumstances.

   (i) MAGI-related Medicaid denials by the FFM.

      a. The following states have delegated MAGI-related Medicaid determinations to the FFM and delegated authority to conduct appeals to CMS – AL, AK, AR, LA, MT, NJ, TN, WV, WY (for MAGI-related Medicaid, not CHIP). When the FFM denies MAGI-related Medicaid to residents of those states who apply to the FFM, they may appeal those denials to the Federal Marketplace Appeals Entity (Marketplace Appeals Center).

      b. Option to Transfer to State Entity. Consumers in these states have a right to have their state entity conduct a Medicaid Fair Hearing. They may request their MAGI-related Medicaid appeal through the Marketplace Appeals Center but can ask that their Fair Hearings be held by their state by checking the appropriate box on their appeal request or otherwise asking for this option. Marketplace Appeals Center will transfer such appeals to the applicable state Medicaid agency Fair Hearing entity. This option does not exist for CHIP appeals.

  (ii) Appeals in Assessment States. For consumers in all other states, the FFM assesses eligibility for MAGI-related Medicaid and CHIP. The state Medicaid agency makes the final eligibility determination and aggrieved consumers may appeal through their state's Fair Hearing process.

 (iii) Non-MAGI-Related Appeals. The FFM does not render eligibility determinations for non-MAGI-related Medicaid. If a state Medicaid agency denies non-MAGI Medicaid, aggrieved consumers may appeal through their state's Fair Hearing process. Consumers whose eligibility is determined on a non-MAGI basis include the aged, blind, or disabled, as well as the medically needy, present or former foster youth, consumers with long-term care needs, and some others.

Consumers who disagree with an eligibility determination made by the FFM may appeal to the Federal Marketplace Appeals Entity (Marketplace Appeals Center) within 90 days of the date of their eligibility notice. Upon receipt, the Marketplace Appeals Center will review the appeal request and validate the appeal based on whether it was submitted within the 90-day timeframe and whether it concerns a matter over which the Marketplace Appeals Center has jurisdiction. For example, if the appeal request is about a matter where no jurisdiction exists, such as a dispute the consumer has with a QHP issuer over a claim denial, the consumer will receive a notice explaining why the appeal request was invalid and what other options the consumer may have. The Marketplace Appeals Center may accept an untimely appeal if a consumer sufficiently demonstrates within a reasonable timeframe that failure to submit the appeal request timely was due to exceptional circumstances that should not preclude the appeal.

Once an appeal has been validated, the Marketplace Appeals Center will review the appeal, including all documentation provided by the consumer and available in the consumer's Marketplace eligibility record. The consumer may be asked in writing to submit additional information or be contacted by phone to discuss the appeal. In many cases, the Marketplace Appeals Center will work with the consumer to resolve the appeal informally. If the consumer is satisfied with the informal resolution, a decision will be sent in the mail. Conversely, if the consumer is not satisfied with the informal resolution, the consumer can request a hearing conducted by telephone of the appeal before a federal hearing officer. After the hearing, the consumer will receive a final appeal decision in the mail. If the appeal decision states that the contested eligibility determination was incorrect, the consumer will be able to choose whether the appeal decision will be effective in the future or retroactively to the coverage effective date associated with the incorrect eligibility determination.

The following rights are afforded to consumers as part of the appeals process:

- Consumers can ask for an expedited appeal review if they believe that they have an immediate need for health services and a delay could seriously jeopardize their health.
- Consumers may have an authorized representative to help them with their appeal. An authorized representative is a person who has the permission of the consumer to talk with the Marketplace Appeals Center about their appeal, see their information, and act for them on matters related to their appeal, including getting information about them and signing their appeal request on their behalf.
- Consumers also can have someone help them with their appeal, including at the hearing like a friend, relative, or lawyer. This person does not have to be formally designated as an authorized representative, but if they are not, they will not be allowed to act for the consumer on matters related to the consumer's appeal.
- Consumers who are appealing a redetermination of eligibility resulting in a loss or reduction of eligibility for advance payments of the premium tax credit and, if applicable, cost-sharing reductions can request a continuation of the previous level of benefits pending their appeal. This is sometimes called "aid-paid- pending." If they do not prevail in their appeal, they would be liable for any advance payments of the premium tax credit that they had received during the appeal, which would be reconciled when they file their taxes.
- Consumers can ask the Marketplace Appeals Center to provide them a copy of their appeal record free of charge.

- Consumers can bring witnesses to testify.
- Consumers may request an auxiliary aid or service and language assistance services to make the appeals process accessible to them.

The sections that follow in this SOP provide guidance on how to assist consumers with requesting an appeal.

B. Procedures

All consumer eligibility determination notices contain instructions on how consumers may request an appeal. Consumers can mail or fax their appeal requests to the Marketplace. The appeal request may either be in the form of a letter or consumers may send a completed and signed appeal request form.

Consumers may receive various notices during the appeals process. **Exhibit B-8** lists sample notices commonly used throughout the appeals process and their corresponding descriptions.

For more information on appeals, assisters and consumers can visit HealthCare.gov/ Marketplace-Appeals.

For an overview of the appeals process, see this presentation on Marketplace Eligibility Appeals. An overview of the appeals process is also available at https://marketplace.cms.gov/technical -assistance-resources/assister-webinars.html.

Additional information is available at https:// marketplace.cms.gov/outreach-and-education /appeals-eligibility-and-health-plan-decisions .pdf and https://marketplace.cms.gov/technical -assistance-resources/logo-and-infographics /steps-for-a-marketplace-appeal.pdf.

C. Next Steps

1. If consumers require further assistance with the appeals process, consider referring them to the Consumer Assistance Program or legal services program available in their state. For more information on Consumer Assistance Programs, visit http://www.CMS.gov/CCIIO/Resources /Consumer-Assistance-Grants. For more information on legal services, visit http:// www.lsc.gov/find-legal-aid.

EXHIBIT B-8 Appeals Notices

Notice Type	Description
Acknowledgment of Your Marketplace Eligibility Appeal	Notice explaining the appeal request has been received.
Notice of Informal Resolution	Notice explaining how CMS proposes to resolve the appeal informally, without a hearing.
Notice of Hearing	Notice explaining a hearing request has been received and details on the hearing (e.g., format, date, and time).
Appeals Decision Notice	Notice explaining the outcome of the hearing.
Notice of Marketplace Eligibility Appeal Dismissal	Notice explaining why the appeal has been dismissed. This notice includes a form to use if the consumer disagrees with the dismissal and wants to request that the appeal be reopened.
Notice Granting (or Denying) Request to Vacate an Appeal Dismissal	Notice explaining whether an appellant demonstrated 'good cause' to reopen an appeal that has been dismissed.

---

2. For more help answering consumers' specific questions, see Appendix A online for Frequently Asked Questions (FAQs) related to SOP - Request an Eligibility Appeal [online].
3. Appellants with questions about their eligibility appeals may call the Marketplace Appeals Center at 1-855-231-1751 (TTY: 1-855-739-2231). The call center is available 7:30 AM to 8:45 PM (EST) Monday through Friday, and 10:00 AM to 5:30 PM (EST) Saturday.

Exemptions

A. Introduction

The Affordable Care Act requires applicable individuals to either have minimum essential coverage (MEC) for the entire year, pay a fee when filing a federal income tax return, or obtain an exemption from the requirement to maintain MEC. Refer to Exhibit B-9 below to learn more about the various exemptions for which consumers may qualify.

Please remember: It's important to remind consumers that you cannot provide tax advice within your capacity as an assister and that you are not acting as a tax adviser or attorney when providing assistance as an assister. However, you should be able to help consumers generally understand that some exemptions can be claimed through the tax filing process and how to request them.

Exemptions that must be claimed through the Marketplace can be claimed at any time during the year. Exemptions available through the federal tax filing process must be claimed when applicants file their federal income taxes for the tax year. The exemption for unaffordable coverage processed by the Marketplace is available prospectively ONLY. After the tax year ends, consumers must claim this exemption on their tax return. For more information on exemptions from the IRS, please visit: https://www.irs.gov/affordable-care-act/individuals-and-families/aca-individual-shared-responsibility-provision-exemptions.

The sections that follow in this SOP provide guidance on how to assist consumers with understanding exemptions and applying for exemptions from the individual responsibility payment that are granted through the Marketplace.

B. Procedures

1. Hardship Exemptions to Purchase Catastrophic Coverage

Consumers may be eligible for an exemption based on financial or other circumstances that

EXHIBIT B-9 Descriptions of Exemptions

When to Use This Exemption	Information Consumers Need When Applying for This Exemption	Link to Exemption Application	How to Claim This Exemption	For More Information on This Exemption
Type of Exemption: Hardship Exemption				
Consumers can use this exemption if they experience a life situation that keeps them from getting health insurance (e.g. homeless, facing eviction or foreclosure, and experienced domestic violence).	• SSNs, if they have them • Information about people in their tax household • Documents that support their claim of hardship (see page 1 of the hardship exemption application), if applying through the Marketplace.	Application for Exemption from the Shared Responsibility Payment for Individuals who Experience Hardships: https://marketplace.cms.gov/applications-and-forms/hardship-exemption.pdf	In most cases, this exemption will be claimed through the Marketplace. Consumers who are ineligible for Medicaid based on a state's decision not to expand Medicaid may apply for this exemption either through the Marketplace or when filing their federal income tax returns.	https://www.healthcare.gov/health-coverage-exemptions/hardship-exemptions/
There are multiple types of categories of hardship exemptions. Hardship exemptions usually cover the month before the hardship, the months of the hardship, and the month after the hardship. But in some cases the Marketplace may provide the exemption for additional months, including up to a full calendar year.	Note: If consumers can't obtain documents to support hardship, call the Marketplace Call Center at 1-800-318-2596. TTY users should call 1-855-889-4325			
Type of Exemption: Membership in a Health Care Sharing Ministry				
Consumers can use this exemption if they are/were members of a health care sharing ministry that is recognized by the Marketplace	• SSNs, if they have them • Information about people in their tax household • If claiming this exemption through the Marketplace, consumers must provide the name and address of the health care sharing ministry of which they are a member.	Application for Exemption from the Shared Responsibility Payment for Members of a Health Care Sharing Ministry: https://marketplace.cms.gov/applications-and-forms/sharing-ministry-exemption.pdf To claim on their federal tax return, consumers should use IRS Form 8965: https://www.irs.gov/pub/irs-pdf/f8965.pdf	Starting September 1, 2016, this exemption may only be obtained by claiming it on an annual federal income tax return through the IRS	https://www.healthcare.gov/exemptions-tool/#/results/2016/details/healthcare-sharing-ministry

(Continues)

Type of Exemption: Income Below the Tax-Filing Threshold		
Consumers can use this exemption if their annual income is below the amount that requires them to file a federal tax return	• Consumer's household income • SSNs, if they have them • Information about people in their tax household	IRS Form 8965: https://www.irs.gov /pub/irs-pdf/f8965.pdf	Consumers who don't have to file a federal income tax return are automatically exempt from the individual shared responsibility pay- ment. However, consumers whose incomes are below the filing thresh- old but who choose to file a federal income tax return anyway can claim the exemption through the tax filing process.	https://www.healthcare.gov /exemptions-tool/#/results/2016 /details/income-below-threshold

Type of Exemption: Membership in a Federally-Recognized Indian Tribe or Eligibility for Services Through an Indian Health Care Provider		
Consumers can use this exemption application if they are either: 1. A member of an federally recog- nized Indian tribe; and/or 2. Eligible for health services through the Indian Health Service, tribes and tribal organizations, or urban Indian organizations.	• SSNs, if they have them • Information about people in their tax household • If claiming this exemption through the Marketplace, consumers must provide documents showing membership in a federally recog- nized Indian tribe or eligibility for services from the Indian Health Service, a tribal health care provider, or an urban Indian health care provider.	Application for Exemption for Ameri- can Indians and Alaska Natives and Other Individuals who are Eligible to Receive Services from an Indian Health Care Provider: http://marketplace.cms. gov/getofficialresources/publications -and-articles/tribal-exemption.pdf To claim on federal tax return use Form 8965: https://www.irs.gov/pub /irs-pdf/f8965.pdf	Starting September 1, 2016, this exemption may only be obtained by claiming them on a federal income tax return through the IRS.	https://www.healthcare.gov /exemptions-tool/#/results/2016 /details/tribal

Consumers qualify for the exemption for any month they had any of these statuses for at least 1 day, or for the full year if they had the status all year. If the consumer was granted this exemption they can use it for future years without submitting another application as long as the membership in the federally recognized tribe or eligibility for services from an Indian health care provider remains unchanged.

Type of Exemption: Incarceration

Consumers can use this exemption application if they were incarcerated (detained or jailed), other than being held pending disposition of charges. Consumers can claim this exemption for any month they were incarcerated for at least 1 day.

- SSNs, if they have them
- Information about people in their tax household
- If claiming this exemption through the Marketplace, consumers must provide documents showing the name and address of the facility where the consumer was incarcerated, and the time periods of incarceration.

Application for Exemption from the Shared Responsibility Payment for Individuals who are Incarcerated (Detained or Jailed): https://marketplace.cms.gov /applications-and-forms /incarceration-exemption.pdf

To claim on federal tax return use Form 8965: https://www.irs.gov/pub /irs-pdf/f8965.pdf

Starting September 1, 2016, this exemption may only be obtained by claiming them on a federal income tax return through the IRS.

https://www.healthcare.gov /exemptions-tool/#/results/2016 /details/incarceration

(Continues)

Type of Exemption: Coverage is Unaffordable

Consumers can use this exemption application if their required contribution for coverage would exceed 8.13% percent of their 2016 household income (for 2015, the threshold was 8.05%).	• SSNs, if they have them • Employer and income information for everyone in their family (for example, from pay stubs, W-2 forms, or wage and tax statements) • Information about any job- related health insurance available to their family • Proof of yearly income for 2015 (examples of documents are found in the exemption application)	Application for Exemption from the Shared Responsibility Payment for Individuals who are Unable to Afford Coverage and are in a State with a Federally Facilitated Marketplace: https://marketplace.cms.gov /applications-and-forms/affordability -ffm-exemption-2015.pdf To claim on their federal tax return, consumers should use IRS Form 8965: https://www.irs.gov/pub/irs-pdf /f8965.pdf	If the consumer needs the exemption for only the months after they sign their exemption application through the end of the tax year, they can submit a Marketplace exemption application or claim it on their tax return. If they need the exemption for the entire tax year or any months before they sign the exemption application, they should claim it on their tax return	https://www.healthcare.gov /exemptions-tool/#/results/2016 /details/marketplace-affordability

Type of Exemption: Membership in a Recognized Religious Sect whose Members Object to Insurance

Consumers can use this exemption if they are a member of a religious sect that is recognized by the Social Security Administration as conscientiously opposed to accepting any insurance benefits, including Social Security and Medicare, and has been in existence since December 31, 1950. Consumers who get this exemption won't have to reapply for an exemption unless they turn 21 or leave their religious sect.	• Name and address of their religious sect • SSNs, if they have them • Copy of an approved IRS Form 4029 with required signatures (Application for Exemption from Social Security and Medicare Taxes and Waiver of Benefits), if they have one	Application for Exemption from the Shared Responsibility Payment for Members of Recognized Religious Sects or Divisions: https://marketplace.cms.gov /applications-and-forms/religious -sect-exemption.pdf	Marketplace exemption application	https://www.healthcare.gov /exemptions-tool/#/results/2016 /details/religion

Type of Exemption: Short Coverage Gap

Consumers can use this exemption if anyone in their tax household experienced a gap in health coverage of no more than 2 consecutive months. If a consumer has more than one short coverage gap during a year, the short coverage gap exemption only applies to the first gap.	• SSNs, if they have them	IRS Form 8965: https://www.irs.gov/pub/irs-pdf/f8965.pdf	Claim on tax return	https://www.healthcare.gov/exemptions-tool/#/results/2016/details/short-gap

Type of Exemption: U.S. Citizens Living Abroad

Consumers can use this exemption if they're a U.S. citizen who either spent at least 330 full days outside of the U.S. during a 12-month period or was a bona fide resident of a foreign country for a full tax year. Consumers can claim the coverage exemption for any month during their tax year that's included in the 12-month period.	• SSNs, if they have them	IRS Form 8965: https://www.irs.gov/pub/irs-pdf/f8965.pdf	Claim on tax return	https://www.healthcare.gov/exemptions-tool/#/results/2016/details/citizen-abroad For more information on the requirements to qualify for this exemption: https://www.irs.gov/individuals/international-taxpayers/foreign-earned-income-exclusion-physical-presence-test

Type of Exemption: Certain Non-U.S. Citizens

Consumers can use this exemption if they are a resident alien who is a citizen or national of a foreign country with which the U.S. has an income tax treaty with a nondiscrimination clause and a bona fide resident of a foreign country for the tax year. Consumers can claim this exemption for the entire year. Consumers who are not lawfully present in the U.S. but who file a tax return can also use this exemption.	• SSNs, if they have them	IRS Form 8965: https://www.irs.gov/pub/irs-pdf/f8965.pdf	Claim on tax return	https://www.healthcare.gov/exemptions-tool/#/results/2016/details/citizen-abroad For more information on the requirements to qualify for this exemption: https://www.irs.gov/individuals/international-taxpayers/foreign-earned-income-exclusion-bona-fide-residence-test

prevented them from obtaining coverage in a QHP. If consumers qualify for and receive one of these hardship exemptions, they may enroll in a catastrophic plan.

Step 1. Consumers should download and fill out the appropriate application for either an affordability exemption or a hardship exemption, depending on the consumer's specific situation. Consumers should mail the application to:

> Health Insurance Marketplace[SM]—Exemption Processing
> 465 Industrial Blvd.
> London, KY 40741

Step 2. The Marketplace will review the exemption application and determine consumers' eligibility for an exemption. The Marketplace may request more information or documentation from consumers as part of this review. The consumer has 90 days from the date the notice is sent to provide additional information if requested by the Marketplace.

Step 3. The Marketplace will mail consumers a notice of the exemption eligibility result. If consumers are granted an exemption, the Marketplace notice will include their unique exemption certificate number (ECN).

Step 4. Consumers should read and understand the notice. Consumers should keep the notice because the ECN will be required when the consumer files their federal income tax return. The notice will direct consumers to view Catastrophic Plan Information or call the Marketplace Call Center at 1-800-318-2596 for assistance with shopping for a plan, if they're interested in purchasing coverage.

Step 5. Assist consumers with contacting the health insurance company of their choice to enroll, if preferred.

2. Hardship Exemptions to Purchase Catastrophic Coverage for Consumers Who Receive Policy Cancellation Notices

If consumers have been notified that their health plan has been cancelled due to lack of compliance with Affordable Care Act standards, and consumers believe that the QHP options available through the individual market in the Marketplace in the area are unaffordable, consumers may be eligible for a hardship exemption and may be able to enroll in catastrophic coverage if it is available in their area. Catastrophic plans are not available in all states. Consumers whose coverage was cancelled may enroll using the steps in the section immediately above or they can choose to enroll in a catastrophic plan directly with the insurer of their choice by following the steps outlined below. For information, QHP options, and insurer contact numbers, visit Catastrophic Plan Information or call 1-866-837-0677, a special phone number for people whose plans have been canceled.

Step 1. Consumers should download and fill out the form for a hardship exemption. Consumers should be sure to answer that their reason for applying is that the consumer's individual policy was canceled and they feel that available coverage is not affordable.

Step 2. Consumers can view a list of catastrophic plans available through HealthCare.gov and should be prepared to submit the following items to an issuer of catastrophic coverage in their area:

a. The hardship exemption form.
b. Supporting documentation indicating that the previous policy was cancelled, such as your cancellation letter.

Step 3. The health insurance issuer will send the consumer's information to CMS; and CMS will verify that the consumer is eligible for the hardship exemption. If the consumer does not submit the supporting documentation with the exemption form, CMS may contact the consumer to notify him or her that the application is incomplete and cannot be processed until the supporting documentation is provided.

Step 4. The consumer can enroll in a plan. Consumers interested in pursuing this option are advised to contact the call center at 1-866-837-0677.

3. Other Exemptions

Depending on the type of exemption, consumers may apply for an exemption via the Marketplace or claim it when filing their federal tax returns.

Use the information and instructions below to help consumers with applying for exemptions.

Step 1. If consumers have not yet started an application for an exemption, they should determine the appropriate exemption application, download the application with the link provided, and determine what information is required to complete the application.

Step 2. The following guidance may be helpful to consumers completing exemption applications:

a. In Step 1 of the application, consumers input their name, address, phone number, preferred language, and other personal information.

b. In Step 2 of the application, consumers input the information required for the specific exemption application, such as information about members of the applicant's tax household (e.g., Social Security number, demographic information, financial information). Be sure to complete a Step 2 page for every person in the consumer's tax household.

c. In Step 3 of the application, consumers should review the information provided, confirm that the answers they provided are accurate, and sign their application.

d. In Step 4 of the application, consumers should review the instructions for mailing their completed application and copies of any supporting documentation. Documentation is required for most exemptions.

e. Depending on the type of exemption application, consumers may need assistance completing additional steps, inputting information in the appendices of the application, or gathering any required supporting documentation. You can provide consumer assistance as needed with applications for exemptions granted through the Marketplace. You can provide general information on exemptions claimed through the tax filing process, and can help consumers access IRS resources on this topic, but should not help consumers claim exemptions on their tax returns or fill out IRS forms.

Step 3. Consumers should mail Marketplace exemption applications and any supporting documentation to:

Health Insurance Marketplace(SM)—Exemption Processing
465 Industrial Blvd.
London, KY 40741

C. Next Steps

1. After consumers submit an exemption application to the Marketplace, the Marketplace will notify them about any additional supporting documentation needed and the status of their exemption application.

2. The consumer has 90 days from the date the notice is sent to provide additional information if requested by the Marketplace.

3. If consumers receive an exemption, they will be assigned an ECN for exemptions granted by the Marketplace. Consumers will need their ECN:

4. If they qualify for a hardship exemption and plan to enroll in a catastrophic health plan in the Marketplace.

5. If they plan to file a federal income tax return, so the IRS knows that they have an exemption. The federal income tax return will include instructions for where consumers should provide their ECN in their federal income tax return forms.

6. Starting with the 2016 tax year, the following exemption types will not be issued an ECN because they will only be available through the tax filing process: Health Care Sharing Ministry, members of Indian tribes and individuals eligible for services from an Indian health care provider and individuals who were incarcerated.

7. If consumers do not receive an exemption, you can assist them with applying for health coverage by referring to SOP - Create an Account.

8. For more help answering consumers' specific questions, see Appendix A for Frequently Asked Questions (FAQs) related to SOP – Exemptions [online].

Report Life Changes

A. Introduction

This SOP provides guidance on how to assist consumers with updating their eligibility application information. Consumers may experience life changes (e.g., marriage, relocation, birth of a child, or change in household income, citizenship or immigration status) during the year. It is important for consumers to report a life change as soon as possible to the Marketplace because (1) this information may change the coverage or savings for which consumers are eligible or (2) consumers may be eligible for a special enrollment period (SEP) as a result of the life change. Consumers must report changes to their application information within 30 days of the change. The Marketplace will re-determine consumer eligibility after any changes are reported and will notify consumers of any resulting changes in eligibility and next steps. If consumers qualify for an SEP, they generally have 60 days to enroll in or change their Marketplace coverage.

B. Procedures

1. Reporting Life Changes

To assist consumers with updates to reflect new life changes, proceed with the following steps:

Step 1. Consumers should log in to their accounts on HealthCare.gov and select the "My Applications & Coverage" tab. Then select the application that needs to be updated to reflect life changes.

Step 2. Consumers should select the "Report a Life Change" tab.

Step 3. Review the types of possible life changes, listed in **Exhibit B-10**, with consumers.

Step 4. Assist consumers with selecting the type of change they would like to report.

Step 5. Assist consumers as they update their application to account for any life changes. Remind consumers that their eligibility results may change as a result of the life change and how this may affect their coverage options.

Step 6. Help consumers submit any required supporting documentation and review updated eligibility results.

2. Special Enrollment Confirmations

The Special Enrollment Confirmation Process requires consumers who apply for coverage outside of the Open Enrollment Period and use certain SEPs to enroll in Marketplace coverage to subsequently provide proof of their eligibility for the SEP to the Marketplace. Consumers should submit required documents to the Marketplace by the deadline date provided in their Eligibility Determination Notice. Consumers will generally have 30 days to submit documentation.

CMS will follow up with consumers by mail and by phone if there is a question or concern about the documents submitted by the consumer. Consumers who submit documents and do not hear back from the Marketplace do not need to take any further action. If consumers don't respond at all, or don't provide sufficient documentation, they could be found ineligible for their SEP and lose their coverage.

Consumers enrolling through 5 common SEPs will need to submit documentation to verify their eligibility to use an SEP. These SEPs are:

- Loss of minimum essential coverage;
- Change in primary place of living if the consumer was enrolled in coverage while living at the original place of residence. Consumers must prove they had qualifying health coverage for one or more days in the 60 days before their move, unless they're moving from a foreign country or United States territory. Note however that moving only for medical treatment or staying somewhere temporarily without intending to reside there (for example, a vacation) doesn't qualify a consumer for a Special Enrollment Period;
- Birth;
- Gaining a dependent through adoption, placement for adoption, placement in foster care, or a child support or other court order; and
- Marriage.

Consumers who applied for Marketplace coverage will be asked to provide documentation to verify eligibility for a special enrollment period.

EXHIBIT B-10 Life Changes

Life Event	Potential Updates
Citizenship/Immigration Status Change	• Change in citizenship or immigration status for a household member needing coverage
Residency Changes	• Report a new residential address
Incarceration Status Change	• Claim current incarceration (in detention or jail) for household member • Claim end of incarceration period for household member
Tax Filing Status Change	• Claim new tax filing status (e.g., married, single, divorced) • Add, remove, or change tax dependents
Pregnancy Status Change	• Claim current pregnancy status • Claim end of pregnancy status
Household Member Change	• Add or remove member of household (including through birth, adoption or placement of child for adoption) • Change household members' names • Update household contact • Correction to date of birth, or Social Security number • Update marital status or other family relationships • Report that a household member has a physical disability or mental health condition that limits their ability to work, attend school, or take care of daily needs • Remove member of household from coverage • Change in status as an American Indian/Alaska Native or tribal member
Change in Request to Lower Health Plan Costs	• Request advance payments of the premium tax credit and cost-sharing reductions • End request for advance payments of the premium tax credit and cost-sharing
Income Change	• Increase or decrease in income
Employer-Sponsored MEC Change	• Changes to job-based coverage (e.g., changes to premiums, coverage no longer offered by employer) • Changes to employment status • Member of the household gets a new offer of job-based coverage
Other MEC Changes	• Gained or lost health coverage (e.g., Medicaid, CHIP, Medicare) in the last 60 days • Will gain or lose health coverage in the next 60 days • Gained eligibility for Medicare coverage on 65th birthday or receives disability benefits

Reproduced from the Center for Medicare and Medicaid Services Marketplace Assister Toolkit

Things You Should Know

- The system may return a list of the supporting documents required depending on the life changes reported. Consumers will see both their previously-uploaded documents and those that they still need to upload.

C. Next Steps

1. If consumers receive a new eligibility determination after reporting life changes, proceed to SOP - Review Eligibility Results.
2. For more help answering consumers' specific questions, see Appendix A for Frequently Asked Questions (FAQs) related to SOP - Report Life Changes [online].

Renew Health Coverage

A. Introduction

As an assister, you can help consumers renew their enrollment in QHPs through the Marketplace.

The process for renewal of health coverage begins with the Marketplace's annual eligibility redetermination process for all consumers who were determined eligible for enrollment in a QHP in the previous year. Consumers are responsible for notifying the Marketplace within 30 days of any changes in their application information during the year. This helps ensure an accurate redetermination of eligibility. Any changes in coverage or eligibility as a result of the annual eligibility redetermination will be effective on January 1 of the next year.

If consumers requested help paying for health coverage, agreed to allow the Marketplace to re-check their tax return information on an annual basis, and have properly reconciled any advance payments of the premium tax credit received for the 2015 benefit year with the IRS, the Marketplace will then check the consumer's income data from the IRS and use it to re-determine their eligibility for help paying for health coverage. For consumers covered by Medicaid or CHIP, their states' Medicaid or CHIP agencies will generally re-determine their eligibility for these programs on an annual basis.

The Marketplace will send consumers a Marketplace Open Enrollment Notice (MOEN) before open enrollment for the coming year. All consumers are encouraged to come back to the Marketplace and log into their HealthCare.gov account to update their application information, compare plan options, and enroll in coverage for the coming year. Consumers should also check to be sure they are receiving the correct amount of help paying for coverage and are still enrolled in the coverage for 2017 that works best for them.

If consumers do not agree to allow the Marketplace to re-check their tax return information on an annual basis when they filed an eligibility application, the Marketplace will still send consumers a notice. The notice will tell consumers that if they want to receive, or continue to receive, advance payments of the premium tax credit (APTC) or income-based cost-sharing reductions (CSRs) for 2017, consumers must contact the Marketplace or go to HealthCare.gov to update their information and select a QHP in time for a January 1 effective date. Otherwise, consumers' advance payments of the premium tax credit or income-based cost-sharing reductions will end on December 31, 2016. Similarly, if a tax filer receiving APTC or income-based CSR in 2014 or 2015, failed to file a 2014 or 2015 tax return (respectively), and did not return to the Marketplace to obtain an updated eligibility determination, enrollees in that tax filer's tax household will lose any help paying for coverage after December 31, 2016.

Most current Marketplace enrollees will be automatically enrolled in coverage for the next benefit year under the re-enrollment guidelines established for the Marketplaces, if they don't do anything. However, if consumers don't return to the Marketplace and select 2017 coverage by December 15, 2016, they could miss out on better deals and cost savings for coverage starting on January 1, 2017. That's why CMS is advising assisters to strongly encourage all consumers—even those who plan to re-enroll in their same plan—to come back to the Marketplace to review their plan options, as well as their application information.

In addition to the Marketplace Open Enrollment Notices, all consumers currently enrolled in a QHP will get a notice from their health insurance company before open enrollment. If the health insurance company does not have information about the estimated APTC amount before it sends the notice, it will provide the information before or during open enrollment.

The plan's renewal letter notice will identify a plan that is the same as or similar to the enrollee's 2017 plan, if available. The plan notice will describe any changes to the enrollee's QHP. If the QHP will be discontinued or coverage in that QHP non-renewed, the issuer will send a notice to tell consumers which plan, if any, the consumers will be enrolled in for 2017 unless they return to the Marketplace and change plans. If the consumer will not have plans offered by their 2016 health insurance issuer available to them through the FFM in 2017, the consumer may be automatically enrolled in a plan with a different health insurance issuer. However, the consumer should be encouraged to return to the

Marketplace to make sure that the new plan with the new health insurance company will meet the consumer's needs—or see if there is another plan that would be a better fit.

The remainder of this SOP provides guidance on how to assist consumers with their annual eligibility redeterminations and completing the renewal process.

B. Procedures

Step 1. All consumers who are currently enrolled in a QHP through the Marketplace for plan year 2016 will be sent a Marketplace Open Enrollment Notice before open enrollment that contains the following information:

a. A note that the open enrollment period begins November 1, 2016 and ends January 31, 2017.
b. A description of the annual eligibility redetermination and renewal process.
c. The requirement to report changes affecting eligibility and the timeframe and channels to report changes.
d. The key dates for ensuring coverage is effective on January 1, 2017.
e. The reconciliation process for consumers receiving advance payments of the premium tax credit and/or cost-sharing reductions.
f. Special instructions for those consumers receiving advance payments of the premium tax credit or cost-sharing reductions. For more information on these instructions, see Step 4.

Step 2. Assist consumers with reviewing their Marketplace Open Enrollment Notice.

Step 3. Explain to consumers that they should update their eligibility application with any new or changed information about themselves or their households. If there are no changes, consumers should still return to their account on HealthCare. gov to review the application and confirm the information is correct and review their financial assistance and plan options.

Step 4. Assist consumers with reporting any changes or new information (e.g., annual household income, household size) to the Marketplace.

Keep in mind the guidance below is based on different consumer scenarios:

a. If consumers who applied for but were determined ineligible for advance payments of the premium tax credits or income-based cost-sharing reductions contact the Marketplace to report any changes or select a new QHP, they will also get an updated eligibility determination based on updated guidelines (e.g., federal poverty levels) for the new plan year.
b. If consumers who are not receiving advance payments of the premium tax credit or income-based cost-sharing reductions do not contact the Marketplace within the specified timeframe, generally, the Marketplace will automatically re-enroll them in the coverage for the next benefit year without advance payments of the premium tax credit or cost-sharing reductions.
c. Consumers who are receiving advance payments of the premium tax credit or income-based cost-sharing reductions and agreed to allow the Marketplace to re-check their tax return information on an annual basis and have filed a 2014 or 2015 tax return (if they received APTC in 2014 or 2015, as applicable) should be aware of the following key points about their annual eligibility redetermination and renewal process:

  i. If consumers have provided updated eligibility information to the Marketplace, the eligibility redetermination notice will be based on their most recent eligibility information on file.
  ii. If consumers have not provided updated eligibility information, the notice will encourage them to contact the Marketplace to get an updated eligibility determination by December 15, 2016.
  iii. If consumers do not update their information, the Marketplace generally will renew their QHP enrollment

for the benefit year with the same level of help selected in the previous year. Income-based cost-sharing reductions and advance payments of the premium tax credit will be updated based on the consumer's most recent income and household size data reported to the Marketplace, updated FPL tables, and plan premiums. The amount of premium tax credits consumers receive in the new plan year depends on their income and the premium cost for the second lowest cost Silver plan available on the Marketplace. However, if data sources show that a consumer's household income is over 500% FPL, the consumer will get a notice that their APTC and CSR will be discontinued unless the consumer takes action. The consumer may still be auto re-enrolled in a health plan on the FFM, but will lose APTC and CSR.

d. Consumers who are receiving advance payments of the premium tax credit or income-based cost-sharing reductions and did not agree to allow the Marketplace to re-check their tax return information on an annual basis should be aware of the following key points about their annual eligibility redetermination and renewal process:

i. The Marketplace Open Enrollment Notice will ask consumers to contact the Marketplace to get an updated eligibility determination.

ii. In general, if consumers do not contact the Marketplace by December 15, their financial assistance (advance payments of premium tax credit or cost-sharing reductions) will end on December 31.

iii. If consumers are still eligible for QHP coverage, the Marketplace generally will renew their coverage for the next benefit year but without financial assistance to help lower costs. Federal

guidance explains how the Marketplace will decide which QHP the consumer will be automatically enrolled in for 2017 coverage. See 45 C.F.R. § 155.335(a)(2).

e. For consumers who are receiving advance payments of the premium tax credit or income-based cost-sharing reductions and did not file a tax return for the 2015 coverage year (and received APTC for 2015), advance payments of the premium tax credit and/or cost-sharing reductions will end on December 31, 2016. Here are key points about their annual eligibility redetermination and renewal process:

i. The Marketplace Open Enrollment Notice will ask consumers to take action to ensure they file a 2015 tax return and then return to the Marketplace to update their application and attest to having filed a tax return. If consumers attest to having filed a tax return by December 15, the Marketplace generally will renew their coverage for the next benefit year.

ii. In general, if consumers do not return to the Marketplace to attest to having filed a tax return or updated information from the IRS does not indicate that they have filed a 2015 tax return by December 15, their financial assistance will end on December 31, 2016.

Step 5. If consumers are unsure if they agreed to allow the Marketplace to re-check their tax return information on an annual basis, tell consumers that they can return to the Marketplace to give this authorization when they update their 2017 eligibility and plan selection.

Step 6. Enrollment.

Changes submitted on a 2017 application generally don't take effect unless consumers complete the process by continuing to enrollment and selecting a plan. If returning consumers want to keep their Marketplace plan for next and it remains available, they should select the plan labeled "YOUR CURRENT PLAN" at the top of the plan results in Plan Compare.

Even if consumers are satisfied with their 2016 plan, it is still a good idea for consumers to compare plans to see what's covered; and whether desired providers, services, and prescription drugs are still covered by the plan; and to compare costs.

C. Next Steps

1. If consumers receive updated eligibility notices, proceed to SOP - Review Eligibility Results.

2. If consumers would like to file an appeals request, proceed to SOP - Request an Eligibility Appeal.

3. If consumers would like to complete an exemption application, proceed to SOP - Exemptions.

4. For more help answering consumers' specific questions, see the Frequently Asked Questions (FAQs) online related to SOP - Renew Health Coverage [online].

State Insurance Regulation

History, Purpose, and Structure

The following is an excerpt. To view the full document, go the following link: http://www.naic .org/documents/consumer_state_reg_brief.pdf

A BRIEF HISTORY

Benjamin Franklin helped found the insurance industry in the United States in 1752 with the Philadelphia Contributionship for the Insurance of Houses from Loss by Fire. The current state insurance regulatory framework has its roots in the 19th century, with New Hampshire appointing the first insurance commissioner in 1851. Insurance regulators' responsibilities grew in scope and complexity as the industry evolved. Congress adopted the McCarran-Ferguson Act in 1945 to declare that states should regulate the business of insurance and to affirm that the continued regulation of the insurance industry by the states was in the public's best interest.

The Financial Modernization Act of 1999—also called Gramm-Leach-Bliley—established a comprehensive framework to permit affiliations among banks, securities firms, and insurance companies. Gramm-Leach-Bliley once again acknowledged that states should regulate the business of insurance. However, Congress also called for state reform to allow insurance companies to compete more effectively in the newly integrated financial service marketplace and to respond with innovation and flexibility to evermore demanding consumer

needs—all while continuing to protect consumers, which is the hallmark of state regulation.

THE ROLE OF THE STATE LEGISLATURES

State legislatures set broad policy for the regulation of insurance. They establish and oversee state insurance departments, regularly review and revise state insurance laws, and approve regulatory budgets. State insurance departments employ 12,500 regulatory personnel. Increases in staff and enhanced automation have allowed regulators to substantially boost the quality and intensity of their financial oversight of insurers and expand consumer protection activities.

State regulation of insurance provides a major source of state revenue. In 2000 states collected more than $10.4 billion in revenues from insurance sources. Of this amount, $880 million—roughly 8.4 percent—went to regulate the business of insurance while the remaining $9.6 billion went to state general funds for other purposes.

NATIONAL ASSOCIATION OF INSURANCE COMMISSIONERS (NAIC)

The NAIC serves as a vehicle for individual state regulators to coordinate their activities and share resources. Established in 1871, the NAIC functions as an advisory body and service provider for state insurance departments. Commissioners use the NAIC to pool scarce resources, to discuss issues of common concern, and to align their oversight of the industry. Each state, however, ultimately determines what actions it will take.

THE PURPOSE AND STRUCTURE OF INSURANCE REGULATION

The fundamental reason for government regulation of insurance is to protect American consumers. State systems are accessible and accountable to the public and sensitive to local social and economic conditions. State regulation has proven that it effectively protects consumers and ensures that promises made by insurers are kept. Insurance regulation is structured around several key functions, including company licensing, producer licensing, product regulation, market conduct, financial regulation, and consumer services.

Company Licensing

State laws require insurers and insurance-related businesses to be licensed before selling their products or services. Currently, there are approximately 7,200 insurers in the United States. All U.S. insurers are subject to regulation in their state of domicile and in the other states where they are licensed to sell insurance.

Insurers who fail to comply with regulatory requirements are subject to license suspension or revocation, and states may exact fines for regulatory violations. In 2000 nearly 300 companies had their licenses suspended or revoked.

The NAIC's Uniform Certificate of Authority Application (UCAA)—a company licensing system—helps states expedite the review process of a new company license. In addition, an NAIC database has been developed to facilitate information sharing on acquisition and merger filings. These databases assist insurance regulators by creating a streamlined and more cost-efficient regulatory process.

Producer Licensing

Insurance agents and brokers, also known as producers, must be licensed to sell insurance and must comply with various state laws and regulations governing their activities. Currently, more than 3.2 million individuals are licensed to provide insurance services in the United States. State insurance departments oversee producer activities in order to protect insurance consumer interests in insurance transactions.

The states administer continuing education programs to ensure that agents meet high professional standards. Producers who fail to comply with regulatory requirements are subject to fines and license suspension or revocation. In 2000, nearly 16,000 insurance producers had their licenses suspended or revoked.

When producers operate in multiple jurisdictions, states must coordinate their efforts to track producers and prevent violations. Special databases are maintained by the NAIC to assist the states in this effort. The National Insurance Producer Registry (NIPR)—a non-profit affiliate of the NAIC—was established to develop and operate a national repository for producer licensing information.

Product Regulation

State regulators protect consumers by ensuring that insurance policy provisions comply with state law, are reasonable and fair, and do not contain major gaps in coverage that might be misunderstood by consumers and leave them unprotected. The nature of the rate review, rating rules, and forms varies somewhat among the states depending on their laws and regulations.

For personal property–casualty lines, about half of the states require insurers to file rates and to receive prior approval before they go into effect. With the exception of workers' compensation and medical malpractice, commercial property–casualty lines in many states are subject to a competitive rating approach. Under such a system, regulators typically retain authority to disapprove rates if they find that competition is not working.

Premiums for life insurance and annuity products generally are not subject to regulatory approval, although regulators may seek to ensure that policy benefits are commensurate with the premiums charged. Many states subject health insurance rates to prior approval—with all other lines using a "file and use" system or no provisions for review.

Financial Regulation

Financial regulation provides crucial safeguards for America's insurance consumers. At the NAIC, the states maintain the world's largest insurance financial database, which provides a 15-year history of annual and quarterly filings on 5,200 insurance companies.

Periodic financial examinations occur on a scheduled basis. State financial examiners investigate a company's accounting methods, procedures, and financial statement presentation. These exams verify and validate what is presented in the company's annual statement to ascertain whether the company is in good financial standing.

When an examination of financial records shows the company to be financially impaired, the state insurance department takes control of the company. Aggressively working with financially troubled companies is a critical part of the regulator's role. In the event the company must be liquidated or becomes insolvent, the states maintain a system of financial guaranty funds that cover consumers' personal losses.

Market Regulation

Market regulation attempts to ensure fair and reasonable insurance prices, products, and trade practices in order to protect consumers. With improved cooperation among states and uniform market conduct examinations, regulators hope to ensure continued consumer protections at the state level.

Market conduct examinations occur on a routine basis, but also can be triggered by complaints against an insurer. These exams review agent-licensing issues, complaints, types of products sold by the company and agents, agent sales practices, proper rating, claims handling, and other market-related aspects of an insurer's operation.

When violations are found, the insurance department makes recommendations to improve the company's operations and to bring the company into compliance with state law. In addition, a company may be subject to civil penalties or license suspension or revocation.

Consumer Services

The states' single most significant challenge is to be vigilant in the protection of consumers, especially in light of the changes taking place in the financial services marketplace. States have established toll-free hotlines, Internet websites, and special consumer services units to receive and handle complaints against insurers and agents. The states also have launched an interactive tool to allow consumers to research company complaints and financial data using the NAIC website.

During 2000, state insurance departments handled 4.5 million consumer inquiries and complaints. As needed, state insurance departments worked together with policyholders and insurers to resolve disputes. In addition, many states sponsor educational seminars and provide consumer brochures on a variety of insurance topics. Some states publish rate comparison guides to help consumers get the best value when they purchase insurance.

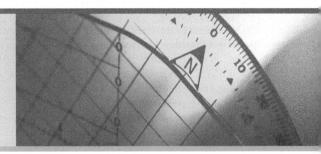

GLOSSARY

Select terms from the Center for Medicare and Medicaid Services.

Accident-only insurance A policy that covers costs related to an accidental injury.

Accountable care organizations (ACOs) Groups of providers—hospitals, physician organizations, and suppliers—responsible for coordinating care for a specified patient population and subject to quality standards.

Actuarial value The estimated proportion of costs covered by an insurer, on average.

Actuarially fair premium The portion of the health insurance premium that is based on enrollees' predicted medical expenses. The remaining portion is the **loading charge**.

Adverse selection A type of sorting (or selection) into health plans that is caused by incomplete or asymmetrical information, e.g. between insurers and enrollees.

Adverse tiering Insurers attempt to dissuade enrollment of high-cost consumers by placing all drugs used to treat high-cost conditions (such as angina, bipolar disorder, or multiple sclerosis) into the same high tier on a formulary.

All-payer rate setting A policy in which the government sets prices for all payers (insurers and employers), rather than allowing payers to negotiate prices with providers

Allowed Amount The negotiated rate for covered health care services, sometimes also called "eligible expense," or "payment allowance." You may be responsible for paying a portion of this rate. See **coinsurance, copayment,** and **deductible**.

Appeal A request for your health insurer or plan to review a decision or a grievance again.

Balance Billing A charge to cover the difference between the provider's fee and the allowed amount (which may be lower than the fee).

Benefit design The costs, conditions, and inclusion and exclusion criteria for benefits coverage in a health care plan.

Benefit mandates Legal requirements that health insurance plans cover specific services or products provided by a specific type of provider, such as a hospital or a physician.

Bundled payment A fixed payment paid to providers for the entire continuum of care, e.g. including pre-operative testing, surgery, and recovery services. Also called **case rate**.

Capitation A flat dollar payment paid to providers per patient per month (sometimes per year).

Case rate See **bundled payment**.

Certificate of coverage (COC) A document in which insurers list the terms, or rules, of an insurance contract. The COC provides comprehensive information about benefits, cost-sharing, coverage limitations, and other plan rules. Also called **evidence of coverage (EOC)**.

Cherry-picking Targeting low-risk or otherwise profitable patients for care; also known as **cream-skimming**.

Closed formulary A type of formulary in which drugs that are not listed are not covered.

Coinsurance A percentage payment for the cost of care, for example 10 percent or 20 percent of the cost of a doctor's visit.

Community-based health insurance An insurance scheme in which members of a village, church or other community (rather than an entire nation) voluntarily contribute premiums. Also called **mutual health insurance**.

Community rating Premiums that are based on spending in the prior year across an entire geographic area, rather than for just one group or individual.

Complications of Pregnancy Conditions due to pregnancy, labor and delivery that require medical care to prevent serious harm to the health of the mother or the fetus. Morning sickness and a non-emergency caesarean section aren't complications of pregnancy.

Concurrent risk adjustment Compensation to providers or insurers based on actual incurred expenses, rather than estimated expenses.

Consumer cost-sharing The portion of health care costs that the insurer does not cover; payments besides the monthly health insurance premium that a consumer makes for medical services or products, such as deductibles, coinsurance, and copayment. Also called **out-of-pocket costs**.

Consumer-directed health plans Plans that impose a high deductible on consumers, sometimes thousands of dollars, usually in exchange for a lower premium.

Coordination of benefits For consumers covered under multiple plans, the rules about which plan pays first in different situations.

Copayment A fixed payment per visit or episode, such as a doctor's visit for hospitalization.

Cost-sharing reduction A subsidy that reduces out-of-pocket costs for health care services, like going to the doctor or filling a prescription.

Coverage exclusions Insurer rules that exclude benefits, such as cosmetic surgery and dental services, from coverage under any circumstance.

Coverage limitations Insurer rules that limit coverage of benefits only to special circumstances, such as with prior authorization.

Cream-skimming See **cherry-picking**.

Critical illness insurance A policy that pays a lump sum in case of a pre-specified disease.

Death spiral The dismantling of the insurance market as a result of adverse selection.

Deductible A fixed amount that the enrollees must pay before insurance covers expenses.

Defined benefit plan A pension plan that guarantee the employee a predefined amount (or benefit) upon retirement.

Defined contribution plan A pension plan in which employees and employers contribute regularly to investment accounts, and benefits depend on the performance of the account.

Diagnosis-related groups (DRG) A Medicare system for paying for inpatient hospitalizations that groups together related diagnoses, then weights payments to these groups by expected resource use and clinical intensity.

Disability income protection A policy that provides reimbursement in case the enrollee cannot work.

Discharge planning Services that assist patients with care they will need at home after a surgery or other hospitalization.

Disease management programs Services that help patients manage chronic conditions by coordinating care among multiple providers, keeping patients on medication regimens, and providing other reminders and tools.

Doughnut hole A gap in a health plan's coverage; particularly in Medicare Part D (prescription drug) coverage.

Drug class Drugs with the same chemical mechanism, generally used to treat the same disease.

Drug formulary A list of prescription drugs covered by a plan.

Dual-eligible beneficiaries Low-income individuals who are eligible for both Medicaid and Medicare.

Durable Medical Equipment (DME) Equipment and supplies ordered by a health care provider for everyday or extended use. Coverage for DME may include: oxygen equipment, wheelchairs, crutches, or blood testing strips for diabetics.

Employer "pay-or-play" mandate A requirement that employers either offer insurance ("play") or contribute towards their employees' health insurance benefits ("pay").

Episode-of-care payment See **bundled payment**.

ERISA The Employee Retirement Income Security Act of 1974, designed to protect the assets of employees enrolled in private retirement plans. As a federal law, ERISA pre-empted most state laws regarding employee benefits, except for health insurance; however, under the "deemer clause," it prohibited states from "deeming" self-funded plans health insurance.

Essential health benefits (EHB) Some insurers are required to cover ten categories of EHB: ambulatory patient services; emergency services; hospitalization; maternity and newborn care; mental health and substance use disorder services, including behavioral health treatment; prescription drugs; rehabilitative and habilitative services and devices; laboratory services; preventive and wellness services and chronic disease management; and pediatric services, including oral and vision care.

Evidence of coverage (EOC) See **certificate of coverage (COC)**.

Exceptions protocols Rules for patient requests for benefits not covered by insurance, such as a non-formulary medication.

Exchanges State or federal health insurance websites where consumers can compare coverage options and determine whether they are eligible for financial help. Also called **marketplaces**.

Exclusive provider organization (EPO) A type of health insurance plan that has a restrictive provider network and limited—if any—out-of-network benefits, but unlike an HMO, usually does not require a primary care gatekeeper.

Experience rating Premiums that are based on spending in the prior year for just one group or individual, rather than across an entire geographic area.

Explanation of benefits (EOB) An evaluation form issued to a patient and health care provider by an insurer after receiving a claim from a provider. The form typically includes the following information: type of service provided, dates of service, charges submitted by the provider, provider discount from charges, amount paid by the insurer to the provider, and remaining patient financial responsibility.

Facility fee For services performed in a hospital, ambulatory surgery center, or other health care facility, the fee paid to the facility (rather than to the physician performing the service).

Fee-for-service Payment for each procedure or service rendered (rather than, for example, the entire continuum of care).

Fee schedule A list of prices used to compensate providers on a fee-for-service basis.

Flexible spending account (FSA) An employer-owned account, jointly funded with pre-tax dollars by the employer and employee to pay for most qualified medical expenses not covered by insurance, also known as a **flexible spending arrangement** (also **FSA**).

Flexible spending arrangement (FSA) See **flexible spending account (FSA)**.

Formulary A list of medications covered by a plan.

Fully insured plan A contract in which an individual or employer pays a state-licensed insurer to take on financial risk and administer benefits.

Global capitation A capitation arrangement (a budget) that encompasses the entire continuum of care for a patient, not just primary care services.

Grievance A complaint communicated to a health insurer or employer.

Group insurance An insurance policy or self-insurance scheme that covers two or more individuals who are not members of the same immediate family, for example two or more employees (but not just two spouses).

Group market The online or brick-and-mortar location where individuals, insurers, and employers buy and sell group insurance policies and administrative services; also, the sum of the consumer preferences, health needs, state policies, regulations, and other conditions that facilitate such exchange of group insurance policies.

Guaranteed issue A requirement to offer coverage to anyone who applies, regardless of health status.

Guaranteed renewability A requirement to renew a policy for anyone who continues to pay premiums, regardless of health status.

Habilitation Services Health care services that help a person keep, learn or improve skills and functioning for daily living.

Health Insurance A contract between an enrollee and a payer, such as a state-licensed health insurer, an employer, or a government, that requires the payer to cover a pre-specified portion of health care costs in exchange for a premium.

Health maintenance organization (HMO) A type of plan that has restrictive provider networks and limited – if any – out-of-network benefits. Beneficiaries are usually required to see a primary care "gatekeeper" before obtaining specialty care

Health reimbursement arrangement (HRA) An employer-owned account, funded with pre-tax dollars by the employer to pay for some pre-specified medical expenses not covered by insurance.

Health savings account (HSA) An individually owned account, funded with pre-tax dollars by the individual and the employer to pay for out-of-pocket expenses associated with a high-deductible health plan. HSAs are "portable," so if the individual changes jobs or leaves the job market, then she may take the HSA with her – she owns the account.

Health systems Structural components that interact with one another to achieve health-related goals, including health status improvement, financial risk protection, and consumer satisfaction with care delivery.

High-deductible health plans (HDHPs) Plans that impose high initial cost-sharing (a high deductible), sometimes thousands of dollars, on consumers, usually in exchange for a lower premium.

High-performance networks A type of **tiered network** in which patients are directed to high-quality or high-value providers, rather than just low-cost providers.

Home Health Care Health care services a person receives at home.

Hospice Services Services to provide comfort and support for persons in the last stages of a terminal illness and their families.

Indemnity A payment to the plan enrollee, usually a fixed amount per hospital day.

Indemnity plan A type of plan that reimburses enrollees, rather than providers, for health care services and supplies. When receiving care, enrollees must pay providers directly, then submit a claim to the plan for reimbursement.

Individual mandate A provision requiring every person to obtain some specified level of health insurance coverage.

Individual market The online or brick-and-mortar location where individuals and insurers buy and sell individual insurance policies (policies that cover just one person or just members of an immediate family); also, the sum of the consumer preferences, health needs, state policies, regulations, and other conditions that facilitate such exchange of individual insurance policies.

In-network providers Physicians, hospitals, medical laboratories, and other medical facilities that have agreed to accept a discounted negotiated price from an private insurer or an administered price from a public insurer. Also called **network providers** or members of a plan's **provider network**.

Insurance A financial guarantee against an unforeseen event. Also see **health insurance**.

Insurer cost-sharing The portion of health care costs that the insurer (or employer) covers, as opposed to the consumer.

Limits With regard to health plans, annual and lifetime ceilings on covered expenses.

List price The menu price reported by providers for health care services and supplies, usually discounted by insurers.

Loading charge The portion of the health insurance premium that covers administrative costs and profit.

Long-term care Assistance with everyday medical and social tasks for individuals with chronic conditions; most is not medical care but instead provides assistance with basic personal tasks of everyday life.

Major medical insurance Comprehensive insurance that covers a wide range of medical services and supplies.

Managed care A set of tools used by managed care plans to reduce spending and improve the quality of health care; these tools include imposing out-of-pocket costs on enrollees, contracting with low-cost providers, and limiting coverage for some types of procedures deemed inappropriate.

Managed care plans Plans, such as HMOs, PPOs, POSs, and EPOs, that utilize managed care techniques, especially by limiting the size of provider networks and managing the utilization of medical resources.

Marketplaces See **exchanges**.

Medicaid Title XIX of the Social Security Act, a health insurance program that provides federal funds for states to provide coverage to people who are low-income or who fall into some category of medical need based on illness or disability.

Medical loss ratio (MLR) The percentage of the health insurance premium paid out in benefits.

Medically necessary A determination by an insurer that a service or product is critical to a particular individual's health, and therefore will be covered by the insurance plan.

Medicare Title XVIII of the Social Security Act, a federal health insurance program that provides coverage to the aged and disabled.

Medicare Administrative Contractor (MAC) A private insurance company that is contracted to process Medicare Part A and B claims or durable medical equipment claims for a geographical area.

Medicare-eligible retirees Persons who retire at age 65 or older.

Medigap Supplemental private insurance that helps pay for out-of-pocket costs (such as deductibles, coinsurance, and copayment) and benefits not covered by Medicare.

Moral hazard Sub-optimal behavior, such as overuse of health care services and more reckless behavior by insured persons, that occurs as a result of financial protection from health insurance.

Mutual health insurance See **community-based health insurance**.

Narrow networks Provider networks that are intentionally very restrictive, in order to negotiate steep price discounts with those providers who are in-network.

Network See **provider Network**.

Network adequacy standards State guidelines that regulate the scope of provider networks.

Network provider See in-network providers.

Non-network provider See out-of-network providers.

Non-preferred brand-name drugs Brand-name drugs for which the insurer cannot obtain a discount, or that are less discounted than preferred drugs.

Non-preferred providers In preferred-provider organizations (PPOs), providers who are out-of-network (have not agreed to accept a discounted price for services).

Open enrollment An established period of time during which consumers may purchase a policy for the following year.

Open formulary A type of formulary in which drugs that are not listed may still be covered, but at a higher rate than those listed on the formulary.

Out-of-network (non-network) providers Physicians, hospitals, medical laboratories, and other medical facilities that have not agreed to accept a discounted negotiated price from an private insurer or an administered price from a public insurer, but rather set their own prices for services.

Out-of-pocket costs See **consumer cost-sharing**.

Out-of-Pocket Limit A ceiling on consumer cost-sharing before an insurer covers 100 percent of costs.

Over-the-counter drugs (OTC drugs) Pharmaceuticals that may be purchased without a prescription.

Panel The set of patients who have selected a physician or practice as their primary care "gatekeeper."

Partial capitation A capitation that covers only certain primary care services, but does not leave the physician at risk for specialty care or hospitalizations.

Per diem A fixed dollar payment per day (e.g. in a hospital or other health care facility), regardless of the intensity of services provided that day.

Pharmacy and therapeutics (P&T) committees Committees that guide insurers' pharmaceutical benefit policies and are responsible for developing and updating formularies, as well as access to medication policies such as prior authorization.

Pharmacy benefit manager (PBM) A third party firm used by health insurers to manage formularies and access to medication policies, process and pay pharmaceutical claims, and contract with local pharmacies and online wholesalers and manufacturers.

Point-of-service (POS) A type of plan that combines aspects of HMOs and PPOs; enrollees are generally assigned a primary care gatekeeper, but may use an out-of-network provider, provided they pay more out of pocket.

Policy The set of terms of a health insurance plan listed in the EOC (evidence of coverage) or COC (certificate of coverage).

Pre-existing conditions Illness or injury that was present before coverage began.

Preferred brand-name drugs Brand-name drugs for which an insurer is able to obtain a discount.

Preferred Provider Organizations (PPO) A type of plan that has a wide network of providers, allows beneficiaries to see out-of-network providers with higher cost-sharing, and does not generally require referrals for specialty care.

Preferred providers In preferred-provider organizations (PPOs), providers who are in-network (have agreed to accept the discounted price for services).

Premium The price, usually monthly, of belonging to an insurance plan.

Premium tax credit A subsidy that reduces the amount that consumers must pay in monthly premiums.

Prescription Drugs Drugs and medications that by law require a prescription.

Prior authorization An example of utilization management, the requirement that enrollees seek approval from an insurer before obtaining medical services. Sometimes also called "preauthorization," or just "authorization."

Private health insurance An agreement that a state-licensed health insurer or a self-funded employee health benefit plan will take on financial risk for health care costs, administer benefits, and pay claims, or contract these functions to a third party, for individuals or groups of individuals, and their families.

Professional fee The fee paid to the physician or other health care professional performing a service.

Prospective attribution A method of assigning patients to an ACO for the upcoming year based on previous health care provider use.

Prospective payment Reimbursement that does not vary with the cost of the patient. Payment can be thought of as a continuum; in other words, payment need not be *either* prospective or retrospective, but rather *more* prospective or *more* retrospective.

Prospective risk adjustment Compensation to providers or insurers based on estimated expenses, rather than actual incurred expenses.

Provider A physician (M.D.–Medical Doctor or D.O.–Doctor of Osteopathic Medicine), health care professional or health care facility licensed, certified or accredited as required by state law.

Provider directories A list (usually online) of a plan's network of providers.

Provider network See **in-network providers**.

Public health insurance An agreement that the government will take on financial risk for health care costs, administer benefits, and pay claims, or contract these functions to a third party, for individuals and their families.

Qualified health plans (QHPs) A plan that is ACA compliant and approved by the state to be sold in the health insurance exchange.

Recall periods How far back a participant must remember to answer a survey question.

Reference pricing (reverse deductible) A cost-sharing structure in which the insurer pays the initial cost-sharing for a service or product, and the consumer is responsible for any remaining cost.

Referral The direction of a patient by a physician (or other clinician) to another physician for specialty care or a second opinion.

Rehabilitation Services Health care services that help a person keep, get back or improve skills and functioning for daily living that have been lost or impaired because a person was sick, hurt or disabled.

Resource-Based Relative Value Scale (RBRVS) Medicare's modified FFS system for paying physicians that assigns higher fees to more intensive services and lower fees to less intensive services.

Retail clinic A clinic located within a pharmacy, grocery store, or other convenient location that provides preventive care and other limited services for conditions that might otherwise be treated in a doctor's office, and generally has hours that extend beyond those of a normal doctor's office.

Retiree health benefits Private or public health care coverage for those who have retired from a job.

Retrospective attribution A method of assigning patients to an ACO for the previous year based on past-year health care provider use.

Retrospective payment Reimbursement that varies with the cost of the patient. Payment can be thought of as a continuum; in other words, payment need not be *either* prospective or retrospective, but rather *more* prospective or *more* retrospective.

Risk adjustment Payment that increases with the estimated cost of an enrollee or patient, intended to make competition more fair among insurers and medical practices by reducing adverse selection.

Risk averse Preferring a certain outcome over an uncertain one.

Risk-loving Preferring an uncertain outcome over a certain one.

Salary A type of reimbursement that is a fixed dollar amount per year.

Selection With regard to health plans, enrollees' sorting into plans based on health status.

Self-funded plan A type of insurance plan in which employers – usually larger, cross-state employers -- take on financial risk by collecting premiums and paying out benefits in-house. Also called a **self-insured plan**.

Self-insured plan See **self-funded plan**.

Service benefit plans A type of insurance plan in which providers are reimbursed for health care services and supplies, in contrast to indemnity plans, in which enrollees must reimburse providers directly and then submit the claim to the insurer.

Service benefits Payments made directly to health care providers for services and supplies.

Skilled Nursing Care Services in one's home or in a nursing home provided by licensed nurses.

Social health insurance An insurance scheme in which workers and their employers make regular tax contributions to the government, which reimburses providers and establishes health care benefits. Contributions are usually based on income to ensure that low-wage workers are not unduly burdened. Those who do not work, such as children, the elderly, and spouses, are covered through general revenues or dependent coverage.

Social Security A federal payroll tax-funded insurance program for retirement income, disability income, and other benefits. Retirees may claim discounted benefits as early as age 62, though full benefits are not available until age 67. Social Security is the primary source of income for the majority of the elderly population, and is therefore an important income source to cover out-of-pocket medical costs.

State Children's Health Insurance Program (SCHIP or CHIP) Title XXI of the Social Security Act, a joint federal-state program in which the federal government provides states with matching funds to expand coverage to low-income children who otherwise would not qualify for Medicaid.

Step therapy An example of utilization management, the requirement that a patient must try other medications before "stepping up" to a more expensive drug.

Summary of benefits and coverage (SBC) A standardized form that summarizes the key features of a plan, including covered benefits, cost-sharing requirements, and coverage limits and exceptions.

Supplier-induced demand consumer use of health care services beyond the volume and intensity that she would prefer if she had full information on the costs and benefits. This phenomenon occurs because of influence from providers.

Surprise medical bill   A bill unexpectedly received from an out-of-network provider.

Sustainable growth rate (SGR)   A formula based on economy-wide growth and the demand for Medicare services, previously used as the basis for annual Medicare physician fee increases.

Tiered formulary   A type of formulary (list of covered drugs) that divides drugs into tiers (levels); drugs on lower tiers have lower cost-sharing, while drugs on higher tiers have of cost-sharing.

Tiered networks   Provider networks in which consumers pay less for providers with steeper discounts or for high-value providers.

UCR (Usual, Customary, and Reasonable)   The mean, median, mode, or otherwise "reasonable" fee for a given service or product in a geographic area, sometimes used by insurers to negotiate prices with providers.

Underinsurance   Insurance that does not provide enough financial protection, e.g. because it does not cover an individual for the entire year, because an individual must switch plans often, because the out-of-pocket costs are unaffordable or because the provider network is too narrow.

Unfunded retiree benefit obligations   The funding gap between what is set aside to pay for retiree benefits and the cost of these benefits.

Universal health coverage   A health care system that provides everyone with access to quality promotive, preventative, curative, and rehabilitative health services, while also protecting people from financial hardship related to paying for these services.

Urgent care centers   A type of **walk-in clinic**, a free-standing facility that treats pressing, but not life-threatening, conditions, and also generally have extended hours.

Utilization management   A broad set of tools that plans use to influence a policyholder's use of covered benefits, such as **prior authorization** and **step therapy**.

Value-based payment (VBP)   A payment strategy that rewards providers for quality and cost containment, rather than volume.

Walk-in clinics   Facilities such as retail clinics and urgent care centers that do not require appointments for visits.

INDEX

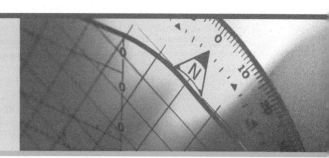

Note: The letters 'f', 't' and 'b' following locators refer to figures, tables and box respectively